The Developmental Relations among Mind, Brain and Education

Michel Ferrari · Ljiljana Vuletic
Editors

The Developmental Relations among Mind, Brain and Education

Essays in Honor of Robbie Case

Springer

Editors
Dr. Michel Ferrari
University of Toronto
Ontario Inst. Studies in
Education
Dept. Human Development &
Applied Psychology
252 Bloor Street West
Toronto ON M5S 1V6
Canada
mferrari@oise.utoronto.ca

Ljiljana Vuletic
University of Toronto
Ontario Inst. Studies in
Education
Dept. Human Development &
Applied Psychology
252 Bloor Street West
Toronto ON M5S 1V6
Canada
lvuletic@oise.utoronto.ca

ISBN 978-90-481-3665-0 e-ISBN 978-90-481-3666-7
DOI 10.1007/978-90-481-3666-7
Springer Dordrecht Heidelberg London New York

Library of Congress Control Number: 2009941544

Printed on acid-free paper

Springer is part of Springer Science+Business Media (www.springer.com)

Acknowledgments

It has been a privilege to work on this volume with so many great scholars and to be able to provide this tribute to Robbie Case. Thanks to our families and to everyone at Springer for their patience and support throughout the completion of the volume.

Contents

Contributors

Alba Agostino Department of Psychology, University of Guelph, Guelph, ON, Canada, agostino@uoguelph.ca

Daniel Ansari Numerical Cognition Laboratory, Department of Psychology and Graduate Program in Neuroscience, University of Western Ontario, London, ON, Canada, daniel.ansari@uwo.ca

Andrew V. Dane Brock University, St. Catharines, ON, Canada, adane@brocku.ca

Andreas Demetriou Department of Psychology, University of Cyprus, Nicosia, Cyprus, ademetriou@ucy.ac.cy

Martha J. Farah Walter H. Annenberg Professor of Natural Sciences and Director of the Center for Cognitive Neuroscience, University of Pennsylvania, PA, USA, mfarah@psych.upenn.edu

Michel Ferrari Department of Human Development and Applied Psychology, Ontario Institute for Studies in Education, University of Toronto, Toronto, ON, Canada, mferrari@oise.utoronto.ca

Kurt W. Fischer Harvard University Graduate School of Education, Cambridge, MA, USA, kurt_fischer@harvard.edu

Isabela Granic Hospital for Sick Children, Toronto, ON, Canada, isabela.granic@sickkids.ca

Stephanie Griffiths Simon Fraser University, Burnaby, BC, Canada, sgriffiths@okanagan.bc.ca

Ian Holloway Numerical Cognition Laboratory, Department of Psychology and Graduate Program in Neuroscience, University of Western Ontario, London, ON, Canada, idholloway@gmail.com

Janice Johnson Department of Psychology, York University, Toronto, ON, Canada, janicej@yorku.ca

Richard E. Kennedy Brock University, St. Catharines, ON, Canada, rk02ae@brocku.ca

Marc Lewis Department of Human Development and Applied Psychology, OISE/University of Toronto, Toronto, ON, Canada, mlewis@oise.utoronto.ca

Zopito Marini Department of Child and Youth Studies, Brock University, St. Catharines, ON, Canada, zmarini@brocku.ca

Anne McKeough Division of Applied Psychology, University of Calgary, Calgary, AL, Canada, mckeough@ucalgary.ca

Antigoni Mouyi Department of Psychology, University of Cyprus, Nicosia, Cyprus, mougi@ucy.ac.cy

Yukari Okamoto Department of Education, University of California, Santa Barbara, CA, USA, yukari@education.ucsb.edu

Juan Pascual-Leone Department of Psychology, York University, Toronto, ON, Canada, juanpl@yorku.ca

Marion Porath The University of British Columbia, Vancouver, BC, Canada, marion.porath@ubc.ca

Gavin Price Numerical Cognition Laboratory, Department of Psychology and Graduate Program in Neuroscience, University of Western Ontario, London, ON, Canada, gavinprice@gmail.com

Marc S. Schwartz University of Texas, Arlington, TX, USA, SCHWARMA@uta.edu

Robert S. Siegler Department of Psychology, Carnegie-Mellon University, Pittsburgh, PA 15213, USA, rs7k@andrew.cmu.edu

George Spanoudis University of Cyprus, Nicosia, Cyprus, spanoud@ucy.ac.cy

Robert W. Thatcher NeuroImaging Laboratory, Applied Neuroscience Research Institute, St. Petersburg, FL, USA, rwthatcher@yahoo.com

Ljiljana Vuletic Department of Human Development and Applied Psychology, Ontario Institute for Studies in Education, University of Toronto, Toronto, ON, Canada, lvuletic@oise.utoronto.ca

About the Authors

Alba Agostino (PhD, 2008, York University) is currently a Post-Doctoral Fellow at the University of Guelph, Guelph, Ontario. Her current research focuses on the development of formal and informal mathematical reasoning; cognitive aspects of non-literal language comprehension; and measurement of executive functions in children.

Daniel Ansari is an Assistant Professor in the Department of Psychology and the Canada Research Chair (Tier II) in Developmental Cognitive Neuroscience at the University of Western Ontario, where he heads the 'Numerical Cognition Laboratory' (where the co-authors of this chapter are graduate students). Before coming to the University of Western Ontario he was an Assistant Professor in the Department of Education at Dartmouth College, USA. He holds a BA in Psychology from the University of Sussex, an MSc in Neuroscience from the University of Oxford and a PhD in Psychology from University College, UK. He is an associate editor for the Journal 'Developmental Science.' In 2009, he was a recipient of the Award for Early Research Contributions from the Society for Research in Child Development (SRCD).

Andrew Dane is an Associate Professor in the Department of Psychology at Brock University, St. Catharines, Canada. His research is focused predominantly on the development of aggressive and antisocial behavior in children and adolescents. He has a particular interest in how parenting, peer relations and temperament combine to differentially predict overt, relational, proactive, and reactive subtypes of aggression.

Another line of his research concerns the identification of predictors that forecast experiences of bullying and victimization, as well as dual involvement in bullying and victimization. In addition, Dr. Dane has applied experience in Clinical Psychology, providing psycho-educational assessments and therapy for children, adolescents and their families.

Andreas Demetriou has a PhD in Psychology (1983) from the Aristotle University of Thessaloniki, Greece. He is a professor of psychology at the University of Cyprus since 1996. He was a professor of developmental psychology at the Aristotle University of Thessaloniki for many years. He has been the Vice and the Acting Rector of the University of Cyprus and the founding President of the Cyprus University of Technology. Currently he is the Minister of Education and Culture of the Republic of Cyprus. His research focuses on cognitive development, the relations between cognitive development and personality, and, currently, the relations between cognitive development and brain development. He advanced a comprehensive theory of intellectual development aiming to integrate research and theory in the traditions of developmental, cognitive, and psychometric psychology. His theory and research is presented in more than 150 articles and books, including The Development of Mental Processing (2002, with C. Christou, G. Spanoudis, and M. Platsidou) in the Monographs of the Society for Research in Child Development and Unity and Modularity in the Mind and the Self (2001, Routledge, with S. Kazis).

Michel Ferrari is Associate Professor in Human Development and Applied Psychology at the University of Toronto. His research focuses on the relations between personal identity and education. He has edited or co-edited several books, most recently Teaching for Wisdom (Springer, 2008, with Georges Potworowski), and is currently preparing a Handbook on Resilience in Children of War (Springer, in press, with Chandi Fernando). In 2002, he edited a special issue of the Journal of Consciousness Studies celebrating the centennial of William James's Varieties of Religious experience and he and Tamara Albertini will edit a special 2011 issue of Intellectual History Review, celebrating the 500th anniversary of Bovelles' Liber de Sapiente. His most recent federally funded research project, with Monika Ardelt and others, involves a cross-cultural study of personal wisdom in China, Ukraine, Serbia, India, the United States, and Canada.

Kurt Fischer is Director of the Mind, Brain, and Education Program and Charles Bigelow Professor at the Harvard Graduate School of Education. In his research, he analyzes cognition, emotion, and learning and their relation to biological development and educational assessment. He has discovered a scale that assesses learning and development in any domain. Leading an international movement to connect biology and cognitive science to education, he is founding editor of the journal Mind, Brain, and Education (Blackwell), which received the award for Best New Journal by the Association of American Publishers. His most recent books include The Educated Brain (Cambridge University Press, 2008).

Isabela Granic, PhD is a research scientist at the Hospital for Sick Children. She works with an interdisciplinary research network that brings together developmental and intervention scientists, neuroscientists, and clinical directors from several Ontario children's mental health agencies. She and her colleagues are studying behavioral changes in parent–child interactions (using direct observation methods) and changes in emotion regulation processes in the brain (using neuroimaging techniques) to identify how treatments help aggressive children and families. They have developed new dynamic systems methods to study change processes in these domains; methods appropriate for both research and clinical purposes (Granic & Hollenstein, 2003; Granic & Lamey, 2002). By integrating brain and behavioral processes to identify what changes when interventions work, they hope to better predict and evaluate treatment effectiveness in community practice, improve outcomes by targeting key psychosocial and neuropsychological mechanisms, and refine interventions to be more sensitive to the needs of different types of youth and families.

Janice Johnson (PhD, 1982, York University) is Associate Professor in the Department of Psychology at York University, Toronto. She has been visiting professor at universities in Italy, the United States, and Chile. Her research interests are in cognitive development, individual differences, and cognitive process analysis. Her current research focuses on culture-fair assessment of cognitive capacity in mainstream and exceptional developmental samples; children's reasoning in mathematics; measurement of cognitive inhibition and executive functions in children and adults; cognitive-developmental factors in metaphor comprehension; and mental arousal/motivation as factors in cognitive performance.

Richard Kennedy is finishing his doctoral degree in Developmental Psychology at Brock University and completing his supervised practice in a private clinic to fulfill the requirements to become a clinical psychologist. His research interests include temperament and aggression subtypes, the additive and interactive roles of parenting and temperament in the prediction of adolescent adjustment, and the roles of such variables as beliefs and attitudes in the prediction of antisocial behavior. He possesses his BA in Psychology (University of Guelph), BEd in Primary/Junior Education (Lakehead University), and MA in Developmental Psychology (Brock University). He has been the recipient of the Early In-Course Scholarship in 1986 and Psychology Faculty Prize in 1986 and 1988, all from the University of Guelph, and an Ontario Graduate Scholarship in 2002 while attending Brock University.

Marc Lewis is a Professor in the Department of Human Development and Applied Psychology and the Neuroscience Program of the University of Toronto. He specializes in the study of personality development and developmental psychopathology as related to emotion and emotion regulation. His work is informed by developmental psychology, affective neuroscience, and a dynamic systems perspective on brain and behavior. His empirical work initially looked at transitions in emotional and cognitive development, and he established a state space grid methodology to facilitate the analysis of socio-emotional behavior over time. More recent work utilizes EEG methods for identifying the neural underpinnings of emotion regulation in normal children and those with aggressive or anxiety disorders. His papers have appeared in highly regarded outlets, including *Child Development, Behavioral and Brain Sciences, Journal of Cognitive Neuroscience, Cognitive Development, and Developmental Science*.

Zopito Marini a developmental and educational psychologist, is a Full Professor of Child and Youth Studies at Brock University, St. Catharines, Canada. Dr. Marini did his graduate work at the University of Toronto with the late Robbie Case, and since 1985 has been at Brock where he was the founding Chair of the Department.

His research interests focus on the area generally known as socio-cognitive development. Dr. Marini does research, writes, and lectures on issues related to family and school conflicts, bullying and victimization, and the development of self-regulation. Using a biopsychosocial perspective, he investigates the cognitive mechanisms and social processes underlying the development of a range of socio-cognitive abilities in typical and atypical children and youths. Projects currently underway in his lab examine psychosocial factors involved in bullying and victimization with a view of developing effective prevention strategies. Other research projects involve an examination of the development of self-regulation and the fostering of civility in teaching and learning. His most recent books include two co-authored publications titled Cognitive Development: Neo-Piagetian Perspectives (Taylor & Francis Group, 2008) and Educational Psychology (McGraw-Hill Ryerson, 2010).

Anne McKeough Professor in the Division of Applied Psychology at The University of Calgary, teaches graduate courses in cognitive development and educational assessment, and undergraduate courses in the Teacher Preparation Program. Anne holds a PhD in Applied Cognitive Science from the Ontario Institute for Studies in Education, University of Toronto. Her research is in the areas of cognitive development and developmentally based instruction, focusing on children's and adolescents' reading and writing. Anne has authored numerous book chapters and articles, and has edited several volumes, including Toward the Practice of Theory Based Instruction, Teaching for Transfer, Schools in Transition, and Literacy Development: A Global View. Anne has also been recognized for her research, teaching, and mentorship locally, nationally, and internationally.

Antigoni Mouyi (PhD, 2008, University of Cyprus, Cyprus) is currently a researcher at the Pedagogical Institute of Cyprus. Her research interests focus on the development of reasoning ability and its dynamic interrelation with various cognitive processes, such as speed and control of processing and working memory, from childhood to early adulthood. She is studying the cognitive profile of individuals at different reasoning levels. She is also interested in the analysis of the complexity of inductive and deductive reasoning tasks. As a PhD candidate she received the *Templeton Prize for Best Student Paper, 2007* at the Conference of the International Society for Intelligence Research.

Yukari Okamoto is a professor in the Department of Education at the University of California, Santa Barbara. She received her PhD from Stanford University, and was a Spencer Post-Doctoral Fellow at the National Academy of Education. She is a developmental psychologist interested in cross-cultural differences in children's thinking, especially in the domains of mathematical, scientific, and spatial thinking. From a neo-Piagetian perspective, she studies children's conceptual development, provides instructional programs, and examines the question of culture and the developing mind. She was a member of the TIMSS video study research team that examined mathematics and science teaching practices in several nations such as Australia, Germany, the Czech Republic, and Japan. Dr. Okamoto co-authored a Monograph with Robbie Case, published by the *Society for Research in Child Development*.

Juan Pascual-Leone (MD, 1957, University of Valencia, Spain; 1960, Neuropsychiatry, C.S. Valdecilla, University of Valladolid, Spain; PhD, 1969, University of Geneva) is Emeritus Professor and Senior Scholar in the Department of Psychology at York University, Toronto. His research concerns cognitive developmental, learning, and individual-difference processes throughout the life span (from infancy to old age) and their neuroscientific foundations. His theoretical interests include organismic–causal theories of high cognition, motivation, and development; constructivist epistemology; and logical/rational methods of process and task analysis. He founded the neo-Piagetian approach to cognitive development. He has been invited visiting professor at universities in France, Italy, Spain, Switzerland, the United States, Israel, South Africa, Argentina, Brazil, Chile, Colombia, and Venezuela. He has been made Fellow of the Foundations' Fund for Research in Psychiatry, the Canadian Psychological Association, and the Van Leer Jerusalem Foundation. In 2006, he received a Doctorate honoris causa in Psychology from the University of Cyprus.

Marion Porath is a Professor in the Department of Educational and Counselling Psychology, and Special Education in the Faculty of Education at The University of British Columbia, Vancouver, Canada. She earned her PhD at the University of Toronto (OISE) in 1988. She was awarded the Killam Prize for teaching excellence at The University of British Columbia in 1998 and is the recipient of numerous research grants. Her research interests include different forms of giftedness, young children's social development, instructional applications of developmental theory, innovative approaches to early childhood education and problem-based learning. Her current research focuses on gifted and gifted/learning disabled students' views of themselves as learners and the roles of intrapersonal and interpersonal competencies in pedagogy.

Marc Schwartz is Professor of Mind, Brain and Education at the University of Texas at Arlington (UTA). At UTA he is currently working on developing the new Southwest Center for Mind, Brain and Education. The Center seeks to identify and support promising research agendas at the intersection of mind, brain and education. Professor Schwartz is a charter member of the International Mind, Brain and Education Society (IMBES) and also an Associate Researcher in the Science Education Department at the Harvard–Smithsonian Center for Astrophysics (CfA). His research at the CfA focuses on how the dynamic enterprise of learning and teaching unfold in physics, chemistry, and biology education.

Robert Siegler is Teresa Heinz Professor of Cognitive Psychology. His research focuses on the development of problem solving and reasoning in general and on the more specific topics of how children learn mathematics and how theoretical understanding of mathematical development can be applied to improving the learning of preschoolers from low-income backgrounds. The theoretically oriented research examines how children's basic representations of numbers influence their ability to learn whole number arithmetic, fractions, and other aspects of mathematics. The topics examined within this work include how representations of numbers change with age and experience, types of mathematical experiences that are especially helpful in producing improvements, the strategies that children use to solve mathematical problems, why some children are more mathematically proficient than others, and how children discover new strategies. This research suggested that certain types of numerical board games would be especially helpful for improving young children's mathematical understanding. Experimental tests of this prediction have yielded encouraging results; playing these board games yields large, rapid, and enduring gains in preschoolers' and young elementary school children's numerical understanding. The gains are especially large with preschoolers from low-income backgrounds. He has published more than 200 articles and chapters, written 8 books, and edited 5 others. His books have been translated into numerous languages, including Japanese, Chinese, Korean, German, French, Greek, and Portuguese.

George Ch. Spanoudis received his BSc and an MSc degree in Developmental Psychology from Aristotle University of Thessaloniki and his PhD degree in Cognitive Psychology with emphasis in developmental and educational Psychology from the University of Cyprus. He is a Lecturer of Psychology at the Psychology Department at the University of Cyprus, Cyprus. His academic interests include developmental psychology, memory, research methods, and learning disabilities. His areas of expertise and research interest include topics related to children's cognitive development, intelligence and language-learning impairments. Dr. Spanoudis is currently investigating age-related changes in intelligence using behavioral and event-related potential (ERP) techniques.

Ljiljana Vuletic is a doctoral candidate in Human Development and Applied Psychology at the University of Toronto. Her main research interests are autism and intentional personal development. She is lead author of *Transfer boy: perspectives on Asperger syndrome* (Jessica Kingsley Publishers, 2005), a case study of an adolescent with Asperger syndrome, and she is currently completing her doctoral thesis looking at intentional personal development in adults with Asperger syndrome.

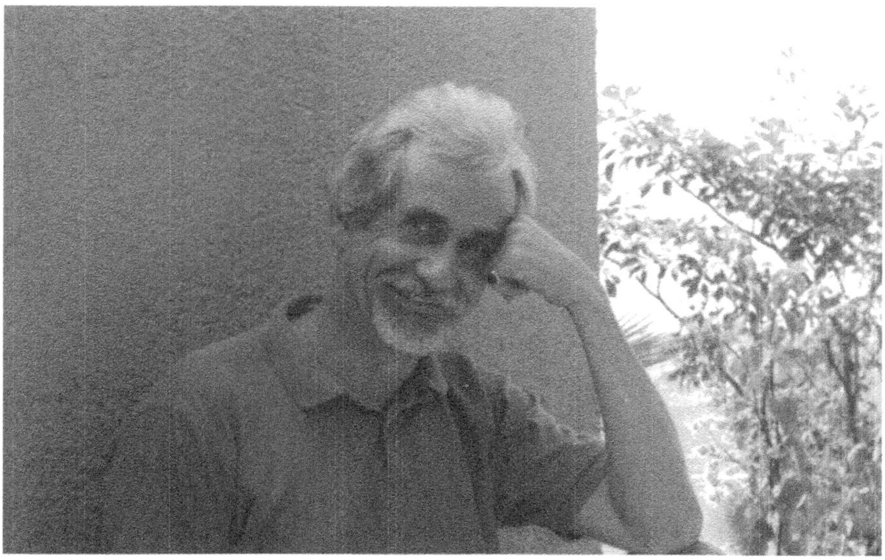

Introduction

Robert S. Siegler

Robbie Case: A Modern Classic

About 15 years ago, Robbie asked me what I thought of a talk we had just heard. I indicated that I hadn't much liked it and noted several serious problems. Robbie agreed with all of the criticisms, but said that he nonetheless liked the talk, because there was one good idea in it that he could use. I agreed with him that the idea was a good one, but it took me a while to understand the wisdom of his position. If there's one useful idea in a talk, then hearing it has been worthwhile, even if the talk also has numerous deficiencies. On that day and on many others, talking with Robbie changed my thinking for the better.

Robbie Case was in many ways a classic developmental psychologist of the old school. The depth and breadth of his theory; the range of age groups, populations, and topics that he studied; and his efforts to connect theory and application are all reminiscent of the greats of the past: Baldwin, Dewey, Piaget, Vygotsky, and Bruner. Like them, Robbie brought a unified developmental perspective to whatever topics, age groups, and populations he studied. Regardless of whether his immediate focus was on general theoretical issues or on more specific issues about working memory, executive functioning, or mathematics learning, Robbie always asked about the sequence of understandings through which children progressed from rudimentary beginnings to mature competence and always strived to find the commonalities in thinking across domains. In an era where analysis has largely trumped synthesis, Robbie's body of work provides a welcome counterweight that depicts the forest as well as the trees and that reminds his readers of the unique contributions that general developmental theories can make. For this service alone, the field owes him a major debt of gratitude.

Alongside this resemblance to the grand developmental theorists of the past was another side of Robbie's thinking, one that was modern, cutting edge, and at times almost futuristic. He was among the first to grasp the implications of progress

R.S. Siegler (✉)
Department of Psychology, Carnegie-Mellon University, Pittsburgh, PA 15213, USA
e-mail: rs7k@andrew.cmu.edu

M. Ferrari, L. Vuletic (eds.), *The Developmental Relations among Mind, Brain and Education*, DOI 10.1007/978-90-481-3666-7_1, © Springer Science+Business Media B.V. 2010

in cognitive neuroscience for understanding of cognitive development. In the late 1980s, when research in cognitive neuroscience was just beginning to accelerate, Robbie was already focusing on the implications of Robert Thatcher's work on the formation of long-distance cortical connections for his own theory of cognitive development. Case's (1992) article "The role of the frontal lobes in the regulation of cognitive development" was one of the first efforts to use neural data to inform a general theory of cognitive development. Similarly, the chapter in Case and Okamato's (1996) *SRCD Monograph*, "Modeling the dynamic interplay between general and specific change in children's conceptual understanding" was among the first efforts to bring dynamic systems modeling techniques to inform stage theories. Robbie's and his students' demonstrations in that same 1996 Monograph and in his 1992 book "The Mind's Staircase" of commonalities within an age group in children's understanding of emotions, drawing, music, social roles, narratives, motor activity, number, space, scientific reasoning, and logical inference remains a remarkable effort to demonstrate unities across these far-flung aspects of cognitive development (Capodilupo, 1992; Case, Hayward, Lewis, & Hurst, 1988; Case & McKeough, 1990; Dennis, 1992; Goldberg-Reitman, 1992; Griffin & Case, 1996; Marini, 1992; Reid, 1992).

Another dimension of Robbie's exceptional breadth of theorizing involves the range of populations to which he extended his theory. He and his collaborators examined the thinking of children from infancy through adolescence (Case & Khanna, 1981); of gifted children (Porath, 1992) and children with learning disabilities (Crammond, 1992); of children from very high and very low SES backgrounds (Griffin & Case, 1996); of children from Portuguese-American, African-American, and European-American backgrounds (Okamoto & Case, 1996); and of children from Africa, Asia, and North America (Fiati, 1992; Okamoto, et al., 1996).

Robbie's efforts to synthesize what was known about cognitive development was encompassing in another sense as well – the variety of theoretical traditions that his theory incorporated. His early research (e.g., Case, 1978; Case & Globerson, 1974) aimed at uniting Piagetian and information processing theory. In particular, he and his colleagues refined and extended to a great many new domains Pascual-Leone's (1969) ideas about how working memory and field independence/dependence influences changes within and between stages of cognitive development. Later, he, Sharon Griffin, and Yukari Okamoto incorporated ideas from socio-cultural theories to account for differences among different groups within Western society and for differences among children in different societies (e.g., Griffin & Case, 1997; Okamoto, Case, Bleiker, & Henderson, 1996). His use of dynamic systems techniques to model stage transitions has already been noted. His efforts to unite different neo-Piagetian theories, including those of Fischer (e.g., 1980), Demetriou (e.g, Demetriou, Efklides, & Platsidou, 1993), Halford (e.g., 1993) and Pascual-Leone (1969) are also noteworthy. In an area that tends to exaggerate small differences among theories, Robbie was noteworthy for adopting a "big tent" approach to identify and build on the commonalities. Ferrari and Vuletic's chapter in the present volume continues this integrative tradition and expands the tent even further; they incorporate not only Piagetian, neo-Piagetian, and socio-cultural perspectives on the development of the self but also perspectives from philosophy, literary studies, biology, neuroscience, psychiatry, and sociology.

Above all, Robbie focused on connecting cognitive development and instruction. His applications of cognitive developmental theory to instructional design remain some of the most insightful and compelling demonstrations that anyone has generated of the value of such applications. Early in his career, he demonstrated the value of precise analyses of the working memory demands of alternative instructional approaches for predicting which approaches could inculcate relatively advanced understanding in young elementary school children. His analysis of how to teach children to solve missing addend problems is a particularly compelling example (Case, 1978). Later, he pursued the more ambitious goal of designing a whole mathematics curriculum that would reflect his cognitive developmental analyses. His and Sharon Griffin's Right Start curriculum was a landmark in demonstrating the remarkably large gains that are possible if preschoolers and kindergartners from low-income backgrounds are provided high-quality instruction based on solid cognitive analyses (Griffin, Case, & Siegler, 1994; Griffin & Case, 1996). His, Bob Sandieson's, Joan Moss', and Mindy Kalchman's subsequent work on teaching older children about rational numbers and mathematical functions was another landmark demonstration of the value of applying cognitive developmental analyses to instruction (Case & Sandieson, 1992; Kalchman, Moss, & Case, 2001; Moss & Case, 1999).

Robbie's role as an educator did not stop with the many preschoolers and elementary school children who have benefited from his and his collaborators' instructional efforts. His role in educating his own PhD students was an equally large contribution, one that has multiplied the impact of his ideas beyond what any one person could accomplish. Part of the reason why Robbie was such a successful advisor was that he looked after his students' social well-being as well as their intellectual development. When I saw him at conferences, I was repeatedly amazed by the gaggle of students he was shepherding around an unfamiliar city and by the high spirits that encompassed the group. When Robbie and I had dinner together, he would often talk about issues confronting his students and how best to deal with them. Some advisors have a few students and know them personally; some advisors have many students and know them only professionally; Robbie was exceptional in finding the time and energy to maintain personal relationships with many students.

The range of Robbie's interests, and his willingness to supervise students with interests far from his own core areas, is evident throughout the present book. Some particularly interesting examples of the long-term evolution of ideas that began in student–advisor interactions with Robbie are seen in Marc Lewis' chapter on emotion regulation, Anne McKeough's chapter on development of understanding of narratives, Marion Porath's chapter on gifted children, Zopito Marini's chapter on bullying, and Yukari Okamoto's chapter on cross-national differences in numerical understanding. Of course, this is only a small sampling of Robbie's PhD students who have gone on to make important contributions on their own after completing their graduate work. A book that included chapters by all of Robbie's students who have gone on to make important contributions would be a weighty tome indeed.

The existence of a number of other chapters in the book reflects the expansive personality that allowed Robbie to maintain positive relations with colleagues who generated competing neo-Piagetian theories: Andreas Demetriou, Kurt Fischer, and Juan Pascual-Leone. Relations among researchers who generate related but distinct theories are inherently complex, and often degenerate into rivalry and resentment. The fact that Robbie and competing neo-Piagetian theorists were able to maintain the type of positive and affectionate relationship that would lead these very busy people to take the time and effort to write chapters relating their work and Robbie's in a book like this speaks well for all of them.

I was one of the many who benefited from Robbie's generosity of spirit. In my book "Emerging Minds" (Siegler, 1996), I used Robbie's metaphor of "the mind's staircase" as a foil to contrast with my own overlapping waves theory. I did this because I highly respected Robbie's approach, and because the many commonalities between our approaches brought the distinctive features of overlapping waves theory into clear relief. Nonetheless, the contrast that I drew could easily have been taken as a rebuke. My main argument was that focusing on variability of thinking within individuals, choices among alternative approaches, and the mechanisms that produce cognitive change results in more accurate depictions of cognitive development than viewing it as a sequence of qualitatively distinct understandings, such as stages or conceptual structures. I therefore felt some trepidation when I sent Robbie a pre-publication version of the relevant chapters for comments. I should have realized that there was no reason for concern. As always, Robbie emphasized what he liked about the chapters, seconded many of the criticisms, argued cogently against others, and encouraged me to complete the book quickly so that others in the field would have a chance to read and discuss it. Instead of harming our friendship, the experience strengthened it.

A central question raised by the present edited book concerns whether neuroscience research can help improve education. In the long run, there seems to be little doubt that it can and will, but with regard to the present and near future, the jury is still out. Certainly, many chapters in the book include intriguing ideas and promising research programs linking neural functioning to thinking and learning. Daniel Ansari's chapter on contributions of neuroimaging data and Martha Farah's chapter on the impact of poverty on brain development are two outstanding examples. Whether these and other early efforts can be translated into improvements in education in the next 10 or 20 years, however, remains unknown. Of course, that's the reaction of a congenital skeptic; Robbie's reaction in all likelihood would have been to praise all of the chapters, to cheer on the strongest efforts, and to point the way toward changes that would make good research even better.

I'd like to close with another anecdote about something I learned from Robbie. Early in both of our careers, I told him that I had received a manuscript of his to review and thought it looked very interesting, but I had returned it because we were too good friends for me to be objective. This was the only time I can remember seeing Robbie really angry. He told me that this was a stupid policy, and provided a reason that permanently changed my thinking. He noted that in academia, a lot of the reason why colleagues become friends is that they have similar ways of thinking about the issues that they care about. Thus, if friends refuse to review each other's manuscripts, it will bias the pool of potential reviewers, because, as Robbie put it, "Your enemies sure as hell won't refuse." Michel Ferrari and Ljiljana Vuletic deserve many thanks for editing this valuable book and reminding both readers and contributors of Robbie Case's enduring impact.

References

Capodilupo, A. M. (1992). A neo-structural analysis of children's response to instruction in the sight-reading of musical notation. In R. Case (Ed.), *The mind's staircase: Exploring the conceptual underpinnings of children's thought and knowledge* (pp. 99–116). Hillsdale, NJ: Erlbaum.

Case, R. (1978). Intellectual development from birth to adulthood: A new-Piagetian investigation. In R. S. Siegler (Ed.), *Children's thinking: What develops?* Hillsdale, NJ: Erlbaum.

Case, R. (1992). The role of the frontal lobes in the regulation of cognitive development. *Brain and Cognition, 20*, 51–73.

Case, R. (1992). *The mind's staircase: Exploring the conceptual underpinnings of children's thought and knowledge*. Hillsdale, NJ: Erlbaum.

Case, R., & Globerson, T. (1974). Field independence and central computing space. *Child Development, 45*, 772–778.

Case, R., Hayward, S., Lewis, M., & Hurst, P. (1988). Toward a neo-Piagetian theory of cognitive and emotional development. *Developmental Review, 8*, 1–51.

Case, R., & Khanna, F. (1981). The missing links: Stages in children's progression from sensorimotor to logical thought. In K. W. Fischer (Ed.), *Cognitive development* (New Directions for Child Development, No. 12). San Francisco: Jossey-Bass.

Case, R., & McKeough, A. (1990). Schooling and the development of central conceptual structures: An example from the domain of children's narrative. *International Journal of Educational Psychology, 8*, 835–855.

Case, R., & Okamoto, Y. (1996). The role of central conceptual structures in the development of children's thought. *Monographs of the Society for Research in Child Development, 61*(1–2).

Case, R., & Sandieson, R. (1992). Testing for the presence of a central quantative structure: Use of the transfer paradigm. In R. Case (Ed.), *The mind's staircase: Exploring the conceptual underpinnings of children's thought and knowledge* (pp. 117–132). Hillsdale, NJ: Erlbaum.

Crammond, J. (1992). Analyzing the basic cognitive-developmental processes of children with specific types of learning disability. In R. Case (Ed.), *The mind's staircase: Exploring the conceptual underpinnings of children's thought and knowledge* (pp. 285–302). Hillsdale, NJ: Erlbaum.

Demetriou, A., Efklides, A., & Platsidou, M. (1993). The architecture and dynamics of developing mind: Experiential structuralism as a frame for unifying cognitive developmental theories. *Monographs of the Society for Research in Child Development, 58*(5–6, Serial No. 234).

Dennis, S. (1992). Stage and structure in the development of children's spatial representations. In R. Case (Ed.), *The mind's staircase: Exploring the conceptual underpinnings of children's thought and knowledge* (pp. 229–246). Hillsdale, NJ: Erlbaum.

Fiati, T. A. (1992). Cross-cultural variation in the structure of children's thought. In R. Case (Ed.), *The mind's staircase: Exploring the conceptual underpinnings of children's thought and knowledge* (pp. 319–342). Hillsdale, NJ: Erlbaum.

Fischer, K. W. (1980). A theory of cognitive development: The control and construction of hierarchies of skills. *Psychological Review, 87*, 477–531.

Goldberg-Reitman, J. (1992). Young girls' conception of their mothers' role: A neo-structural analysis. In R. Case (Ed.), *The mind's staircase: Exploring the conceptual underpinnings of children's thought and knowledge* (pp. 135–152). Hillsdale, NJ: Erlbaum.

Griffin, S., & Case, R. (1996). Evaluating the breadth and depth of training effects when central conceptual structures are taught. In R. Case & Y. Okamoto (Eds.), The role of central conceptual structures in the development of children's thought. *Monographs of the Society for Research in Child Development, 61*(1–2), 83–101.

Griffin, S., & Case, R. (1997). Rethinking the primary school math curriculum: An approach based on cognitive science. *Issues in Education, 3*, 1–65.

Griffin, S., Case, R., & Siegler, R. S. (1994). Rightstart: Providing the central conceptual prerequisites for first formal learning of arithmetic to students at risk for school failure. In K. McGilly (Ed.), *Classroom lessons: Integrating cognitive theory and classroom practice* (pp. 25–49). Cambridge, MA: MIT Press.

Halford, G. S. (1993). *Children's understanding: The development of mental models*. Hillsdale, NJ: Erlbaum.

Kalchman, M., Moss, J., & Case, R. (2001). Psychological models for the development of mathematical understanding: Rational numbers and functions. In S. M. Carver & D. Klahr (Eds.), *Cognition and instruction: Twenty-five years of progress* (pp. 1–38). Mahwah, NJ: Lawrence Erlbaum Associates Publishers.

Marini, Z. A. (1992). Synchrony and asynchrony in the development of children's scientific reasoning. In R. Case (Ed.), *The mind's staircase: Exploring the conceptual underpinnings of children's thought and knowledge* (pp. 55–74). Hillsdale, NJ: Erlbaum.

Moss, J., & Case, R. (1999). Developing children's understanding of rational numbers: A new model and experimental curriculum. *Journal for Research in Mathematics Education, 30*, 122–147.

Okamoto, Y., & Case, R. (1996). Exploring the microstructure of children's central conceptual structures in the domain of number. In R. Case & Y. Okamoto (Eds.), The role of central conceptual structures in the development of children's thought. *Monographs of the Society for Research in Child Development, 61*(1–2, Serial No. 246), 27–58.

Okamoto, Y., Case, R., Bleiker, C., & Henderson, B. (1996). Cross cultural investigations. In R. Case & Y. Okamoto (Eds.), The role of central conceptual structures in the development of children's thought. *Monographs of the Society for Research in Child Development, 61*(1–2, Serial No. 246), 131–155.

Pascual-Leone, J. (1969). *Cognitive development and cognitive style*. Unpublished doctoral dissertation, University of Geneva.

Porath, M. (1992). Stage and structure in the development of children with various types of "giftedness". In R. Case (Ed.), *The mind's staircase: Exploring the conceptual underpinnings of children's thought and knowledge* (pp. 303–318). Hillsdale, NJ: Erlbaum.

Reid, T. R. (1992). Horizontal and vertical structure: Stages and substages in children's motor development. In R. Case (Ed.), *The mind's staircase: Exploring the conceptual underpinnings of children's thought and knowledge* (pp. 247–266). Hillsdale, NJ: Erlbaum.

Siegler, R. S. (1996). *Emerging minds: The process of change in children's thinking*. New York: Oxford University Press.

Part I
Developing Mind and Brain

A Three-Level Model of the Developing Mind: Functional and Neuronal Substantiation and Educational Implications

Andreas Demetriou, George Spanoudis, and Antigoni Mouyi

This chapter summarizes a comprehensive theory of developing the self-aware and self-regulated human mind that integrates the three traditions in psychology that have focused on it since the end of the 19th century – the traditions of cognitive, differential, and developmental psychology. As such, this theory provides answers to the questions following:

1. *What* is the general architecture of the developing mind? That is, what are the main functions and dimensions involved in the mind and how are they interrelated?
2. What is the condition of the various functions and processes at different phases of development?
3. *How* do they change with age? That is, what are the mechanisms responsible for their transformation with growth into higher levels of functioning?
4. What are the causal factors underlying their change? That is, *why* do these dimensions and functions change with age?
5. What are the factors responsible for individual differences in cognitive architecture and development?

It is beyond the scope of the present chapter to answer all of these questions. Our focus will mainly be on the first three questions and touch upon the other two. We will also try to show how the general architecture and dynamics of the mind map onto our recent knowledge of the organization and development of the brain.

The Architecture and Development of the Human Mind

We propose that the mind is organized in three levels, two of them comprising general-purpose mechanisms and processes and one comprising specialized systems of thought and problem solving. These levels are distinguished from each other on the basis of functional criteria. Each of the levels is itself a complex network of

A. Demetriou (✉)
Department of Psychology, University of Cyprus, Nicosia, Cyprus
e-mail: ademetriou@ucy.ac.cy

M. Ferrari, L. Vuletic (eds.), *The Developmental Relations among Mind, Brain and Education*, DOI 10.1007/978-90-481-3666-7_2, © Springer Science+Business Media B.V. 2010

processes and systems involving multiple dimensions and tiers of organization that may be uncovered if appropriately examined. The most basic of these levels involves general processes and functions that define the processing potentials available at a given time. Thus, the condition of the processes comprising this level constrains the condition and functioning of the systems included in the other two levels. The other two are *knowing* levels, in that they involve systems and functions underlying understanding and problem solving. One of these two *knowing* levels is primarily directed to the environment. It involves systems of cognitive functions and abilities specializing in the representation and processing of the different aspects of the physical and the social environment. The other *knowing* level is directed to the self. That is, it involves processes underlying self-monitoring, self-representation, and self-regulation. In other words, this level comprises processes underlying awareness and consciousness, intentionality, and self-control. Understanding, learning, or performing any task, at a particular point in time, is a mixture of the processes involved in all three levels. Figure 1 shows an illustration of this model. In the section below we first outline this architecture and present supporting empirical evidence. Then, the discussion focuses on the development of and the dynamic interrelations between the various constructs.

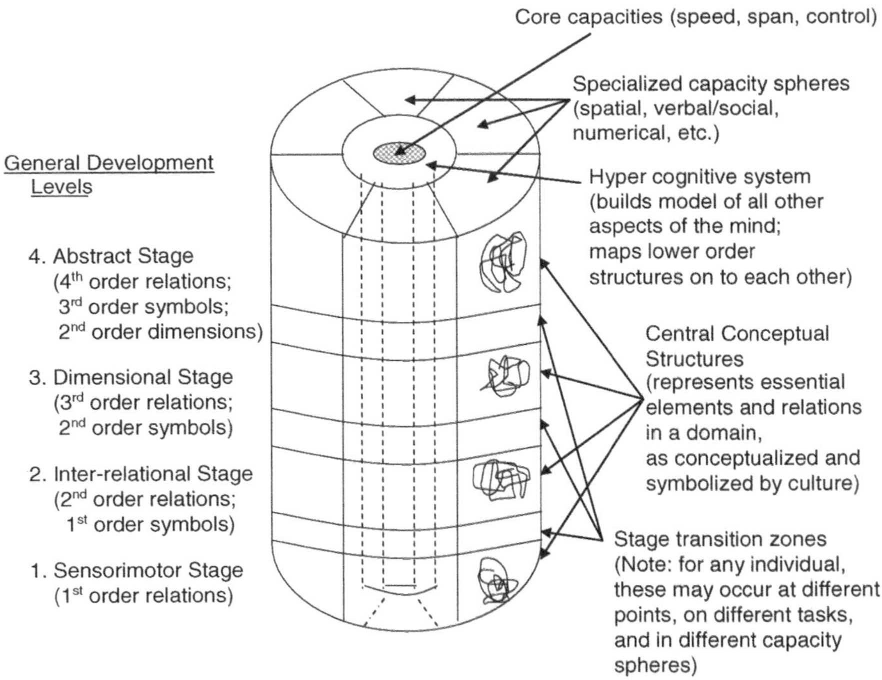

Fig. 1 The general model of the architecture of the developing mind integrating concepts from the theories of Demetriou and Case.
Note: Based on Fig. 13 in Demetriou, Efklides, and Platsidou (1993)

Processing Potentials

Cognitive (Baddeley, 2007; Cowan, 1999, 2001; Engle, 2002), psychometric (Deary, 2000; Jensen, 1998), and developmental psychologists (Case, 1992a; Halford, 1993; Pascual-Leone, 1970) concur that humans always operate under conditions of limited resources for representing and processing information about the environment and the self. In this model, processing potentials are specified in terms of three dimensions: *speed of processing*, *control of processing*, and *representational capacity*.

Speed of Processing

It basically refers to the maximum speed at which a given mental act may be efficiently executed. Usually, in tests of speed of processing, the individual is asked to recognize a simple stimulus as quickly as possible, such as locating or identifying a geometrical figure, a letter, or a word. Under these conditions, speed of processing indicates the time needed by the system to record and give meaning to information. Traditionally, the faster an individual can recognize a stimulus, the more efficient information processor is thought to be (Posner & Peterson, 1990; McLeod, 1991; Sternberg, 1966). This is due to the very nature of the human brain. That is, the neural traces of stimuli encountered at a given moment tend to decay rapidly or to be overwritten by the traces of information encountered at the next moment (Nelson, de Haan, & Thomas, 2006). Therefore, fast processing ensures that the goals of a particular step of processing will be met before the initiation of a new step that will impose its own competing demands on the system (Salthouse, 1996).

Control of Processing

The information of relevance at a particular moment usually co-exists with other non-relevant information. Also, information that is relevant at a certain moment may not be relevant soon after. Therefore, efficient processing requires a mechanism that would enable the thinker to keep control of processing so that she stays focused on the information of interest while filtering out interfering and goal-irrelevant information and shifting focus to other information, if this is required (McLeod, 1991; Navon, 1977; Neil, Valdes, & Terry, 1995; Posner & Boies, 1971). Therefore, control of processing is usually tested under conditions that can generate conflicting interpretations, such as the well-known Stroop phenomenon (Stroop, 1935). In this test, words denoting color are written with a different ink color (e.g., the word "red" written with blue ink), and the individual is asked to name the ink color as quickly as possible. These conditions accurately test control of processing, because the individual is required to inhibit a dominant but irrelevant response (to read the word) in order to select and emit a weaker but relevant response (name the ink color) (Demetriou, Efklides, & Platsidou, 1993; Dempster & Brainerd, 1995).

Representational Capacity

Representational capacity is defined as the maximum amount of information and mental acts that the mind can efficiently activate simultaneously at a given moment. In the current psychological literature, working memory is regarded as the functional manifestation of representational capacity. It is generally accepted that working memory involves central executive processes that are common across domains and modality-specific storage specializing in the representation of different types of information. Baddeley's (2007) model is exemplary for this type of architecture of working memory. According to this model, working memory involves two general systems, the central executive system and the episodic buffer, and two specialized storage buffers, one specializing in the storage of phonological and one specializing in the storage of visuo-spatial information.

Specialized Domains of Thought

Specialized processes refer to mental operations and problem-solving skills that are suitable for the handling (i.e., the comparison, combination, transformation) of different types of information, relations, and problems. We propose that to qualify for the status of a domain of thought, a block of mental operations must satisfy the following criteria. First, it must serve an identifiable *special function or purpose* vis-à-vis the organism's adaptational needs. Second, it must be responsible for the representation and processing of a particular *type of objects and relations* between environmental entities. In fact, the special function of the system is to enable the organism to deal with a particular type of environmental relations. Third, it must involve *specialized operations and processes* that are appropriate for the representation and processing of the type of relations concerned. In a sense, the operations and processes of a domain of thought are the mental analogs of the type of relations concerned. Fourth, it must be *biased to a particular symbol system* that is better appropriate than other symbol systems to represent the type of relations concerned and facilitate the execution of the operations concerned.

Each of the domains involves two types of processes: core processes and mental operations and processing skills. The functioning of these processes generates domain-specific knowledge and beliefs but we will not embark on this issue in the present chapter. Core processes are very fundamental processes that ground each of the domains into its respective environmental realm. We suggest that these processes are the result of our evolution as a species, and they somehow characterize the cognitive functioning of other species as well (Rumbaugh & Washburn, 2003). During development, core processes are the first manifestations of the systems, and they are predominantly action and perception bound. If a minimum set of conditions is present in the input, they are activated and provide an interpretation of the input, which is consistent with their organization. In other words, core processes are inferential traps within each of the systems that respond to informational structures with core-specific interpretations that have adaptive value and "meaning" for the organism.

Operations and processing skills are systems of mental (or, frequently, physical) actions that are used to purposefully deal with information and relations in each of the domains. From the point of view of development, core processes constitute the starting points for the construction of operations and skills included in each of the domains. That is, at the initial phases of development, operations, skills, and knowledge arise through interactions between domain-specific core processes, the environment, and the executive and self-monitoring and self-regulation processes of the hypercognitive system. That is, the systems of operations and processes within each domain emerge as a process of differentiation and expansion of the core processes when these do not suffice to meet the understanding and problem-solving needs of the moment. In other words, the initial inferential traps are gradually transformed into inference that is increasingly self-guided and reflected upon.

The Domains

Our research has uncovered six domains of thought that satisfy the criteria summarized above. These are the domains of categorical, quantitative, spatial, causal, social, and verbal thought (Demetriou, 2000; Demetriou & Efklides, 1985, Demetriou, Efklides, & Platsidou, 1993; Demetriou, Efklides, Papadaki, Papantoniou, & Economou, 1993; Demetriou, Pachaury, Metallidou, & Kazi, 1996; Demetriou & Kazi, 2001; Kargopoulos & Demetriou, 1998).

According to many studies conducted in our laboratory both at the Aristotle University of Thessaloniki, Greece, in the 1980s and the early 1990s and at the University of Cyprus in the recent years, all six domains do come out as distinct factors in factor analysis (Case, 1992a; Case, Demetriou, Platsidou, & Kazi, 2001; Demetriou & Kyriakides, 2006). One such study, which is drawn from a recent study (Stavrinidis, 2005), is illustrated in Fig. 2.

This study involved tasks addressed to all six domains and it included participants from 12 to 18 years of age who were tested by a large number of tasks addressed to each of the six domains. Specifically, the domains of categorical, quantitative, causal, spatial, verbal, and social reasoning were examined by problems addressed to classification and Raven-like matrices, proportionality and algebra, hypothesis testing and understanding of causal relations, mental rotation and co-ordination of perspectives, inductive and deductive reasoning, and understanding intentions and socio-political issues, respectively. Performance on the tasks addressed to each domain was reduced to two mean scores, standing for performance on the domain components mentioned above. A confirmatory factor analysis was performed, where each pair of scores addressed to a domain was related to a different factor and the six domain-specific factors were regressed on a common second-order factor. The fit of this model was excellent, indicating that the six domains do stand as separate but related dimensions of performance. Obviously, the second-order factor in

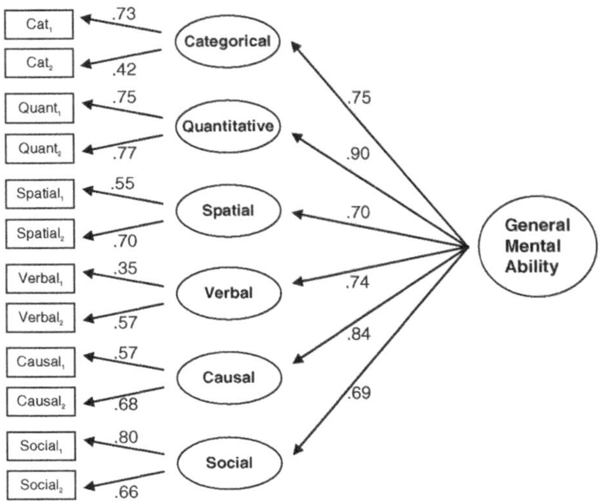

Fig. 2 The hierarchical structure of the six domains of thought as revealed by the confirmatory factor analysis.
Note: Model fit was excellent (χ^2/df = 71.053/48 = 1.48; p <.02, CFI = .97, RMSEA = .03, RMR = .01)

this model stands for *g* in psychometric models. In terms of the present theory, this factor is very generic and involves all sorts of general processes, such as processing efficiency, general inference, and the processes involved in working hypercognition.

In terms of Case's (1992a) analysis of central conceptual structures, which, by and large, coincide with most of the domains analyzed here, each of them involves its own semantic networks for the representation of domain-specific information and relevant actions and operations from the part of the person. Moreover, it must be noted that an analysis of these systems from the point of view of their logical composition suggests that each operates according to its own logical principles (Kargopoulos & Demetriou, 1998). These semantic and logical differences between the domains suggest that they are cognitively distinct from each other in addition to being dimensions of systematic individual differences, as suggested by their factorial autonomy. Therefore, it is clear that the psychometric methods of classical and modern confirmatory factor analysis that capture dimensions of individual differences converge with the cognitive methods of logical and semantic analysis that capture the formal and mental composition of cognitive domains.

Categorical Reasoning

Categorical reasoning specializes in the handling of relations of similarity and difference between objects. The primary function of categorical reasoning is to reduce unnecessary complexity by building concepts about the world that would facilitate future encounters on the basis of objects already encountered. Processes related to categorical perception according to color are examples of the core elements involved in this system. Infants are able to draw inductive inferences based on perceptual similarity from the very first days of life, if not at birth. Thus, the core processes in this domain are the seeds of inductive inference. At the second level of organization, this domain involves operations enabling the person to systematically represent and process similarities and differences between objects. For example, it involves classification skills and strategies enabling the individual to construct and process categories and classes. Our conceptions and misconceptions about the world, such as the concepts that we have about physical phenomena, living beings in general, or different types of persons, constitute the third level of organization in this system.

Quantitative Reasoning

All elements of reality can potentially undergo quantitative transformations. Things aggregate or separate so that they increase, decrease, split, or multiply in space or time for many different reasons. Subitization is an example of the core processes involved in this system. Subitization refers to our ability to specify the number of elements in small sets (smaller than three or four elements) by simply looking at them. At the second level of organization, quantitative reasoning involves operations enabling the thinker to deal with the various quantitative transformations mentioned above. Prominent among these operations are counting, pointing, bringing in, and removing and sharing, and their internalized mental counterparts, that is, the four arithmetic operations.

Spatial Reasoning

Spatial reasoning enables thinking about objects and episodes as such, and orientation and movement in space. Therefore, in this domain, spatial relations within objects (the composition and structure of objects) and between objects (relative distances, directions, and orientations) acquire prominence because they are crucial in the representation of the objects themselves, their location in space, and the space that surrounds them, as such. Formation of mental images and processes, such as perception of size, depth, and orientation of objects, is examples of this system's core processes. To be able to represent them, operate on them, and move between them, the thinker needs operations, such as mental rotation or direction tracking and reckoning, which honor these relations, thereby enabling the thinker to visualize objects and space from the perspective needed so as to be able to recognize and locate them and efficiently move between or toward them.

Causal Reasoning

Objects and people are very often dynamically related, sometimes functioning as the cause of changes and other times as the recipients of causal effects. Causal reasoning enables the grasp of dynamic interactions between objects or persons. Perception of fundamental causal relationships, such as when there is a direct transfer of energy from one object to another (e.g., we push something to move it), are examples of the core processes involved in this system. At the second level of organization, causal reasoning involves operations enabling the thinker to manipulate and represent causal relations. Prominent among these is trial and error manipulation aiming to uncover the causal role of objects. Isolation of variables (or systematic experimentation) is a more elaborate process employed to systematically manipulate dynamic causal relations (Demetriou, Elfklides, Papadaki, Papantoniou, & Economou, 1993).

Social Reasoning

Social reasoning deals with the understanding of social relationships and interactions. These range from the dynamics concerned with ongoing inter-personal interactions and relationships between individuals to general rules and principles governing the relationships between individuals and social or cultural institutions. In this latter case, one may refer to the moral principles and conventions regulating what is permissible in a given society at particular historical times or the rules governing the political organization of society. Core processes in this system involve the recognition of conspecifics (i.e., recognition of the members of the same species), such as the infant's preference for the human face as contrasted to other objects, or the recognition of particular emotionally laden facial expressions, such as a smile or growl, which are adaptively important for the individual. At the second level of organization, there are operations and processes that enable the individual to decipher the mental and emotional states and the intentions of others and organize his or her actions toward others accordingly. Imitation, actual or mental, decentering and taking the other's perspective, are examples of operations involved in understanding and handling social interactions.

Verbal Reasoning

There are three main functions of verbal reasoning: to facilitate interaction between persons, guide action, and organize inference across different domains and occasions. As a facilitator of inter-personal interactions, verbal reasoning enables persons to share information, cooperate, and check for consistency in the information provided and thus avoid deception, if present (Cosmides & Tooby, 1994). As a guide of action, it enables persons to specify the results of their possible actions from the beginning and thus choose between alternative courses of action according to the goals selected. As an inference organizer, it enhances mental economy and efficiency by generating mental tools that can readily be called upon in the future.

Core processes in this system underlie the ability to use the grammatical and syntactical structures of language (e.g., "*if* this *then* that," "*either* this *or* that") in order to infer the relations between the events or situations mentioned in a sequence of sentences (Braine, 1990). At the second level of organization, operations and processes in this domain are primarily directed to the truth and validity relations between verbal statements so that the person may judge the accuracy of the information received, decipher deception, etc. Two types of skills are used to attain these aims. First, there are grammatical and syntactical skills enabling the individual to interpret and interrelate the components in verbal statements so that information may be abstracted in goal-relevant, meaningful, and coherent ways. Second, there are skills enabling one to differentiate the contextual from the formal elements in a series of statements and operate on the latter. For example, focusing on verbs such as "is" or "belongs to" or conjunctions such as "and," "if," and "or" directs thinking to the relationships between the statements, rather than simply the statements themselves. These processes enable one to construct and express the basic logical relations of conjunction (... and... and...), disjunction (either... or), and implication (if... then). When available, these relations can be invoked for the sake of dealing with problems in any of the other domains. With development and experience, facility in intentionally calling upon these relations for the sake of the functioning of different domains increases.

The Hypercognitive System

Obviously, problem-solving creatures other than humans, such as animals, can draw inferences, and they possess many domain-specific abilities, such as orientation in space, object recognition, quantification. Even modern robots possess these abilities. However, possession of these abilities is not sufficient to credit these creatures with a mind. For this to be possible, a cognitive system must be capable of *self-mapping*. That is, it must be able to record its own cognitive experiences and keep maps of them that can be used in the future, if the need arises (Demetriou, 2000; Demetriou, Elfklides, & Platsidou, 1993; Demetriou & Kazi, 2001). Positing this principle implies that creatures capable of self-mapping possess a second-order level of knowing. In our terms, this is the *hypercognitive system*. The input to this system is information coming from the other levels of the mind (sensations, feelings, and conceptions caused by mental activity). This information is organized into the maps or models of mental functions to be described below. These are used to guide the control of the functioning of the domain-specific systems and the processing potentials available. The hypercognitive system involves *working hypercognition* and *long-term hypercognition*.

Working hypercognition revolves around a strong directive-executive function (DEF) that is responsible for setting and pursuing mental and behavioral goals until they are attained. Specifically, DEF involves processes enabling the person to (i) set the mind's current goals, (ii) plan the steps needed to attain the goal, (iii) monitor ongoing mental activity, (iv) register discrepancies between the present state and the goal and suggest corrective actions and, finally, (v) evaluate each step's processing demands vis-à-vis the available structural possibilities and skills. These processes operate recursively, so that goals and subgoals may be renewed according to every moment's evaluation of the system's distance from its ultimate objective (Demetriou, 2000; Demetriou & Efklides, 1985; Demetriou & Kazi, 2001).

Long-term hypercognition. Consciousness is an integral part of the hypercognitive system. That is, the very process of setting mental goals, planning their attainment, monitoring action vis-à-vis both the goals and the plans, and regulating real or mental action requires a system that can remember and review and therefore know itself. Therefore, conscious awareness and all ensuing functions, such as a self-concept (that is, awareness of one's own mental characteristics, functions, and mental states) and a theory of mind (that is, awareness of others' mental functions and states) are part of the very construction of the system. In fact, long-term hypercognition comprises the models and representations concerning past cognitive experiences that result from the functioning of working hypercognition. These models involve descriptions about the general structural and dynamic characteristics of the mind – for example, that there are different cognitive functions, such as perception, attention, and memory, and different cognitive structures, such as the domain-specific systems to be described below. Moreover, these models involve prescriptions and rules about the efficient use of the functions – for instance, that excessive information requires organization if it is to be retained in memory or that rehearsal is needed if one is to learn quickly and permanently. Research on theory of mind (e.g., Flavell, Green, & Flavell, 1986; Wellman, 1990) sheds light on this aspect of long-term hypercognition. Moreover, research on self-evaluation and self-representation with regard to intellectual functioning is related to the evaluative and regulatory aspects of hypercognition (Demetriou & Kazi, 2001; Harter, 1999).

Therefore, working hypercognition involves the control and executive functions ascribed by Baddeley's model to the central executive and the episodic buffer of working memory or by experimental researchers to functions underlying control of processing, inhibition, and selective attention. The ascription of these functions to the hypercognitive system rather than to working memory or control of processing conveys our assumption that self-awareness and control emanate from a higher-order system that specializes in the surveillance and regulation of cognitive functions oriented to the environment. This system may have evolved from primary inhibition and control mechanisms associated with perception and automated action sequences (Gibson, 1966).

Relations Between the Levels of Mind

The three-level architecture. The model presented in Fig. 2 above is consistent with our assumptions about the organization of domains, but it does not directly speak about the three-level architecture, which includes processing potentials as such, the domains, and hypercognition, which generates self-awareness and self-regulation. Several studies satisfy this requirement (Demetriou & Kazi, 2001, 2006). One of them will be summarized here.

This study addressed all three dimensions of *processing potentials* (a series of Stroop-like tasks addressed speed and control of processing) and *representational capacity* (phonological, visual, and executive working memory), three *domains of reasoning* (i.e., a series of tasks addressed verbal, quantitative, and spatial reasoning) and *self-awareness* about the domains of reasoning mentioned above. These tasks were given to 11- to 15-year-old adolescents. Therefore, this study can show how all three important dimensions of the human mind, namely processing efficiency and representational power, reasoning or psychometric *g*, and self-awareness, contribute to the formation of general intelligence. In other words, this study can show if a fundamental aspect of *g*, processing efficiency, and representational power, that is supposed to be the engine of fluid intelligence, shares variance not only with inferential processes, which is now taken for granted by all researchers of intelligence, but also with self-awareness about them. To our knowledge, no previous study has examined these relations. The model that captures performance on these tasks is shown in Fig. 3.

It can be seen that this model includes a first-order factor standing for processing efficiency and another first-order factor standing for working memory. These two factors are related to a second-order factor that stands for general mental capacity. Also, there were three first-order factors standing for performance on quantitative, verbal, and visuo-spatial reasoning. These three factors relate to another second-order factor that stands for general reasoning processes. Finally, there are three first-order factors standing for self-representation in each of the three reasoning domains. The three factors relate to another second-order factor that stands for general perceived competence. Obviously, these three factors stand for the three main levels of the mental architecture described here. These three second-order factors were regressed on a third-order factor, the $\mathbf{G}_{grand}$. Attention is drawn to the relations between the three second-order factors and the $\mathbf{G}_{grand}$ factor. They are all very high (all > 0.82), clearly suggesting that processing efficiency and capacity, inferential and problem-solving processes, and self-representation about them, are all complementary and very strong components of *g*. All in all, this study shows clearly that all three types of processes are equally strong constituents of the human mind.

Dynamic Relations Between Processes and Systems

The relations between the general and the specialized processes are complex and bi-directional. On the one hand, general processes set the limits for the construction, the operation, and the development of the domain-specific systems. On the other hand, specialized processes provide the frame and raw material for the functioning of general processes. Thus, variations from the general forms across persons and domains reflect, to a large extent, differences between the specialized processes.

The models of the effects of general processes on specialized processes adopt a reductionist or bottom-up approach. That is, they assume that lower-level and thus more general-purpose processes constrain the condition of more complex and thus more specialized processes (Fry & Hale, 2000; Kail, 1991; Kyllonen & Christal, 1990). To validate this model, we (Demetriou, Mouyi, & Spanoudis, 2008) designed tasks addressed to the following processes: speed of processing (SP), perceptual discrimination (PD), perceptual control (PC), conceptual control (CC), working memory (WM), information integration (InfI), and reasoning (Reason).

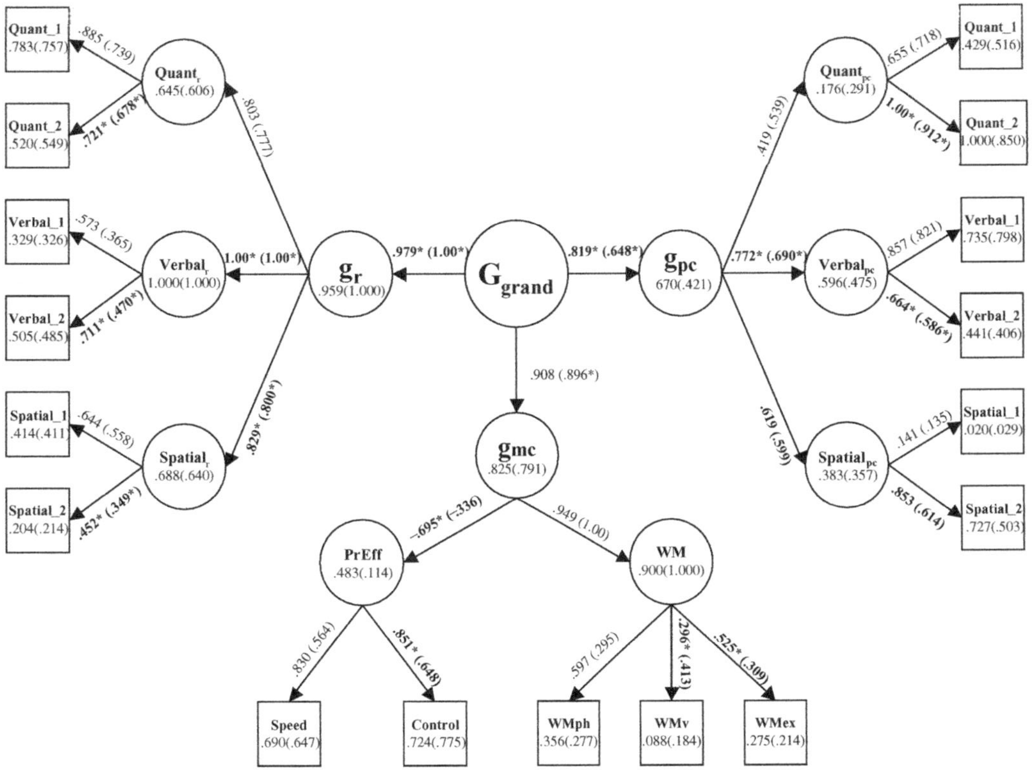

Fig. 3 The confirmatory factor analysis for processing efficiency and capacity, and self-representation of the cognitive processes.
Notes: 1. The first and second coefficient in each pair represent relations before and after partialling out age.
2. Free parameters are denoted by bold characters.
3. Significant coefficients are denoted by an asterisk.
4. Numbers in squares and circles indicate variance accounted for

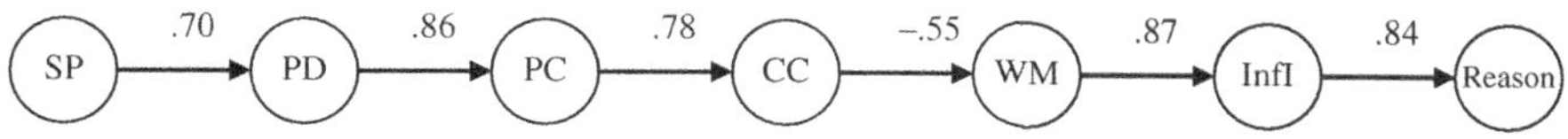

Fig. 4 The simplex model of the structural relations between factors in the Demetriou et al. (2008) study

We postulate that these tasks require processes embedded in each other so that PD includes speed together of perceptual discrimination processes. Perceptual control includes these two types of processes plus processes allowing the control of perceptual interference. Conceptual control involves all of the processes above together with processes allowing the control of conceptual interference. Working memory involves all of these processes together with storage and retrieval processes. Information integration involves all of these processes together with processes allowing to integrate information according to plan. Finally, reasoning includes all of the processes above together with processes allowing to draw valid conclusions from premises. These tasks were given to 140 children, about equally drawn from the six primary school grades, that is, 6.5- to 11.5-year-old children.

To test the model capturing the structural relations between the various processes specified above, a series of structural equation models were evaluated. One of these models is presented in Fig. 4. These models are built on the assumption that processes are hierarchically organized so that the processes at each level in the hierarchy are largely based on the processes of the previous levels together with processes specific to this level. In the present case, the various processes were represented by seven first-order factors. Specifically, speed of processing, perceptual discrimination, perceptual control, conceptual control, working memory, information integration, and reasoning were identified by relating each of the corresponding sets of measures to a separate factor. These factors were regressed on each other in the cascade fashion shown in Fig. 4. The fit of this model was excellent (χ^2 (143) = 166.741, $p = 0.085$, CFI = 0.974, RMSEA = 0.045).

It can be seen that all structural relations were significant and high. Therefore, it is clear that cognitive processes are hierarchically organized so that effects are carried over from the one level of organization to the other where new processes are constructed in a level-specific fashion.

General Developmental Patterns

All of the processes mentioned above develop systematically with age. The structural models summarized suggest that there are strong developmental relations between the various processes, such that changes at any level of organization of the mind open the way for changes in other levels. Specifically, the simplex cascade models above suggest that changes in speed of processing open the way for changes in the various forms of control of processing. These, in turn, open the way for the enhancement of working-memory capacity, which open the way for development in inferential processes as such. Eventually, all of these changes result in the development of the various specialized domains through the reorganization of domain-specific skills, strategies, and knowledge and the acquisition of new ones. Other studies, not presented here, show that there is top-down escalation of change as well but space considerations do not allow expanding on this aspect of development (Demetriou, Christou, Spanoudis, & Platsidou, 2002). We summarize below the basic developmental trends in each of the main levels of the mind.

Processing Efficiency

Our research shows that reaction times decrease with age in all of the processing efficiency functions described below (see Fig. 5). Although absolute values vary depending upon the complexity of the process concerned, the pattern of change is the same. Specifically, change in processing efficiency is exponential. That is, it is fast at the beginning (i.e., from early to middle childhood) and it decelerates systematically (from early adolescence onward) until it attains its maximum capacity in early adulthood. According to Kail (1991), what is common between the different tasks is the person's cycle time – that is, the time needed to execute each step or mental operation in the sequence of operations needed to attain a goal. Thus, any speed difference between a child and an adult solving the same task is due to the fact that the child's cycle times are longer than those of the adult. As cycle times decrease, processing becomes faster until reaching its maximum capacity.

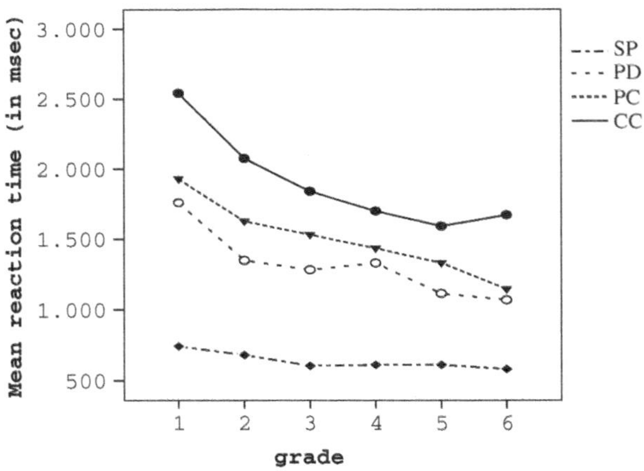

Fig. 5 Processing efficiency as a function of age and process

Working Memory

There are many ways to measure the capacity of working memory. This explains why scholars differ in their specification of the capacity of working memory at different periods of life. Pascual-Leone (1970), for example, maintained that the sheer capacity for holding information in focus is one unit at the age of 3 years and it then increases by one unit every second year until to reach the maximum of seven units at the age of 15 years. Unlike Pascual-Leone, however, Case (1992a) maintained that total representational capacity does not change with development. Only the relationship between operating space, which is occupied by executive control processes, and short-term storage space change. That is, Case asserted that, with development, the quantity of mental resources required by operating space decreases due to increasing processing efficiency. The space left free because of these changes is used by the short-term storage space. Thus, short-term storage space increases as processing efficiency increases. Case maintained that the capacity of short-term storage space is 1, 2, 3, and 4 schemes, at the four levels constituting each of the four main cycles of development, that is, sensorimotor, relational, dimensional, and vectorial thought, respectively.

However, Case's position is not accepted by many because there is strong evidence that there indeed is expansion of actual working-memory capacity independent of other processes (Halford, 1993). According to our studies, all components of working memory (i.e., executive processes, phonological storage, and visual storage) increase with age (Demetriou, Elfklides, & Platsidou, 1993; Demetriou et al., 2002). In fact, the development of all three components seems to follow the same pattern of change and can be described by a logistic curve which is very similar to the exponential curve that describes the change of processing efficiency (see below). This pattern of change of working memory is illustrated in Fig. 6.

The quantitative task here required more executive control than the spatial task. It can be seen that there indeed (Case, 1992a) is an inverse trade-off between the central executive and the storage buffers, so that the higher the involvement of

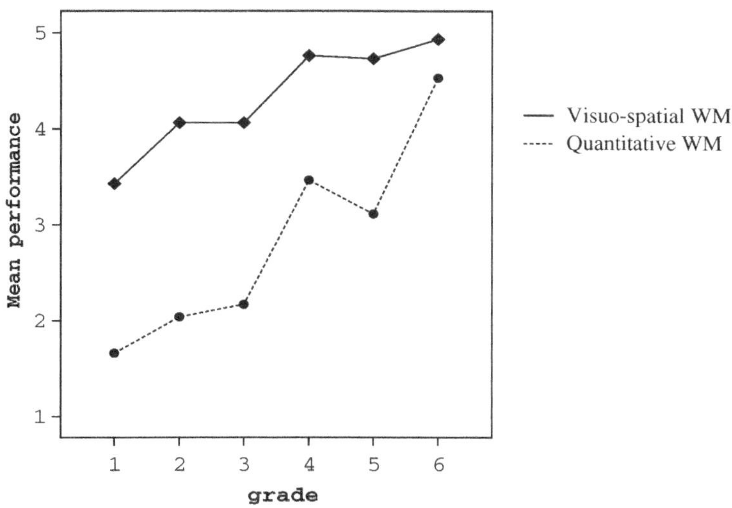

Fig. 6 Visuo-spatial and quantitative memory as a function of age

executive processes, the less the manifest capacity of the modality-specific buffers. This is so because the executive operations themselves consume part of the available processing recourses. However, with age, executive operations and information are chunked into integrated units. As a result, with development, the person can store increasingly more complex units of information. For instance, children of primary school age can remember single numbers, whereas adolescents can store the products of operations applied on numbers.

To account for this evidence, we proposed the functional shift model (Demetriou, Efklides, & Platsidou, 1993). This model presumes that when the mental units of a given level reach a maximum degree of complexity, the mind tends to reorganize these units at a higher level of representation or integration so as to make them more manageable. Having created a new mental unit, the mind prefers to work with this rather than the previous units due to its functional advantages. An example in the verbal domain would be the shift from words to sentences and in the quantitative domain from natural numbers to algebraic representations of numbers of numerical relations. The model suggests that working memory cannot be disentangled completely from its content. By definition, then, working memory is representational in nature.

Development of the Specialized Domains

Explicating the development of each of the six specialized domains is far beyond the scope of the present chapter. Thus, we will only outline here the general trends of development across the various domains and present the modal characteristics of each domain from the age of 3 through the age of 15 years in a very condensed way in Table 1.

Inspection of Table 1 suggests that with development each of the domains moves from fewer and reality-referenced to more and reciprocally referenced representations. As a result, concepts in each of the domains become increasingly defined in reference to rules and principles bridging more local concepts which may be specified in reference to observable characteristics of the objects concerned. Moreover, understanding and problem solving in each of the domains evolve from global and less integrated to differentiated, but better integrated, mental operations. As a result, planning and operation from alternatives becomes increasingly part of the person's modus operandi. This offers flexibility in cognitive functioning and problem solving across a broad spectrum of domains. Finally, as we will show in the next section, increasing reflection on cognitive and problem-solving processes, self-guidance, and self-awareness become part of the system.

Hypercognition

Hypercognition develops along a number of different fronts, including the various functions of working hypercognition, such as DEF and self-evaluation, and the various dimensions of long-term hypercognition, such as the theory of mind, implicit theories of cognition and intelligence, and the self-concept. Space considerations do not allow a complete discussion of development along all of these fronts. Discussion

Table 1 Modal characteristics of the specialized domains with development

Age	Class	Number	Cause	Space	Verbal	Hyper
3–4	Proto-categories	Proto-quantitative schemes	Proto-causal schemes	Global images	Primary reasoning	Differentiation between modalities (perception vs. knowing)
5–6	Single criterion classes	Co-ordination of proto-quantitative schemes	Co-ordination of proto-causal schemes	Single spatial dimensions or operations	Permission rules	Understanding the stream of consciousness and inner speech
7–8	Logical multiplication	Number concepts and quantitative dimensions	Experience-based proto-theories	"Fluent" mental imagery	Explicit inference	Grasp of the constructive nature of thought
9–10	Logical multiplication on unfamiliar context	Construction of simple math relations (e.g., $a + 5 = 8$)	Testable theories in action	Representation of complex realities	Logical necessity	Differentiation between cognitive functions (memory vs. attention)
11–12	Flexible logical multiplication	Proportional reasoning. Co-ordination of symbolic *structures*	Suppositions, isolation of variables	Imagination of the non real	Logical validity of propositions	Differentiation between clearly different domains (space vs. maths)
13–14	Strategic classification including relevant–irrelevant information	Algebraic reasoning based on mutually specified symbol systems	Hypothesis driven experimentation	Originality in mental images	Grasp of formal relations	Awareness of specialized mental operations within a domain
15–16	Multilevel classes Networks of classification criteria	Generalized concept of variable	Integrated theory building	Personal imaginal worlds, aesthetic criteria	Reasoning on reasoning	Integrated cognitive theory

here focuses on the development of awareness of cognitive processes because they are instrumental in the functioning and development of the other levels of the mind.

One of our studies (Demetriou & Kazi, 2006) examined if 3- to 7-year-old children are aware of the cognitive processes involved in tasks addressed to three domains of reasoning – that is, spatial, quantitative, and categorical reasoning. Specifically, children were presented with pairs of cards, each of which showed a child trying to solve a task, and they were asked to evaluate if the tasks of the two children were similar to each other and explain their answers. In some pairs, these model children were required to use the same processes, applied either on the same or on different objects. For example, two of the pairs addressed classification (the two children were trying to classify the same objects in the first pair and different objects in the second pair), two addressed counting (the same objects in the first pair and different in the second), and two addressed visuo-spatial reasoning (reproduction of a model figure in the first pair and puzzle construction in the second). Finally, there were pairs where the two children were required to use different mental processes. Specifically, one of the children was supposed to classify and the other to count, one of the children was supposed to classify and the other to reproduce a model figure, or one of the children was supposed to count and the other to reproduce a figure. It was found that the judgments of similarity between processes in these self-awareness tasks moved, with age, from the perceptual characteristics of the tasks to the mental operations involved. Specifically, from the age of 3–5 years, the majority of children based their judgments on perceptual similarity across all nine task pairs. More than half of 6-year-old children and more than the two thirds of the 7-year-old children were able to recognize that the three task pairs involving tasks belonging to a different domain require different mental processes. However, it was only at the age of 7 that the majority of children were able to recognize the mental process required by similar process tasks where the objects of application of the process differed. This pattern suggests that the development of self-awareness about mental processes develops with the development of reasoning processes as such (Demetriou & Kazi, 2006).

In another study (Demetriou & Kazi, 2006), 11- to 17-year-old adolescents were examined by tasks addressed to four domains: quantitative reasoning, causal reasoning, social reasoning, and drawing. In addition to solving the various tasks addressed to each of these domains, participants were asked to evaluate their performance on the tasks and to answer a general self-representation inventory probing their general self-concept related to each of the domains (e.g., "I can easily derive the mathematical rules behind many specific examples," "To find out which of my guesses is correct, I proceed to methodically consider each time only the things my guess proposes," "I understand easily the intentions of others before they express them," "I can draw a person very accurately").

We found that the relation of self-evaluation and reasoning is very low and nonsignificant at the age of 11 years and it then steadily and systematically increases until approaching unity at the age of 15–16 years (0.97). Interestingly, the relation of self-concept and reasoning does follow the same trend but with a considerable age lag. That is, it is very low until the age of 13, it rises to moderate and significant at the age of 14 (0.34), and to high (0.55) at the age of 15–16 years. In a similar fashion, the relation of self-concept and self-evaluation is very low until the age of 13 years, it rises to moderate and significant at the age of 14 (–0.30) and to very high at the age of 15–16 years (–0.80). The negative relation here implies that with increasing accuracy in self-evaluations, adolescents become more conservative and strict in their self-representation (Demetriou & Kazi, 2006).

The findings above suggest that self-awareness and self-evaluation of cognitive processes develop in a recycling fashion, which involves three major cycles: 3–7, 8–12, and 13–18. That is, within each phase of development, self-evaluation and self-awareness concerning the relevant mental operations are very low and inaccurate at the beginning but they tend to increase and become more accurate with development until the end of the phase. Entering the next phase resets both of them to an initial low level, from where they gradually take off again with the development of the new phase-specific problem-solving operations and skills. This pattern of change indicates, on the one hand, that the thinker needs time and experience to acquire knowledge and sensitivity to the condition of the operations and processes of the new phase. On the other hand, it also indicates, as shown in the study summarized in Fig. 3, that increasing self-awareness of cognitive processes becomes part of the very functioning of the processes concerned. We try to show below that this intertwining of cognitive functioning with awareness about it, which makes metarepresentation or, in other words, the explicit representation of cognitive processes possible, is in fact a very robust mechanism of cognitive development.

Metarepresentation as a Mechanism of Cognitive Development

Metarepresentation is a hypercognitive process which looks for, codifies, and typifies similarities between mental experiences (past or present) to enhance understanding and problem-solving efficiency. So defined, metarepresentation is the constructive aspect of working hypercognition that integrates the contents of the episodic buffer, in Baddeley's (2007) terms, or the screen of conscience, in James's terms (1890), thereby generating new mental schemes and operations. In a sense, metarepresentation is the inductive inference applied to mental experiences, representations, or operations, rather than to environmental stimuli and information as such. We will explicate this process here in reference to the development of logical reasoning itself.

According to many theorists, reasoning reflects a universal language of thought that comprises a limited set of ready-made inference patterns. For example, Braine (1990) argued for a number of fundamental inference schemas corresponding to particular patterns of events and occurrences in the environment. The most common of these patterns are *joint iteration*, which refers to repetitions of actions, events, or objects, *iteration of alternatives*, which applies to a situation wherein one event or object is present and another event or object may or may not be present, and *contingencies*, which refer to time-dependent sequences which may or may not be causal.

Learning spoken language, according to these theorists, is equivalent to learning a translation into the language of thought. In other words, learning the connectives *and*, *or*, and *if*, in their native language, which correspond to the three patterns mentioned above, is equivalent to mapping them onto the corresponding connectives of the language of thought. Obviously, the three schemas correspond to the logical relations of conjunction, disjunction, and implication, which were examined in most of the studies summarized above. Both psychometric and developmental theorists would feel perfectly happy with the assumption of a universal language of thought. For psychometric theorists, it maps onto their construct of fluid intelligence as a system of general reasoning processes, such as Spearman's (1904) eduction of relations and correlates. For developmental theorists, it maps onto operative intelligence (Piaget, 1970), executive control structures (Case, 1992a), skill structures (Fischer, 1980), or structure mappings (Halford, 1993).

We maintain that these general inference patterns do not exist at the beginning. Instead, they are constructed by mapping domain-specific inference patterns onto each other. Therefore, a general language of thought is an emergent product of guided and reflected upon domain-specific functioning. For example, joint iteration in the categorical domain (e.g., property A is present in this object, *and* in this object, *and* in this object, *and*...) is equivalent to recognition of perceptual similarity. That is, it signifies a generality that may be associated with a class of objects defined by this particular property A. Joint iteration in the quantitative domain (e.g., I see this object, *and* this object, *and* this object, *and* ...) signifies an amount that may be associated with a particular number. At the beginning, there is nothing recognizably common between these two variations of joint iteration. They are just implicitly applied within each of the two domains leading to domain-specific meaning making: perceptual similarity in the categorical domain that generates concepts of objects and subitization that generates number representations. Gradually, however, joint iteration in the categorical domain generates self-directed class reasoning and classification skills, and joint iteration in the quantitative domain generates number concepts and counting skills. Likewise, when a child realizes that the sequencing of the *if...then* connectives in language is associated with situations in which the event or thing preceded by *if* always comes first and that it produces the event or thing introduced by *then*, this child is actually formulating an inference schema that leads to predictions and interpretations specific to this schema. When abstracted over many different occasions and somehow tagged (or symbolized) in the mind, it becomes the frame which guides reasoning by implication.

A general language of thought is gradually constructed when these patterns of thought are compared across domains and reduced to schemes that can be intentionally activated across domains. A good sign of the state of this general language of thought is logical necessity. That is, taking the conclusion of an inferential scheme as logically necessary implies that this scheme has been lifted from a context-bound processing frame to an advanced rule-bound organizer of relations, which does not allow any exceptions. Therefore, this general language of thought is a construction that gradually expands and stabilizes through the interaction between domain-specific processing and executive, self-awareness, and self-regulation processes of the hypercognitive system. Obviously, natural language has a privileged relation with this emergent universal language of thought, because it is the main symbol system that can be used to express and manipulate its constructions. Thus, natural language and the emergent language of thought are gradually intertwined and increasingly used to guide and facilitate inference and processing within each of the domains. Structural modeling shows that the relations between propositional reasoning as such and the other domains of thought become stronger with age. However, these relations always deviate considerably from unity, suggesting that there are other processes in these domains in addition to propositional reasoning (Demetriou et al., 2002). Thus, there is a dynamic interaction such that the functioning of domains feeds in the development of general inferential processes and these, once in place, guide and facilitate the functioning of the domains.

In conclusion, according to this theory, metarepresentation is the mechanism that drives the development of reasoning from automated or stimulus-driven inference to explicit logical reasoning. Obviously, metarepresentation reminds one of Piaget's (2001) reflective abstraction and Karmiloff-Smith's (1992) representational redescription. Like reflective abstraction, it abstracts general patterns from different mental functions or activities. Like representational redescription, it reorganizes them at a higher, more efficient representational level. However, its primary constituent is self-awareness. Although its accuracy and degree of involvement varies from age to age, self-awareness is always part of the abstraction and reconstruction processes which generate new concepts and schemes out of old ones. In fact, our studies about self-evaluation and self-awareness summarized above suggest that moving across developmental phases is a product of increasing binding between actual cognitive processing and the awareness about it. Moreover, there is accruing evidence that self-awareness and executive control are part of the learning process and that the efficiency of learning changes in development because of changes in them (Kuhn & Pease, 2006). These processes ensure that future use of the new construction is under the intentional control of the thinker and not just under the control of external stimuli.

Mapping the Mind–Brain Architectures

We can imagine human mind and human brain as the two sides of the same coin. The human brain is the underlying biological mechanism of the human mind. In other words, the mind in all of its expressions emerges from the structure and functioning of the brain. Research in cognitive neuroscience in both its empirical (Kandel, Schwartz, & Jessell, 1995) and its computational (O' Reilly & Munakata, 2000) branches has blossomed in recent years. The guiding question of this research is simple: What are the neuronal underpinnings of the various functions and processes modeled by theories of intelligence and intellectual development? In this section we will review research on the brain that shows what the neuronal analog of the architecture proposed here might be and why we can proceed in order to link neuroscience data with education.

However, a note of caution is in order here, because simple questions do not always have simple answers. Specifically, we must bear in mind that psychological and brain functions reside on different levels of analysis and involve different "research objects." The objects of psychological research include (i) observable responses (ranging from reaction times to various types of stimuli to solutions to various types of problems) and (ii) subjective experiences and related reports. The objects of neuroscience research include biological entities, such as the nature, volume, and organization of neuronal matter itself and the responses and correlates of neuronal matter. This last type of objects is extremely variable, including (i) blood supply and glucose consumption of different brain areas, (ii) the electrochemical activity of neuronal networks, (iii) pattern of chemical responses related to the communication between neurons through the release and use of neurotransmitters, and, (iv) at a more basic level, various types of protein synthesis which, under the direction of genes, express the responses of the brain to ongoing cognitive needs raised by the environment. We still do not know how to map the different levels of analysis onto each other. In fact, the lack of a commonly accepted language for describing each of these levels renders their mapping onto each other difficult.

With this caution in mind, from the perspective of our theory, we can outline the questions that neuroscience must answer:

1. Is the architecture of mind specified by our theory reflected in the various levels of the organization and functioning of the brain? Specifically, are the various structures reflected in models such as those shown in Figs. 2, 3, and 4 also present at the various levels of the organization and functioning of the brain? For example, are the various environment-oriented systems of thought represented by different regions or networks in the brain? If this is the case, do the neural structures serving different systems of thought function differently? Alternatively, is local differentiation enough to ensure functional differentiation? In case the networks differ in functioning, how does each of them carry on its own job (e.g., in terms of rate coding and type of neurotransmitters used)?
2. What entities and conditions in the brain stand for the second- and third-order factors of the models shown in Figs. 2 and 3? That is, are there actual structural analogs in the brain for each of the second-order factors that stand for levels of organization in the mind, such as general inferential processes related to fluid intelligence and general self-representation? Is there any structural analog for the third-order factor that stands for whatever is common between all kinds of cognitive activity? If yes, what are they and how does each of them function? If not, how are they served (e.g., by different patterns of activity)? What are these patterns? How do they differ from each other? In any case, how do structures, networks, and/or patterns interact with each other (e.g., in terms of temporal coding)? How are they integrated into a final solution or experience (e.g., in terms of synchronization)?

3. How are different networks differentiated subjectively so that intentional decisions can be made in advance about their activation? What other regions are involved when processing surfaces to consciousness? Does awareness emerge from particular structures or networks or does it result from particular coactivation patterns than may involve alternative networks?
4. Brain has evolved to handle change and variation in the environment. We have shown above that each of the systems modeled by our theory changes as a result of learning and development. How is learning in each of the domains reflected in changes in the associated neural networks? What is the neuronal analog of learning transfer and generalization?
5. Brain itself changes ontogenetically for genetically controlled reasons (such as increases in neuronal volume, myelination, and neuronal pruning within particular time windows). These changes are, to a large extent, although not completely, independent from the environment. How are these changes related to the changes of the various cognitive processes described here? For example, what might be the neuronal analog of the chain of changes suggested by the model shown in Fig. 4? This model suggests that brain development would have to proceed as follows: First there should be changes in aspects of the brain related to general speed of processing, such as myelination. Then there should be changes in brain networks related to control, such as the prefrontal cortex. These changes must then lead to changes to structures related to working memory, such as the hippocampus and several areas of the prefrontal cortex. Eventually, do all of these changes have to be followed by changes in networks serving specialized thought domains?

Obviously, the grand neuro-cognitive developmental theory of intelligence to come would have to answer the questions above thereby integrating brain with functional and subjective maps of mental functions into a common landscape. We review below recent research and theorizing in cognitive and developmental neuroscience to show that the structural and functional organization of the brain can indeed be mapped on the general levels and tiers of mind described by the present model. In recent years, neuroscientists believe that the brain is organized along two seemingly conflicting principles: segregation and integration (Sporns, Chialvo, Kaiser, & Hilgetag, 2004). On the one hand, segregation refers to the fact that the brain consists of different types of neurons (i.e., afferent neurons, which carry information in the system; efferent neurons, which carry instructions to other systems such as the muscular system; and interneurons, which integrate and process information and instructions) and different areas (layers, lobes, circuits), which subserve different tasks and functions, such as vision, audition, inference. In other words, according to this principle, the brain consists of systems that are anatomically and functionally specialized. On the other hand, integration refers to the fact that the brain functions as a whole. That is, the brain's products (perception, motor behaviors, cognition) emerge from the interactions among specialized neuronal populations. We trust that this chapter has demonstrated that these two major organizational principles of brain organization and functioning describe the organization and functioning of the mind as well. According to our theory, the mind is also segregated into specialized cognitive systems and subsystems which are integrated at different levels to produce coherent understanding and problem solving and a coherent sense of experience. We try to show in this section how the organization and functioning of the mind might correspond to organization and functioning of the brain.

Brain–Mind Maps

The study of brain activation by modern neuroimaging methods, mainly PET and fMRI, has blossomed in the recent years. As a result, there is considerable evidence about the relations between cognitive processes and brain functioning. In a recent review of a large number of neuroimaging and lesion studies, Jung and Haier (2007) attempted to synthesize this evidence into an integrated model associating brain functioning with the theory of general intelligence, which they called the parieto-frontal integration theory (P-FIT) of general intelligence. According to this theory, information is first registered and processed in regions of the cortex which specialize to deal with different types of sensory information, such as the visual (BA 18, 19) and the auditory cortex (BA 22). From there, information is then fed forward to several regions in the parietal cortex (BA 7, 39, 40) for symbolism, abstraction, and elaboration. Then there is an interaction of these regions with frontal regions (BA 6, 9, 10, 45–47) for the conception and hypothesis testing of alternative solutions to the problem at hand. Finally, the anterior cingulate (BA 32) is engaged to constrain response selection and inhibit alternative responses. If interference is caused by the fact that the same neural networks are activated by different blocks of information (Gruber & von Cramon, 2003; Klingberg, 1998), the anterior cingulate may be conceived as a conductor orchestrating when different players must come into play. Individual differences in the volume, quality, efficiency, and connectivity of these neuronal ensembles and the underlying white matter are associated with individual differences in general IQ.

Mapping the P-FIT onto our model suggests some interesting isomorphisms are related to the first two of the questions posed above. Overall, there are indeed brain structures related to the mind structures uncovered by our research. Specifically, the sensory areas involved in the P-FIT model as well as other information-specific networks may be more related to the domain-specific processes represented by first-order factors in the present model, such as verbal and spatial reasoning. The parietal areas of the P-FIT model may be related to the information integration, meaning making, and inferential processes applied on domain-specific information and emerging as second-order factors in structural models. The frontal areas of the P-FIT model may be related to working memory, attention, and executive control as reflected by the working memory and the control factors of the present model. Finally, the anterior cingulate of the P-FIT model may be related to intentional planning, inhibition, and conscious selection of responses included in the hypercognitive system of the present model.

What are the specific brain networks serving the specialized reasoning domains? The clearest differentiation in neuronal infrastructure supporting the functioning of different cognitive processes is between verbal and visuo-spatial information. In recent years there has been a clear substantiation of this differentiation in regard to the short-term storage of verbal and visuo-spatial storage of information. That is, neuroimaging shows that verbal storage is served by two distinct circuits, one specializing in verbal rehearsal as such (i.e., a left-lateralized premotor-parietal network) and another one subserving nonarticulatory maintenance of phonological information (i.e., a bilateral anterior-prefrontal/inferior parietal network). In contrast, visuo-spatial storage relies on only one bilateral brain system (i.e., the posterior parts of the superior frontal sulcus and the entire interparietal sulcus). Some brain regions are activated during processing of both, the verbal and the visuo-spatial tasks, which is in line with the assumption that a central episodic buffer may exist (i.e., right middle frontal gyrus and the pre_SMA as well as bilaterally in the deep frontal opercular cortex and the cortex along anterior and middle parts of the intraparietal sulcus).

At the level of reasoning processes as such, there is evidence showing that different types of reasoning are served by different neural networks, in addition to the P-FIT networks mentioned above. According to Osherson et al. (1998), inductive and deductive reasoning are served by different but partially overlapping neural networks (frontal gyrus and the right insular cortex for inductive reasoning and associative visual areas, the right superior parietal lobule and thalamus, and the right anterior cingulate for deductive reasoning). Even the same type of reasoning, such as deductive reasoning, activates different networks depending upon the information to be integrated (Goel, Buchel, Frith, & Dolan, 2000). Specifically, content-based propositions activate temporal (BA 21, 22) and frontal regions (BA 44, 8, 9). Formal propositions activate occipital (BA 18, 19), left parietal (BA 40), bilateral dorsal frontal (BA 6), left frontal (BA 44, 8, 10), and right frontal (BA 46) regions, suggesting the construction of visual mental models of the relations implied by the formal propositions. Quantitative information is processed in the inferior parietal cortex, particularly its posterior convolution called the angular gyrus (BA 39) (Dehaene, 1997). Understanding of causal relations between objects is processed in the medial and dorsal part of the superior frontal cortex whereas perception of causality is served by visual cortices, such as V5 (Fonlupt, 2003). Crucial aspects of social understanding are related to the activation of the medial prefrontal cortex, the superior temporal sulcus, and the temporal poles bilaterally. Processing of categorical information is very closely related to language understanding and it is thus associated with the entire superior temporal gyrus which analyzes the "object" properties of auditory signals (Galaburda, 2002).

The discussion about consciousness and awareness is related to the third of the questions raised above. There is no consensus as to the brain bases of consciousness and self-awareness. According to some scholars, these distinctive functions of the human mind do not reside in a particular locus of the brain. Specifically, according to Edelman and Tononi (2000) and Lamme (2006), there is evidence showing that awareness emerges from brain functioning as such rather than from any particular brain region dedicated to it. Specifically, it is assumed that awareness emerges from two characteristics of the brain functioning: recurrent activation of the same network and co-ordinated activation of complementary networks. That is, the person becomes aware of stimuli and processes whose processing is re-cycled over the same neuronal networks so that they are co-ordinated or tuned to each other thereby producing an experience of functioning, so to speak.

This interpretation of consciousness has been questioned by Crick and Koch (2005). These scholars have recently argued that consciousness emerges from the functioning of particular brain structure which is connected to all sensory and motor regions of the cortex and the amygdala which is related to emotion. This small structure, the claustrum, is located below the cortex. According to Crick and Koch (2005), it functions as the spot of attention as it receives input from all areas activated at a particular moment and binds them together.

The reader is reminded that it was argued above that consciousness emerges from directive-executive functions because these functions are recursive. In a sense, then, mind maps of cognitive functions, such as those shown in Fig. 3, are representations of maps of recurrent brain activity that gradually become explicitly represented. Our studies on self-evaluation and self-representation show that explicit representation of cognitive processes is a slow process that grows side by side with the development of the cognitive processes themselves, slightly lacking behind them and recycling with them. An important task for future research is to provide crucial evidence about these models of the neuronal bases of consciousness. That is, is moment to moment self-awareness, the coherent self-representation which emerges from the unification of moment to moment self-awareness in time, and the ensuing self-evaluations that are produced by applying self-representations on on-line activity the result of (i) increasing co-ordination of different distributed networks in the brain, as suggested by the Edelman's model or (ii) the functioning of a particular brain nucleus, as suggested by Crick and Koch's model, or (iii) both, that is a combination of these two models – that is a single structure such as the claustrum orchestrates the co-ordination of different networks?

The structural equation and development models presented in this chapter lean toward the third option. That is, the presence of domain-specific factors at both the performance and the self-representation levels of the model may be taken to correspond to the networks that carry the different types of processing and their registration in awareness and self-representation as such. The presence of level-specific factors (such as the general reasoning and the general self-representation factors) may be taken to correspond to general patterns of neuronal activity that run through each of these levels, that is, patterns related to processing as such (e.g., general associative and inferential mechanisms) and patterns related to self-monitoring and self-awareness as such (i.e., general self-observation processes), respectively. Finally, the presence of a grand factor binding the general performance and self-representation factors may reflect the operation of a common central neuronal structure binding everything together and pulling the strings of different systems at different levels.

The reader may have noticed that a very powerful factor in models of intellectual functioning and development, that is, speed of processing, is not mentioned above. We suggest that this factor stands for general qualities of the brain networks involved, or even the brain as a whole, rather than for a particular region or network. These qualities may be the sheer neuronal volume, myelination, and connectivity between and within regions. Efficiency of operation and response to environmental demands by building the required neural networks may also be important parameters of this general quality. Garlick (2002) proposed that the underlying neural correlate of general intelligence might be the plasticity of the nervous system to respond appropriately to stimulation and build the required networks that may be spatially differentiated and distributed for different kinds of tasks. For instance, there is evidence indicating that individuals who are more intelligent use less brain volume and therefore less energy to process a task than individuals of average intelligence do (Jausovec & Jausovec, 2004). Thus, higher speed may reflect plasticity and flexibility in the construction and use of the networks needed to deal with cognitive tasks (Neubauer, Grabner, Freuddenthaler, Beckman, & Guthke, 2004).

In line with these findings, genetic research suggests that a large part of variance in intelligence (50% or more) is accounted for by shared genes (Grigorenko, 2002). It seems that specific genes are responsible for differences in the size and general plasticity of the brain to respond efficiently to information by building the required networks as specified above (Kovas & Plomin, 2006; Posthuma & de Geous, 2006). It may be noted, however, that in addition to these general qualities of the brain, special networks that participate in the complex described above are directly linked to the genetic makeup of the individual. Specifically, there is evidence that particular genes are responsible for individual differences in brain networks related to attention and executive control (Posner, Rothbart, & Sheese, 2007).

Brain–Mind Development

The last two of the questions posed above refer to the possible equivalent of the developmental patterns described by our model to the developmental changes in the organization and functioning of the brain. Case (1992b) has suggested that increases in the myelination of neuronal axons, which protect the transmission of electrical signaling along the axons from leakage, are related to changes in general processes efficiency. This, in turn, enhances the capacity of working memory, thereby facilitating transition across the stages of cognitive development. Thatcher (1992) maintained that changes within stages of cognitive development are associated with improvements in neuronal networking within brain regions whereas transitions across stages are associated with improvements in networking between brain regions. These findings are consistent with connectionist modeling of cognitive development, suggesting that limited changes are associated with strengthening the connections between the existing networks subserving a particular behavior or skill.

Major changes leading to higher levels of cognitive development (e.g., increasingly abstract cognitive structures in different domains) are associated with the gradual construction of intervening higher level hidden units (new neural networks) that encode and compact the functioning of lower-level information-specific networks already in existence (Shultz, 2003).

A recent study of the relations between intelligence and cortical development suggests that the brain expression of intelligence is dynamic. Specifically, this study (Shaw et al., 2006) showed that the trajectory of change in the thickness of the cerebral cortex rather that thickness itself is most closely related to the level of intelligence. That is, more intelligent children demonstrate a very plastic cortex, particularly in the frontal regions, with an initial accelerated and prolonged phase of cortical increase followed by an equally vigorous cortical thinning in early adolescence. Moreover, other research suggests that developmental changes in patterns of brain activity appear to involve a shift from diffuse to more focal activation, which probably represents a fine-tuning of relevant neural systems with experience. That is, these changes reflect an increasing efficiency in the selection of the right networks and the deactivation of the less relevant or proper ones (Durston & Casey, 2006). Moreover, Bunge and Zelazo (2006) show that there is a correspondence in the developmental levels of mastering rules of increasing complexity in executive tasks and the maturation of different regions in the prefrontal cortex (orbitofrontal first, followed by ventrolateral, and then by the dorsolateral prefrontal cortex). These patterns of brain development explain both increasing speed and control efficiency. That is, blocks of neurons that are not used are pruned, yielding faster, more focused, and efficient processing. In turn, these changes make possible the increasing intertwining of networks as directed by experience thereby increasing the person's storage, integration, and reasoning capabilities.

The isomorphisms between the cognitive model presented here and the neuronal model emerging from neuroscience research is encouraging and justifies further research. Overall, it is clear that cognitive structures are associated with different brain structures and different levels of cognitive organization are associated with different levels in the organization of the brain. Moreover, changes in structures, their functioning, and their connectivity are clearly associated with both intellectual growth and differentiation. However, this research has many unanswered questions and problems to solve. In fact, none of the five groups of questions raised above is fully answered.

Implications and Applications for Education

Mapping Mind Science onto Educational Science

Any theory of the developing mind is, by definition, relevant to education, because they are both concerned with the same basic questions. Theories of mind describe and explain how the mind is organized and how it changes in time. Education systematically attempts to cause changes in different subject matters in as many individuals, and in an as effective way, as possible. Therefore, a satisfactory explication of the organization and change of the human mind may be a useful frame that can guide education as to what can be taught, when, and how.

We believe that our theory can meet the expectations of educators more than other theories and can provide answers to their concerns because of its very representation of the developing mind. Specifically, the recognition of several domain-general and domain-specific constructs and of their interrelations during development does justice to the whole range of factors that influence learning and school performance. That is, the specification of the dimensions of processing efficiency and their role in cognitive functioning and development may allow the educator to capture the general constrains of learning that may operate across the wide spectrum of the different school subjects, and tune the rate of presentation, the volume of information to be presented, and its level of inferential complexity so that it is appropriate for each age and each individual within age groups. The specification of self-monitoring and self-regulation processes and the ensuing metarepresentation processes may direct the education as to how to differentiate between the teaching of general self-management and reasoning processes and skills from the development of management and reasoning processes and skills related to specific domains of understanding and knowledge. Moreover, learning experiences in specific domains generate and develop general reasoning and problem-solving ability since general inferential schemes and patterns emerge from the metarepresentational and reflective processes related to self-awareness and self-regulation. In Perkins' (1992) terms, these processes constitute the royal road to knowledge transfer, which has always been of primary concern to education. Finally, the specification of six different domains of thought allows the educator to understand inter- and intra-individual differences in learning in different domains and appropriately design teaching and intervention programs so that it is apt for each particular domain in terms of content requiring processing and in terms of thinking processes and skills.

Moreover, it is suggested that the correspondence noted above between the functional architecture and the development of the mind, on the one hand, and the architecture and development of the brain, on the other hand, provide a strong biological basis for the theory of instruction. The main message to be drawn from this correspondence is that learning is possible at all levels and dimensions because the brain is a system with great plasticity that evolved for learning and problem solving. Actually, learning and problem solving are the evolutionary functions of the brain. The brain imposes constraints on learning that represent the constraints of evolutionary engineering that shaped its development over the millennia. Core processes are the foundational, experience-expectant processes that are easily learned early in development once the relevant stimulation is made available. Operations and processing skills are structurally and conceptually based on the core processes. Therefore, they are, by definition, functionally more complicated and more difficult to teach or learn. The teaching of mental operations and skills should start from the domain's core elements and should be viewed as a result of their interaction with relevant experience and knowledge in the domain concerned. Furthermore, teaching must ascent to increasingly higher abstraction levels where the acquired knowledge and skills are distilled into general inference patterns. Obviously, these inferential schemas are the most difficult to construct. Nevertheless, their construction is possible if teaching honors their natural abstraction hierarchy, however condensed it may be in time. This is so because these three kinds of learning are related to brain networks and systems that are separated by millions of years in evolution (perception specific networks, inference-specific networks, and self-awareness and reflection-specific networks, respectively). These constrains are captured by our theory in the maps of the mental architecture and development. Therefore, this theory can guide learning in a way that is brain-sensitive and relevant.

How Are Developing Mind, School Performance, and Learning Interrelated?

How justified are the claims above? A first step in the direction of demonstrating the power of the claims above would be to show that the various dimensions of mind specified by the theory do predict performance at school. The model shown in Fig. 7 is an answer to this question (χ^2 (281) = 420.285, $p = 0.00$, CFI = 0.942, RMSEA = 0.08). This model summarizes a study which addressed speed of processing, working memory, and problem solving in three domains, namely, quantitative, verbal, and spatial reasoning. In addition, school performance in mathematics, science, and Greek language, as evaluated by the teachers, was recorded. In this model, the factors standing for performance on each of these three school subjects was regressed on all three factors standing for the dimensions of mind mentioned above.

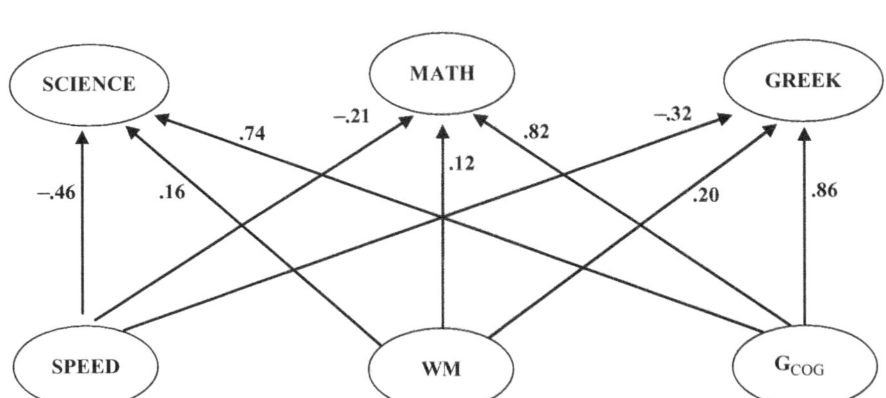

Fig. 7 School performance as a function of speed, WM, and thinking (for the ages of 7–12 years)

It can be seen that a very large part of the variance of each school subject is highly accounted for by these three dimensions of the mind's architecture (79% in science, 72% in mathematics, and 88% in Greek). Of the three dimensions, the strongest predictor was always the general reasoning factor (55% in science, 67% in mathematics, and 74% in Greek). The effect of processing speed, although considerably lower (21% in science, 4% in mathematics, and 10% in Greek), was always significant. The effect of working memory was very weak (lower than 4% in all cases). It is clear therefore that the inferential processes activated by the three domains are very much involved in everyday school learning. Speed of processing is also involved and it adds extra predictive power to our ability to understand learning in the classroom.

A second study (Demetriou, Christou, Spanoudis, Pittalis, & Mousoulides, 2007) aimed to assist learning in mathematics and specify the involvement of the various dimensions of mind, as they were presented above. Specifically, this study involved 9- and 11-year-old students who were first examined on processing speed and control, working memory, and reasoning in the domains of quantitative, spatial, and verbal thought. Moreover, they have been examined on various aspects of self-representation, self-monitoring, and problem-solving styles. These children were then allocated into three groups. The main experimental group received 20 1-hour sessions addressed to mathematics aiming to develop both, specific mathematical skills for dealing with different types of problems such as proportionality and algebra, and general problem-solving skills. Training took place by specifically trained teachers who used specifically designed material. A second experimental group was simply exposed to the training material. That is, they were given the material and they were asked to study it and solve the problems involved. Finally there was a control group. All three groups were tested on all measures both before and after the end of the training phase. Figure summarizes the results of pre-test and post-test performance on mathematics.

It can be seen in panel A that there has been no progress in the control group and that both the main and the "material-only" experimental group progressed significantly and equally. Should we have stopped the analysis here, we would have had to conclude that the material used was sufficient to cause progress and that the intervention as such exerted no effect whatsoever on learning. However, this is half of the story told by this study. The other half is shown in panel B. This panel compares the three groups after statistically partialling out the effect of processing speed and working memory. It can be seen that, under this manipulation, the pre- and post-test difference of the main experimental group remained significant but it vanished almost completely in the "material-only" experimental group. The message that this study conveys for learning is very clear: When the learning environment is well structured and systematic every one can profit because structuring the learning environment compensates for weakness in processing efficiency. In other words, on the one hand, a well-scaffolded learning environment enables the students who are weak in their processing and representational capabilities to learn despite their weaknesses. On the other hand, the students who are strong in processing and representational capacity can themselves compensate for the shortcomings in their learning environment because they learn fast and efficiently thereby discovering and constructing by themselves the relations and concepts that float, so to speak, in the information provided. Moreover, appropriate modeling showed that the gains from learning transferred from the domain of maths to general inferential processes. In fact, a third study has recently focused on the impact of self-awareness on leaning. This study showed clearly that the more reflective and self-aware a person is the more the person profits from training. These studies show, in agreement with research by other scholars, that when properly targeted, domain-specific learning can affect general-purpose learning mechanisms, such as metarepresentation. (Shayer & Adey, 2002; Shayer & Adhami, 2007).

General Principles for Cognitively Guided Instruction

In asking precisely what it is that is enhanced by Cognitive Acceleration, the most obvious answer is some kind of cognitive structures such as those proposed by Piaget as the active meaning-makers of informational input. These "structures" remain ill-defined, and do not find a specific place within current models of intellectual development. In terms of our model, this far transfer seems to offer strong support for the operation of general intellectual mechanisms which can be enhanced in one context but then become available to be deployed in quite different contexts. Specifically, we believe that the directed learning experience provided in these experiments affects the metarepresentational processes which extract, shape, and stabilize general reasoning patterns and generate cognitive self-management strategies and skills. Moreover, the experience of success on cognitively demanding tasks generates a positive attitude toward problem solving: problems are solvable once the right approach and reasoning patterns are adopted. All of these acquisitions are transferable. It needs to be stressed, however, that domain-specific skills and action patterns are not and need not be transferable across domains. For example, we found that teaching experimentation skills does not generalize to mathematical problem solving and vice-versa (Demetriou, Efklides, & Platsidou, 1993).

In fact, the ideal for learning is twofold: On the one hand, it must generate, strengthen, and enhance general reasoning patterns and problem-solving skills so as to optimize the use of available processing resources at a particular point in time. On the other hand, it must sharpen and refine the operation of domain-specific processing and problem-solving skills so that each problem is tackled with the right mixture of domain-general and domain-specific inferential, processing, and problem-solving processes and activities.

To approach this ideal, the following principles must be implemented in any program for learning based on our theory.

1. To support metarepresentation and facilitate the emergence of general reasoning patterns from domain-specific processing, teaching must continually raise awareness in students of what may be abstracted from any particular domain-specific

learning. Specifically, the student must be led to become aware of the underlying relations that surpass content differences and of the very mental processes used while handling them (for instance, elaborate on how particular core inference schemas, such as joint iteration, operate in different domains).

2. The student must acquire awareness of the processing demands of mental labor. Therefore, the student must note factors in the target concept, such as the organization or the quantity of information that cause difficulties in representing and processing. That is, teaching must build awareness about limitations of what and how much can be represented and processed, with an aim of finding strategies that can ameliorate the problem. Reorganizing and re-chunking information, specifying information that can be dropped without damaging understanding, or problem solving could be such effective strategies.
3. We must lead the student to take control of the thinking and learning processes as such, thereby transferring mental power from the teacher to the thinker. In other words, the student gradually must become self-reliant and self-regulating, rather than depending on the teacher to continually monitor and guide his or her thinking. This implies that problem-solving strategies and processes must be reworked so that they can run smoothly.
4. Each learning experience needs to be connected to the concept space and the learning space of the past. That is, the person should be able to identify whether similar concepts are already mastered and how each newly acquired experience relates to the previously acquired. Furthermore, the person should be able to recognize how the learning of these other concepts was handled in the past. Finally, a person should capitalize on the experience accumulated through the various difficulties faced during the learning process of a concept, check if these difficulties are specific to this concept, to all concepts similar to it, or to any concept.
5. The application range of the concept and skills learned must be specified. That is, the student must first understand that learning within each of the domains is to one or another degree domain-specific. Therefore, it needs domain-specific input and practice if learning is to take place and when it does it does not automatically affect the other domains. Moreover, even within the same domain, generalizability varies depending upon the domain-specific structure affected. It is reminded that the environment-oriented systems involve both core elements and component processes which represent and process particular types of relations from environmental input. For example, in mathematical thought, the principle of number succession and the four basic arithmetic operations are involved in most types of quantitative processing. In the same domain, the range of applicability of concepts, such as ratio and proportionality, is narrower than the range of the processes mentioned above but wider than the range of more specialized processes, such as the principles for transposing elements from one part of an algebraic equation to the other. Thus, our theory suggests that the transfer of domain-specific learning within an environment-oriented system would be proportionate to the status of the affected component within the system. In general, learning which involves very basic processes would transfer more easily and expand more quickly than learning which involves processes specific to a

particular component of the domain. The second type of learning requires effort and practice. All in all, the student must be led to understand domain boundaries within which the newly learned unit can be applied.

Even if everything stated in this section would be verified, we would like to note that there is no one-to-one correspondence between the architecture and development of mind and the structure of knowledge or the curriculum. Although our theory suggests that there may be a rough correspondence between the systems and levels of mind and different knowledge domains represented in the curriculum (such as the causal system–science correspondence or the quantitative system–mathematics correspondence), the various fields of study in education are usually complex domains which require the co-ordinated application of various systems. Moreover, the hypercognitive system is variously involved in school performance across different subject areas (Demetriou, Gustafsson, Efklides, & Platsidou, 1992).

Conclusions

This chapter aimed to integrate findings and postulates from cognitive, differential, and developmental models of the human mind into an overarching model that would be able at one and the same time to describe and explain the architecture of the mind, its development, and individual differences in regard to both architecture and development. As such, the model is based on studies specifically designed to empirically substantiate it. As far as architecture is concerned, it seems clear that both general and specialized capabilities and processes do exist, which are organized hierarchically so that more complex and specialized processes include more simple or general processes. This type of architecture, which is the culmination of more than a century of psychometric research (Carroll, 1993; Jensen, 1998), is largely consistent with findings in both the cognitive and the developmental approach (Case et al., 2001; Demetriou et al., 2002). Specifically, a large part of what is defined as *g* in psychometric theory (that is, the factors that are responsible for the fact that all mental tests correlate positively with each other) can be reduced to mechanisms underlying processing efficiency, processing capacity, and directive-executive control, which have been the primary target of research and theory in cognitive psychology. In fact, these very mechanisms seem able to explain, to a considerable extent, the state of understanding and problem solving at successive age levels, which is the object of developmental psychology and individual differences in regard to it.

In this common model, the definition of intelligence boils down to a simple function: The more mentally efficient (that is, the faster and more focused on goal), capable (that is, the more information one can hold in mind at a given moment), foresighted (that is, the more clearly one can specify his goals and plan how to achieve them), and flexible (that is, the more one can introduce variations in the concepts and mental operations one already possesses) a person is, the more intelligent (both in regard to other individuals and in regard to a general developmental hierarchy) this person will prove to be. In other words, excelling and developing in understanding, learning, reasoning, and problem solving is, to a considerable extent, a function of increase in mental efficiency, capacity, planning, and flexibility. In psychometric terms, this is tantamount to saying that differences in the processes associated with *g* cause differences in general inferential and reasoning mechanisms. In developmental terms, this is tantamount to saying that changes in the processes underlying *g* result in the qualitative transformation of the general structures of thought underlying understanding and reasoning at successive ages so that more complex and less familiar problems can be solved and more abstract concepts can be constructed. This is so because the missing links in the abstract or unfamiliar problems and concepts can be constructed ad hoc or introduced by the thinker from other realms or from the thinkers' experiences. The advantage of the person in these processes provides a relative advantage in learning and self-directed problem solving.

It is highly interesting that modern research on the organization and functioning of the brain lends support to this architecture. The evidence summarized above suggests that some general aspects of the brain, such as myelination, plasticity, and neuronal connectivity, are related to some dimensions of general intelligence, such as speed of processing and learning efficiency. Moreover, there are brain regions, located mainly in the frontal and parietal cortices that subserve functions that are central to all cognitive processing, such as control, and working memory. Also, there are many neural networks that specialize in the representation of different types of information such as spatial, causal, quantitative, social, and categorical. In fact, it is highly interesting that new mental schemes emerge from the interaction and integration of existing schemes in a way that is reminiscent of the fact that consciousness may emerge from the dialog between overlapping neuronal networks and/or through the co-ordinating operation of neuronal structures orchestrating this dialog.

As far as change is concerned, the three traditions also seem to melt into this overarching model. Specifically, on the one hand, transition mechanisms specified by developmental theory are useful for differential theory, because they highlight why and how change in mental age occurs. On the other hand, mechanisms of change as specified in the cognitive theory, which underlie the automation of performance, highlight how newly acquired developmental structures in a given phase get established and consolidated, thereby preparing the way for the transition to the next phase of development. Moreover, both kinds of mechanisms of change explain individual differences in IQ, because they underlie changes in mental age.

The differentiation of development across domains is an integral part of the organization and functioning of the human mind. This is so because in each of the domains there are constraints directly coming from the particularities in the mental operations, the representations, and the skills that characterize each of the domains. That is, performance within and across persons may vary even if general processes are kept constant, because the dynamics of functioning and development differ across domains, and the mastering of this dynamics depends on both special domain-specific disposition and domain-specific experience. Domain-specific disposition is a multiplier of general potentials. If domain-specific disposition falls short of general potentials in a given domain, obviously attainment in this domain will prove to fall below the level of general potentials. For instance, visuo-spatial ability will fall below general potentials in the blind, even if general potentials are very high. If domain-specific disposition is high, such as a special proclivity in visualization, visuo-spatial ability will exceed the level expected on the basis of the condition of general potentials. Domain-specific experience is needed to give the chance to the developing person to customize, so to speak, the general possibilities and processes to particularities and constrains of each of the domains. Obviously, practice to the extreme in a domain will elevate this domain to the upper limit of general potentials. Overall, the particular combination of general potentials, domain-specific disposition, and domain-specific experience determines the momentum, the stability, and the direction of development in the individual.

It is hoped that this chapter suggests clearly that neither Gardner-like theories (e.g., Gardner, 1983), which postulate the existence of autonomous multiple intelligences, nor Jensen-like theories (e.g., Jensen, 1998), which stress the primacy of general processes, do justice to the complexity of the human mind. The human mind involves both general and specialized abilities, each of which functions as a dimension of intra- and inter-individual differences during both on-line functioning and developmental time. That is, general processes are everywhere, but they can never be seen alone, and specialized domains are the interfaces through which the mind interleaves with the different realms of the world, but specialized processes involve general processes as part of their construction and they need them for their functioning and development. Developmental dynamics provide the melting pot where general and specialized processes get integrated and refined into world-relevant systems of understanding and action.

Education needs to take this reality into account if it is to be efficient and achieve the maximum of its goals. Specifically, each student's potentials associated with general intelligence must be taken into account. That implies that the teacher must be sensitive to both her classroom modal *g* level and each student's condition relative to this modal *g* level. One may not necessarily need to measure speed as such or working-memory capacity as such. The traditional language of cognitive development theory may serve this purpose to a very large extent. At the same time, the teacher needs to remember that *g* level is characterized by its plasticity and it is therefore malleable. We have summarized here a general plan of action in this direction. Directly addressing the dimensions of *g* today greatly facilitates and elevates what can be learned tomorrow because it directly changes the general learning potential. At the same time, most of learning is domain-specific. Mathematics needs understanding, mastering, and using mathematical knowledge and skills. Physics needs understanding, mastering, and using mathematical knowledge and skills. Therefore, the developmental and individual proclivities and dispositions for each domain need to be respected and used as the starting point for any teaching attempt that aspires to be successful. Properly managing domain-specific learning, by way of the methods summarized here, enhances general intellectual capacities as much as the enhancement of general intellectual capacities modifies domain-specific learning.

References

Baddeley, A. D. (2007). *Working memory, thought, and action*. Oxford: Oxford University Press.

Braine, M. D. S. (1990). The "natural logic" approach to reasoning. In W. F. Overton (Ed.), *Reasoning, necessity, and logic: Developmental perspectives* (pp. 133–157). Hillsdale, NJ: Erlbaum.

Bunge, S. A., & Zelazo, D. P. (2006). A brain-based account of the development of rule use in childhood. *Current Directions in Psychological Science, 15*, 118–121.

Carroll, J. B. (1993). *Human cognitive abilities: A survey of factor-analytic studies*. New York: Cambridge University Press.

Case, R. (1992a). *The mind's staircase: Exploring the conceptual underpinnings of children's thought and knowledge*. Hillsdale, NJ: Erlbaum.

Case, R. (1992b). The role of the frontal lobes in the regulation of cognitive development. *Brain and Cognition, 20*, 51–73.

Case, R., Demetriou, A., Platsidou, M., & Kazi, S. (2001). Integrating concepts and tests of intelligence from the differential and the developmental traditions. *Intelligence, 29*, 307–336.

Cosmides, L., & Tooby, J. (1994). Beyond intuition and instinct blindness: Toward an evolutionarily rigorous cognitive science. *Cognition, 50*, 41–77.

Cowan, N. (1999). An embedded-processes model of working memory. In A. Miyake & P. Shah (Eds.), *Models of working memory: Mechanisms of active maintenance and executive control* (pp. 62–101). Cambridge: Cambridge University Press.

Cowan, N. (2001). The magical number 4 in short-term memory: A reconsideration of mental storage capacity. *Brain and Behavioral Sciences, 24*, 87–114.

Crick, F. C., & Koch, C. (2005). What is the function of the claustrum? *Philosophical Transactions of the Royal Society: Brain and Biological Sciences, 30*, 1271–1279.

Deary, I. J. (2000). Simple information processing and intelligence. In R. J. Sternberg (Ed.), *Handbook of intelligence* (pp. 267–284). Cambridge: Cambridge University Press.

Dehaene, S. (1997). *The number sense*. New York: Oxford University Press.

Demetriou, A., (2000). Organization and development of self-understanding and self-regulation: Toward a general theory. In M. Boekaerts, P. R. Pintrich, & M. Zeidner (Eds.), *Handbook of self-regulation* (pp. 209–251). San Diego, CA: Academic Press.

Demetriou, A., Christou, C., Spanoudis, G., Pittalis, M., & Mousoulides, N. (2007). Processing, working memory, and problem solving requirements for mathematics learning. In preparation.

Demetriou, A., Christou, C., Spanoudis, G., & Platsidou, M. (2002). The development of mental processing: Efficiency, working memory, and thinking. *Monographs of the Society of Research in Child Development, 67*, Serial Number 268.

Demetriou, A., & Efklides, A. (1985). Structure and sequence of formal and postformal thought: General patterns and individual differences. *Child Development, 56*, 1062–1091.

Demetriou, A., Efklides, E., Papadaki, M., Papantoniou, A., & Economou, A. (1993). The structure and development of causal-experimental thought. *Developmental Psychology, 29*, 480–497.

Demetriou, A., Efklides, A., & Platsidou, M. (1993). The architecture and dynamics of developing mind: Experiential structuralism as a frame for unifying cognitive developmental theories. *Monographs of the Society for Research in Child Development, 58*(5–6), Serial No. 234.

Demetriou, A., Gustafsson, J.-E., Efklides, A., & Platsidou, M. (1992). Structural systems in developing cognition, science, and education. In A. Demetriou, M. Shayer, & A. Efklides (Eds.), *The neo-Piagetian theories of cognitive development go to school: Implications and applications for education* (pp. 79–103). London: Routledge.

Demetriou, A., & Kazi, S. (2001). *Unity and modularity in the mind and the self: Studies on the relationships between self-awareness, personality, and intellectual development from childhood to adolescence*. London: Routledge.

Demetriou, A., & Kazi, S. (2006). Self-awareness in g (with processing efficiency and reasoning). *Intelligence, 34*, 297–317.

Demetriou, A., & Kyriakides, L. (2006). A Rasch-measurement model analysis of cognitive developmental sequences: Validating a comprehensive theory of cognitive development. *British Journal of Educational Psychology, 76*, 209–242.
Demetriou, A., Mouyi, A., & Spanoudis, G. (2008). Modelling the structure and development of g. *Intelligence, 5*, 437–454.
Demetriou, A., Pachaury, A., Metallidou, Y., & Kazi, S. (1996). Universal and specificities in the structure and development of quantitative-relational thought: A cross-cultural study in Greece and India. *International Journal of Behavioral Development, 19*, 255–290.
Dempster, F. N., & Brainerd, C. J. (Eds). (1995). *Interference and inhibition in cognition*. New York: Academic Press.
Durston, S., & Casey, B. J. (2006). What have we learned about cognitive development from neuroimaging? *Neuropsychologia, 44*, 2149–2157.
Edelman, G. M., & Tononi, G. A. (2000). *Universe of consciousness*. New York: Basic Books.
Engle, R. W. (2002). Working memory capacity as executive attention. *Current Directions in Psychological Science, 11*, 19–23.
Fischer, K. W. (1980). A theory of cognitive development: The control and construction of hierarchies of skills. *Psychological Review, 87*, 477–531.
Flavell, J. H., Green, F. L., & Flavell, E. R. (1986). Development of knowledge about the appearance-reality distinction. *Monographs of the Society for Research in Child Development, 51* (1), Serial No. 212.
Fonlupt, P. (2003). Perception and judgement of physical causality involve different brain structures. *Cognitive Brain Research, 17*, 248–254.
Fry, A. F., & Hale, S. (2000). Relationships among processing speed, working memory, and fluid intelligence in children. *Biological Psychology, 54*, 1–34.
Galaburda, A. M. (2002). The neuroanatomy of categories. In A. M. Galaburda, S. M. Kosslyn, & Y. Christen (Eds.), *The languages of the brain* (pp. 23–42). Cambridge, MA: Harvard University Press.
Gardner, H. (1983). *Frames of mind. The theory of multiple intelligences*. New York: Basic Books.
Garlick, D. (2002). Understanding the nature of the general factor of intelligence: the role of individual differences in neural plasticity as an explanatory mechanism. *Psychological Review, 109*, 116–136.
Gibson, J. J. (1966). *The senses considered as perceptual systems*. London: Allen & Unwin.
Goel, V., Buchel, C., Frith, C., & Dolan, R. J. (2000). Dissociation of mechanisms underlying syllogistic reasoning. *NeuroImage, 12*, 504–514.
Grigorenko, E. L. (2002). Other than g: The values of persistence. In R. J. Sternberg & E. L. Grigorenko (Eds.), *The general factor of intelligence: How general is it?* (pp. 299–327). Mahwah, NJ: Lawrence Erlbaum Associates.
Gruber, O., & von Cramon, D. Y. (2003). The functional neuroanatomy of human working memory revisited – evidence from 3T-fMRI studies using classical domain-specific interference tasks. *NeuroImage, 19*, 797–809.
Halford, G. S. (1993). *Children's understanding: The development of mental models*. Hillsdale, NJ: Erlbaum.
Harter, S. (1999). *The construction of the self*. New York: The Guilford Press.
James, W. (1890). *The principles of psychology* (Vol. 1). New York: Hold.
Jausovec, N., & Jasovec, K. (2004). Differences in induced brain activity during performance of learning and working memory tasks related to intelligence. *Brain and Cognition, 54*, 65–74.
Jensen, A. R. (1998). *The G factor: The science of mental ability*. New York: Praeger.
Jung R. E. & Haier, R. J. (2007). The Parieto-Frontal integration theory (P-FIT) of intelligence: Converging neuroimaging evidence. *Behavioral and Brain Sciences, 30*, 135–154.
Kail, R. (1991). Developmental functions for speed of processing during childhood and adolescence. *Psychological Bulletin, 109*, 490–501.
Kandel, E. R., Schwartz, J. H., & Jessell, T. M. (1995). *Essentials of neural science and behavior*. New York: Appleton & Lange.

Kargopoulos, P., & Demetriou, A. (1998). What, why, and whence logic? A response to the commentators. *New Ideas in Psychology, 16*, 125–139.

Karmiloff-Smith, A. (1992). *Beyond modularity: A developmental perspective on cognitive science*. Cambridge, MA: MIT Press.

Klingberg, T. (1998). Concurrent performance of two working memory tasks: Potential mechanisms of interference. *Cerebral Cortex, 8*, 593–601.

Kovas, Y., & Plomin, R. (2006). Generalist genes: Implications for the cognitive sciences. *Trends in Cognitive Sciences, 10*, 198–203.

Kuhn, D., & Pease, M. (2006). Do children and adults learn differently? *Journal of Cognition and Development, 7*, 279–293.

Kyllonen, P., & Christal, R. E. (1990). Reasoning ability is (little more than) working-memory capacity? *Intelligence, 14*, 389–433.

Lamme, V. A. F. (2006). Towards a true neural stance on consciousness. *Trends in Cognitive Science, 10*, 494–501.

McLeod, C. M. (1991). Half a century of research on the Stroop effect: An integrative review. *Psychological Bulletin, 109*, 163–203.

Navon, D. (1977). Forest before trees: The precedence of global features in visual perception. *Cognitive Psychology, 9*, 353–383.

Neil, W. T., Valdes, L. A., & Terry, K. M. (1995). Selective attention and inhibitory control of cognition. In F. N. Dempster, & C. J. Brainerd (Eds.), *Interference and inhibition in cognition* (pp. 207–263). New York: Academic Press.

Nelson, C. A., de Haan, M., & Thomas, M. M. (2006). *Neuroscience of cognitive development: The role of experience and the developing brain*. New Jersey, NY. Wiley & Sons.

Neubauer, A. C., Grabner, R. H., Freuddenthaler, H. H., Beckman, J. F., & Guthke, J. (2004). Intelligence and individual differences in becoming neurally efficient. *Acta Psychologica, 116*, 55–74.

O' Reilly, R. C., & Munakata, Y. (2000). *Computational explorations in cognitive neuroscience: Understanding the mind by simulating the brain*. Cambridge, MA: MIT Press.

Osherson, D., Perani, D., Cappa, S., Schnur, T., Grassi, F., & Fazio, F. (1998). Distinct brain loci in deductive versus probabilistic reasoning. *Neuropsychologia, 36*, 369–376.

Pascual-Leone, J. (1970). A mathematical model for the transition rule in Piaget's developmental stages. *Acta Psychologica, 32*, 301–345.

Perkins, D. (1992). *Smart schools: From training memories to educating minds*: New York: The Free Press.

Piaget, J. (1970). Piaget's theory. In P. H. Mussen, (Ed.), *Carmichael's handbook of child development* (pp. 703–732). New York: Wiley.

Piaget, J. (2001). *Studies in reflecting abstraction*. London: Psychology Press.

Posner, M. I., & Boies, S. J. (1971). Components of attention. *Psychological Review, 78*, 391–408.

Posner, M. I., & Peterson, S. E. (1990). The attention system of the human brain. *Annual Review of Neuroscience, 13*, 25–42.

Posner, M. I., Rothbart, M. K., & Sheese, B. E. (2007). Attention genes. *Developmental Science, 10*, 24–29.

Posthuma, D., & de Geous, E. J. C. (2006). Progress in the molecular-genetic study of intelligence. *Current Directions in Psychological Science, 15*, 151–155.

Rumbaugh, D. M., & Washburn, D. A. (2003). *Intelligence of apes and other rational beings*. New Haven, CT: Yale University Press.

Salthouse, T. A. (1996). The processing-speed theory of adult age differences in cognition. *Psychological Review, 103*, 403–428.

Shaw, P., Greenstein, D., Lerch, J., Clasen, L., Lenroot, R., Gogtay, A., et al. (2006). Intellectual ability and cortical development in children and adolescents. *Nature, 440*, 676–679.

Shayer, M., & P. Adey, Eds. (2002). *Learning intelligence: Cognitive acceleration across the curriculum from 5 to 15 years*. Milton Keynes, Open University Press.

Shayer, M., & Adhami, M. (2007). Fostering Cognitive Development through the context of Mathematics: Results of the CAME Project. *Educational Studies in Mathematics, 64*, 265–291.
Shultz, T. R. (2003). *Computational developmental psychology*. Cambridge, MA: CMIT Press.
Spearman, C. (1904). "General intelligence" objectively determined and measured. *American Journal of Psychology, 15*, 201–293.
Sporns, O., Chialvo, D. R., Kaiser, M., & Hilgetag, C. C. (2004). Organization, development and function of complex brain networks. *Trends in Cognitive Sciences, 8*, 418–425.
Stavrinides, P. (2005). *The formation and the effects of parental involvement on the child's cognitive development and psychological adjustment*. Unpublished doctoral dissertation, University of Cyprus, Nicosia, Cyprus.
Sternberg, S. (1966). High-speed scanning in human memory. *Science, 153*, 652–654.
Stroop, J. R. (1935). Studies of interference in serial verbal reactions. *Journal of Experimental Psychology, 18*, 643–662.
Thatcher, R. W. (1992). Cyclic cortical reorganization during early childhood. *Brain and Cognition, 20*, 24–50.
Wellman, H. M. (1990). *The child's theory of mind*. Cambridge, MA: MIT Press.

Mental Attention, Multiplicative Structures, and the Causal Problems of Cognitive Development

Juan Pascual-Leone, Janice Johnson, and Alba Agostino

Cognitive development traditionally has been characterized in terms of qualitatively distinct typical performance patterns that are tied chronologically (in their onset and course) to specified moments or periods of children's normal growth. Collections of these *typical performance patterns* serve to characterize *stages of development*. Using his logical analytical models, Piaget recognized that these typical performance patterns are functionally *nested into* psycho-genetic *sequences* that serve as landmarks stipulating course of development within particular types of situations (or *paradigms*). These types of situations are characteristic of cognitive growth in various areas of interest. Piaget was first to define developmental stages in terms of collections of these context-sensitive (i.e., situation- or paradigm-specific) typical sequences. He also emphasized that stages are functionally nested into invariant sequences that exhibit the progressive complexification of performance from young childhood to adulthood. The best known example of these sequences of typical behaviors is described by Piaget in the context of appraising conservation of quantities under various manipulations or physical transformations. In the case of so-called continuous quantities (e.g., plasticine or clay whose shape is being transformed), Piaget and Inhelder (1974) described the *conservation of substance* at about 7–8 years of age, which was followed by *conservation of weight* at about 9–10 years, and *conservation of volume* at about 11–12 years.

The paradigm of conservation of substance involves visual appraisal of amount in the distal object that is symbolized by a make-believe situation – for instance, two equal balls of plasticine *that stand for candy*, one of which is transformed by rolling into (e.g.) a long sausage. The child then is asked which piece of candy (plasticine) contains more amount of substance as a distal object in the goal-directed activity of eating the piece of candy (distal objects always emerge in the context of praxis). Piaget did not explicitly use these terms. A *proximal or perceptual object* is the object as it appears to the here-and-now perceptual appraisal: In perceptual appraisal, the sausage appears to be much longer and to have more amount than

J. Pascual-Leone (✉)
Department of Psychology, York University, Toronto, ON, Canada
e-mail: juanpl@yorku.ca

M. Ferrari, L. Vuletic (eds.), *The Developmental Relations among Mind, Brain and Education*, DOI 10.1007/978-90-481-3666-7_3, © Springer Science+Business Media B.V. 2010

the ball, due to a common perceptual (Gestalt-field) illusion. A *distal or intellective object* is an object as it appears in goal-directed activities that aim to obtain some intended result (this is often called *agency* or, when conscious, *praxis*). Symbolically represented in the paradigm of substance conservation, this is *the future act* of eating the "candy" the sausage stands for. Thus conservation of substance appears as ability to withstand misleading perceptual appearances and uphold valid appraisal of future distal-object possibilities. It exhibits a victory of intellective processes over perceptual processes.

Remarkably, however, 8-year-olds who may pass conservation of substance often fail in *conservation of weight*, when the child is asked to anticipate whether or how a two-plate balance scale would tip if one placed the sausage on the first plate and the other ball on the second. The qualitative patterns of performance exhibited by 8-year-olds who fail conservation of weight are similar to those of 6-year-olds who fail conservation of substance. The same happens with 9- or 10-year-olds who often fail *conservation of volume*: when they are asked whether or not the water level would rise the same in two glasses, if the sausage were placed inside one full glass of water and the ball inside another full glass. Error patterns of performance are again in this case similar to those of 6-year-olds in conservation of substance and 8-year-olds in conservation of weight.

This recurrence of qualitative stage patterns within a paradigm as the *complexity* of the situation is increased often is found in child development in different qualitative forms and across content domains.[1] Robbie Case maintained a keen eye for this recurrence of typical qualitative patterns across domains. He also noticed its recurrence within domains, and his theory highlights these points. What often is not recognized, however, is what the recurrence of typical stage patterns as a function of increasing complexity suggests: Qualitative patterns of performance often are not a causal determinant in cognitive development. Rather, they frequently are manifestations of a deep quantitative dimension of variation. Indeed, as Engels (Marx, Engels, & Lenin, 1977) and many others have emphasized, within dialectical or dynamic processes quantity often transforms itself into quality, and vice-versa. This principle appears, for instance, in "the importance of the size of mental-attentional capacity/working memory in determining the patterns of performance that the subject is capable of producing. [. . .] But conversion of quantity into quality is perceived as a problem only by those who see difficulties in the demarcation of the *unit of analysis* (i.e., schemes, structures) during the quantitative evaluation of complexity; and by those who [do not][2] recognize in the organism's constitution of psychological units, proof that it is capable of *dynamic/creative syntheses*[3] – syntheses which

[1]Notice that in addition to the complexity of conservation of substance, conservation of weight requires an understanding of the balance scale's functioning; and conservation of volume requires an understanding that "heavy" solids sink into water and that concurrently the water rises forced by the object as it sinks.

[2]The words in square brackets were omitted by error from the printed version of the article.

[3]Footnote in the original 1987 paper: "Dynamic/creative syntheses are the little understood processes that enable the organism to produce *truly-novel*, behavioral or mental, performances that

endogenously construct the units in question as an 'inner language' of the brain." (Pascual-Leone, 1987, p. 537). In other words: Qualitative patterns in performance express the working of the organism as a functionally organized totality. A change in functional qualitative patterns, therefore, expresses a change (often initially quantitative) within some organismic processes that codetermine this qualitative performance.

Notice that such causal analysis involves shifting from one epistemological level of description (i.e., behavioral performance) to another level of description (i.e., the organismic–neuropsychological processes whose functioning codetermines the qualitative performance in question). In what follows we say, for the sake of simplicity, that qualitative causal components (or *units*) of performance, for example, psychological schemes or structures *are* organismic neural circuits or networks. Strictly speaking this is not correct, because one cannot categorically equate theoretical entities defined at one *epistemological level* with theoretical entities defined at a very different (deeper and finer) level. More accurately, schemes *epistemologically* (i.e., semantic-pragmatically vis-à-vis performance) *correspond to* the neural circuits in question, and this correspondence is not deterministic but rather is intrinsically situated and probabilistic – intrinsically because the brain's informational correspondence to behavioral patterns is, by its own nature, relative to the contextual situation (i.e., is *situated*) and probabilistic. This intrinsic probabilistic functioning (e.g., neuronal summation and spreading of activation, overdetermination of neuronal activation) is well recognized in current neuronal modeling of behavior (e.g., Edelman & Tononi, 2000; Freeman, 1995).

These units of performance (e.g., schemes) are, probabilistically speaking, dynamically constituted neuronal circuits or networks; circuits in which neurons are cofunctional and often co-activated, as an emergent or synthesized totality. Working memory, or mental/focal attention, currently is considered (e.g., Cowan, 2005) a key brain mechanism that serves to activate (i.e., add purely internal information-processing *enhancement* to) task-relevant processes – a mechanism that may be instrumental for success within task-misleading situations. Current views on the centrality of *mental attention* for the emergence of stage-typical patterns of activity (often phrased in terms of executive- or affect-driven working memory) agree with Pascual-Leone's (1970, 1987) original developmental view – a view that William James (1966) and a few others (e.g., Spearman, 1927) pioneered in a non-developmental perspective.

Because mental attention so conceived is an endogenous process that increases with chronological age as a function of maturation, development and its qualitative stages can be seen to result from causal dialectical interactions (i.e., intertwining, trade-off relations) between maturation (*maturational development*, i.e., development in the narrow sense – as Piaget liked to say) and *learning*. Pascual-Leone and Johnson (2005), in a model of developmental stages adapted from Robbie Case and

---

were never learned, are not computationally implied by the combinatorial possibilities of the repertoire, nor are, properly speaking, innate or prewired."

reproduced below, show how the qualitative substages of Case and Piaget can be indexed and causally explained by the intertwining of learning with the endogenous developmental growth of mental-attentional capacity – a quantitative parameter hidden in the organism, whose maturational incrementation works as "transition rule" for passing from one qualitative stage to the next (Pascual-Leone, 1970). This is so because such incrementation enables synthesis of more complex truly novel performances that can then be learned. From this perspective it is clear, as the late Piaget (e.g., 1980) may have recognized, that there is a dialectical relation of complementarity, in the sense formulated by modern physics (Bohr, 1961), between maturational development and learning proper. Indeed, both causal factors are needed to explain development as manifested, but they cannot be investigated within the same research paradigm or situation: Any attempt to experimentally clarify one member of this pair will tend to prevent/confuse clear observation of the other.

For instance, with each act of learning the repertoire of psychological processing units of the child will change, and with it the qualitative patterns (and often the sophistication) of her or his performance. When maturation brings an incrementation in the child's mental capacity, however, the same repertoire of units (schemes, or structures – i.e., schemes of schemes of schemes) will be used much more efficiently, because the added mental attention will allow more encompassing scheme coordinations (i.e., dynamic *syntheses* produced via overdetermination) to take place. As new mental-attentional capacity is being endogenously acquired, performance improves due to the possibility of more encompassing syntheses of truly novel performances; and these syntheses in turn bring the occasion for more learning of processing units.

In this chapter we illustrate the relationship between maturational development and learning, both theoretically and empirically. We do so in the context of the acquisition of multiplicative structures, to honor Robbie Case who made important contributions to the study of elementary mathematics in children. We first summarize our theoretical organismic model, to make clear the distinction between causal constructs (e.g., schemes, hidden operators) and descriptive ones (e.g., typical performances, stages).

A Brief on the Theory of Constructive Operators (TCO)

Schemes as Psychological Units

Information is carried or mediated by distinct collections of neurons, often distributed over the brain, that are cofunctional (vis-à-vis certain activities) and co-activated in some tasks. These functional collections epistemologically correspond to psychological *schemes*. To simplify, we also call schemes these collections of cofunctional neuronal circuits (Arbib, Erdi, & Szentagothai, 1998; Hunt, 1961).

Psychological schemes are distinct, situation specific (i.e., *situated*) causal factors that *overdetermine* manifest performance. Schemes overdetermine performance because they are *self-propelling* (Piaget's *assimilation* function) and tend to *apply* to the situation (i.e., fire as collections of neurons) under minimal conditions of activation. Each scheme is a functional *package of qualitative relational characteristics* that can inform (i.e., inject form into) experience when the scheme applies to codetermine performance. Proper recognition of schemes facilitates process and task analysis (Pascual-Leone, 1970, 1995; Pascual-Leone & Goodman, 1979; Pascual-Leone & Johnson, 1991, 2005; Pascual-Leone, Johnson, Baskind, Dworsky, & Severtson, 2000).

Piaget said that a scheme is like *an association* between a releasing response (the behaviorist "stimulus") and an effective response (the action-response) that *also embodies an expectancy*. Indeed, our theory claims that a scheme (Sc) can be recognized by the conjunction of four components: (Sc1) an antecedent contextual pattern or patterns (which we call *releasing component*); (Sc2) a semantic-pragmatic expectancy of what the scheme does when it applies (which we call *functional component*); (Sc3) a description of how the scheme produces its effect when it is applied (called *effecting component*); and (Sc4) a probabilistically stable coordination of Sc1⇔Sc2⇔Sc3, which gets written in the repertoire (long term memory) as a probabilistic functional *invariant* that expresses an expectancy and/or strategy. All schemes have this form, and by identifying these four components one can diagnose the schemes that contribute to an individual's performance within a given context across a set of situations. For instance, I sit in a car's driver's seat (Sc1) and take the car key (Sc1). I anticipate that the car will start (Sc2) when I place the key in the ignition keyhole and turn the key (Sc3). If this anticipation reliably occurs within the same context across cars and situations (Sc 4), I have demarcated one such executive scheme (the overall sequence) and several coordinated action schemes (the actual distinct steps). *Executive schemes* embody plans of action, implemented by (perceptual/figurative and motor/operative) *action schemes*.

This diagnostic procedure works even when the most abstract sort of schemes, executive schemes, unexpectedly intrudes in our behavior, because (under good releasing conditions) schemes are self-propelling. Consider *executive schemes* in the motor domain. Practitioners of Judo learn to fall safely without hurting themselves, even when they fall head first, because they learn the plan of tumbling in the air and, thus, hit the ground rolling on their backs (their impact is attenuated by shoulders and arms that in passing actively beat the ground to discharge onto it much of the body's kinetic impulse). This complex safe-falling strategy is difficult to learn, because one must let oneself fall softly while rolling on one's head without rigidity. One of us (JPL) learned this strategy as a young man practicing Judo for 4 years. For close to 50 years afterward, JPL did not practice any Judo. Recently, walking fast on a city sidewalk, JPL tripped on a crack and found himself falling forward head first. Automatically, to his astonishment, his body implemented the Judo frontal safe-falling routine, and he landed on the ground safely after softly rolling forward.

How can we explain this improbable saving reaction? He had in his repertoire, dormant after nearly 50 years, the learned Judo safe-falling executive. It is an executive, and not just a fixed automatized routine, because the pattern of falling was clearly adjusted to the present truly new circumstances: Action schemes were coordinated under this monitoring executive process to synthesize the truly novel performance. The executive was released by the experience of falling forward (Sc1), and it carried the implicit expectancy (Sc2) that the body would hit the ground softly if the appropriate relaxed head-on body rolling was implemented. The operative schemes for implementing this strategy were still available in the repertoire and were recruited (Sc3); and the resulting performance was recognized after the fact by JPL as being a learned *invariant*: an adequate Judo safe-falling performance (Sc4). These automatized executive processes, which are capable of synthesizing truly novel adaptive performances by recruiting and then monitoring the appropriate action schemes, are abundant albeit often not recognized. They are common in all complex sports, martial arts, creative dancing, creative arts, expert problem solving, science, complex or charismatic writing or talking. Creativity would not be possible without many executives, learned in the past and stored in the repertoire, ready to be elicited unexpectedly in novel situations.

Schemes are like recursive procedures and can be learned: It is common to have scheme hierarchies (i.e., schemes of schemes of schemes, etc.), which we call *structures* or *schemas* (e.g., the coordinated "program" or "script" that governs our behavior in restaurants or within familiar sorts of problem solving). Schemes are abstracted across situations for a given sort of praxis, and must be internally consistent to be formed. Their contextual conditions and/or effects can in turn be constituted by (copies of) other schemes. Experiences are possible only because compatible schemes accommodate to situations, or apply (Piaget's assimilation) to structure them. Long term memory corresponds to a manifold repertoire of schemes or structures sorted in kinds: *executive* schemes (prefrontal), *operative* schemes (frontal), *figurative* schemes (i.e., perceptual or representational or linguistic – occipital, parietal, or temporal), coordinated packages of automatized *operative/motor* schemes (frontal right hemisphere, basal ganglia, and cerebellum), *affective/emotion* schemes (broadly defined limbic system), *analytical* schemes *produced with mental*-attentional *effort* (initially in the left hemisphere), *global or holistic automatized* schemes (right hemisphere), etc.

Note that *action schemes* (i.e., schemes that can instantiate plans embodied by executive schemes) are first and foremost experiential and geared to praxis (i.e., goal-directed activity). The three main kinds of action schemes are operatives, figuratives, and parameters. *Operatives* are schemes that stand for procedures, in the sense that they carry "blueprints" of operations (behavioral or mental) that must be performed to obtain a certain result. When an operative scheme applies on a figurative scheme (i.e., a physical or mental object representation) it changes some figurative characteristics, thus setting conditions for a different figurative to apply and represent the outcome. Note that (as their frontal-lobe cortical location suggests), executive schemes are a special, distinct and more abstract, kind of operative. Ordinary operative action schemes carry out actual operations, transformations, or procedures by applying onto figuratives, often under the monitoring of executives. *Figuratives* are schemes that embody characteristics of physical or mental objects, and stand cognitively for these objects. When logically symbolized, figuratives often correspond to predicates or to compound-predicate functors that categorize the input (or the internal stream of thought) representing objects on which operations can apply. *Parameters* are relational, adjunct-information figuratives, which stipulate boundary conditions that will enable a given operative to apply successfully onto a given figurative.

Consider again the example of starting a car. The perception of sitting in the driver's seat is caused by a *complex figurative* that applies to categorize the actual situation. Taking the car key and placing it inside the ignition keyhole is carried out by one or two *operatives* in coordination with *figuratives*. Placing the key inside the keyhole is a boundary condition for starting the car, if the key is properly turned in its keyhole. Another boundary condition (among many others) is to have a working battery. The figurative schemes that stand for these two conditions can therefore be recognized as *parameters* of the overall executive scheme, starting the car.

Conceptual schemes (when concepts are narrowly and properly defined) are metacognitive abstractions, mediated by language, that epistemologically reflect (generically) experiential schemes, when they are not imaginative anticipations of to-be-learned truly novel experiential schemes. For this reason, all schemes (even proper conceptual schemes) are situated constructs: They all have their releasing contextual conditions, and at times their parameters, that stipulate types of situation where they can be applied (boundary conditions that function as their releasers and demarcate their applicability). In contrast, hidden "brain hardware" operators, to which we now turn, are truly content-free, because they do not have (external, situational) releasing conditions, nor are they information-bearing processes.

The Hidden Operators of the Mind's Brain

The theory of schemes alone cannot explain *general* organismic constraints (i.e., those applying across kinds of schemes) such as "central" working memory capacity limits, or "central" inhibitory mechanisms, or structural versus content learning, or "central" resolution of schemes' *competition* in the network, or the emergence of truly novel performances via unplanned dynamic syntheses. We propose that the brain, in addition to a repertoire of schemes, has a small set of general-purpose functional resources that we call *hidden* or silent *operators* (Pascual-Leone, 1987, 1995, 2000; Pascual-Leone & Johnson, 1991, 2005; Pascual-Leone et al., 2000). We call them *operators*, because they are functional mechanisms of brain "hardware," defined as molar procedures whose computational details are unspecified, and which apply on (constrain) schemes to change or produce new schemes, or to synthesize truly novel performances. These operators are *hidden* because, unlike schemes, they lack "substantive" content referents and so do not convey information as schemes do. Instead, operators express purely relational multivariate constraints – surprising patterns or "anomalies" that a pure theory of schemes cannot explain. As

Table 1 TCO's hidden operators listed in order of their likely evolutionary emergence

Operator	Description	Brain region
A	Set of **affective** processes that intervene in motivation and attentive arousal.	Limbic lobes
C	Both the process of **content** learning and the schemes derived from associative content learning.	Brodmann primary and secondary areas
F	The **field** operator, which acts as the brain's binding mechanism that brings closure to mental representations in a neo-Gestaltist manner.	All areas
LC	The process of automatized **logical-structural** learning derived from **C-learning** through overpractice.	Right hemisphere
T	**Temporarily** and effortlessly collates **sequences** of schemes, thus facilitating the coordination that constitutes distal objects.	Occipito-temporal
S	By coordinating relations of coexistence among activated schemes, effortlessly within the situation, it facilitates emergence of **spatial** schemes or schemas.	Occipito-parietal
I	The attentional **interrupt**, which corresponds to the power of central active inhibition of unwanted schemes activated in the situation.	Prefrontal
M	**Mental**-attentional capacity of the individual.	Prefrontal
LM	**Logical-structural learning** caused by the effortful use of mental-attentional capacity	Left hemisphere tertiary areas
E	**Executive** schemes in the person's repertoire, for the task at hand.	Prefrontal

constructs, operators reflect purely organismic constraints, which the brain's cortical architecture imposes on psychological processes and behavior.

We currently propose 10 hidden operators, which we present in Table 1, ordered by their supposed evolutionary emergence (Table 1 is modified from Arsalidou, 2003, with permission; see also Pascual-Leone & Johnson, 2005). Mental (*M*-) attentional capacity is the key operator underlying the maturational (non-learning) component of working memory. *M*-capacity appears empirically as a purely relational pattern relating the task complexity variable to the subjects' age when they first solve the task. As we parametrically increase the number of aspects in the task to be entertained simultaneously (thus increasing the task's mental complexity), the age of children capable of passing the task (or item) increases predictably. *M*-capacity (often called working memory by neo-Piagetians) increases endogenously with chronological age till adolescence (e.g., Case, 1995, 1998; Johnson, Fabian, & Pascual-Leone, 1989; Pascual-Leone, 1970, 1987, 2001; Pascual-Leone & Baillargeon, 1994).

Development of *M* explains the endogenous growth of mental attention. In our theory *mental* (i.e., endogenous, executive) *attention* results from dynamic interactions among four different sorts of processes: *M*-operator (the scheme-activation resource), *I*-operator (attentional interrupt, "central" inhibition mechanism), *F*-operator (neo-Gestaltist internal-field mechanism, often known as Minimum-Principle or Stimulus-Response compatibility), and *E*-operator (the currently dominant set of executive schemes – *E* allocates *M* or *I* to relevant/irrelevant schemes). *M, I,* and *E* are prefrontal functions. We believe *F* results from local lateral-inhibition processes in the cortex.[4] This system <*E*, *M*, *I*, *F*> is our model for mental attention. Note that this mental-attentional system combines a capacity construct with constructs similar to those other researchers would call central executive (Baddeley & Hitch, 2000) or controlled focal attention (e.g., Cowan, 2005; Heitz, Unsworth, & Engle, 2005).

To explain cognitive development, other hidden operators are needed as well. For instance, there is a Content (i.e., substantive) learning or *C* operator, and a Logical-structural/relational learning or *L*-operator. The *L*-operator encompasses at least two varieties: one obtained by automatization from *C*-learning, called *LC* learning, and another obtained from repeated acts of mental attention (*M*), which we call *LM* learning or effortful learning.

Unfolding of Developmental Intelligence: Case's Staircase Model

Piaget was aware that changing levels of analysis (in the epistemological sense) was difficult, because to do so children had to avoid (actively inhibit) the perceptual saliencies or "figural traps" created by schemes that applied to constitute the initial level. Piaget knew that this growing mobility of (mental) decentration was a major indicator of cognitive growth. He thus formulated his theory of development in terms of the progressive emergence, via decentration, of hierarchically organized schemes or structures that constitute distinct coordinated levels of processing, and which in turn represent new emergent levels of experienced reality. In Piaget's sense, *decentration* is changing the focus of mental attention or *centration*, whether the level of processing is changed or not. He called the cognitive-learning processes that caused these decentrations *regulations*. He labeled as *reflective abstraction* the mechanisms that permit emergence, via cognitive learning, of new more complex structures of various stages of development (i.e., sensorimotor, preoperational, concrete operational, formal operational) and of substages within each of them (Piaget, 1985; Vuyk, 1981).

---

[4] According to Edelman (1987) this lateral inhibition, i.e., activity by local inhibitory neurons that sharpen and segregate dynamic responses of the more highly activated neurons against other competing activated neurons, takes place in layer 4 of the neocortex. Edelman (1987, pp. 163–173) offers a model of how this happens.

Some neo-Piagetians, pioneered by Pascual-Leone, have introduced a new form of causal theorizing about developmental stages (e.g., Case, 1992, 1998; Demetriou, Christou, Spanoudis, & Platsidou, 2002; Halford, 1993; Morra, 2000; Pascual-Leone, 1969, 1970). Their two key assumptions are as follows: (1) stages of development are not universal (i.e., are only locally developed with experience, when endogenous mechanisms support them), and (2) Piaget's reflective abstraction and the transition into new stages have as a key mechanism either endogenous growth of mental attention (e.g., Case, 1998; de Ribaupierre & Bayeux, 1994; Halford, 1993; Morra, 2000; Pascual-Leone, 1970) or greater efficiency in both use of mental attention and automatization (or chunking) of schemes (e.g., Case, 1985; Demetriou et al., 2002; Fischer & Bidell, 1998; Lautrey, 2002; Mounoud, 1986; Siegler, 1996).

From a neo-Piagetian perspective Case (1985, 1992, 1998) has offered a suitable general descriptive model of stages: The *staircase model*, which we present in Fig. 1. We have modified this figure to show the correspondence between Case's substages (which agree with Piaget's) and the growth of *M-capacity* (endogenous or mental attention) prescribed by our theory. Notice that in our view *stable* stages appear *only* within misleading situations. A situation is *misleading* when it elicits schemes that are unsuitable for the task at hand and whose application would lower the probability of activation of task-relevant schemes (Pascual-Leone, 1969, 1987, 1989; Pascual-Leone & Baillargeon, 1994; Pascual-Leone & Johnson, 2005). In *misleading situations*, the unsuitable schemes or strategy must be averted by using active, central inhibition (i.e., mental-attentional interruption – our *I*-operator), and task-relevant schemes must be boosted by mobilizing mental attention (*M*-operator). *Facilitating situations,* in contrast, are those in which only task-relevant schemes are activated. Note that familiarity or practice may transform (via learning) misleading situations into facilitating ones, and thus any developmental stage could in principle be changed, with practice, in its local expression. That is, maturational development and learning maintain a *dialectical relation of complementarity* with each other: Both are jointly needed, but each tends to obscure the clear manifestation of the other.

Within each stage there are substages, each of which uses the maturational growth of mental attention (noticeably of *M*-power and *I*-interruption or central inhibition) as a bootstrap that impacts on a subject's ability to learn, given a suitable learning environment. In Fig. 1 we write the initial, sensorimotor levels of *M*-power (i.e., *M-levels*) as *Me* to signify that these *sensorimotor units* of *M*-capacity are later used to activate basic (well-learned) executive schemes relevant to the task at hand. We write the *mental-processing units* of *M*-capacity following the form $M = \mathbf{e} + \mathbf{k}$. By the term *mental-processing unit* we mean the quantum or amount of *M*-capacity needed to hyperactivate one scheme. We call *hyperactivation* the activation of a scheme (neural circuit) to its normal maximum, so that no higher level of activation can be expected.

Sensorimotor schemes should necessitate much less capacity to be hyperactivated than the more complex mental (e.g., symbolic, representational, conceptual) schemes. We therefore distinguish two distinct quantitative components (or implicit

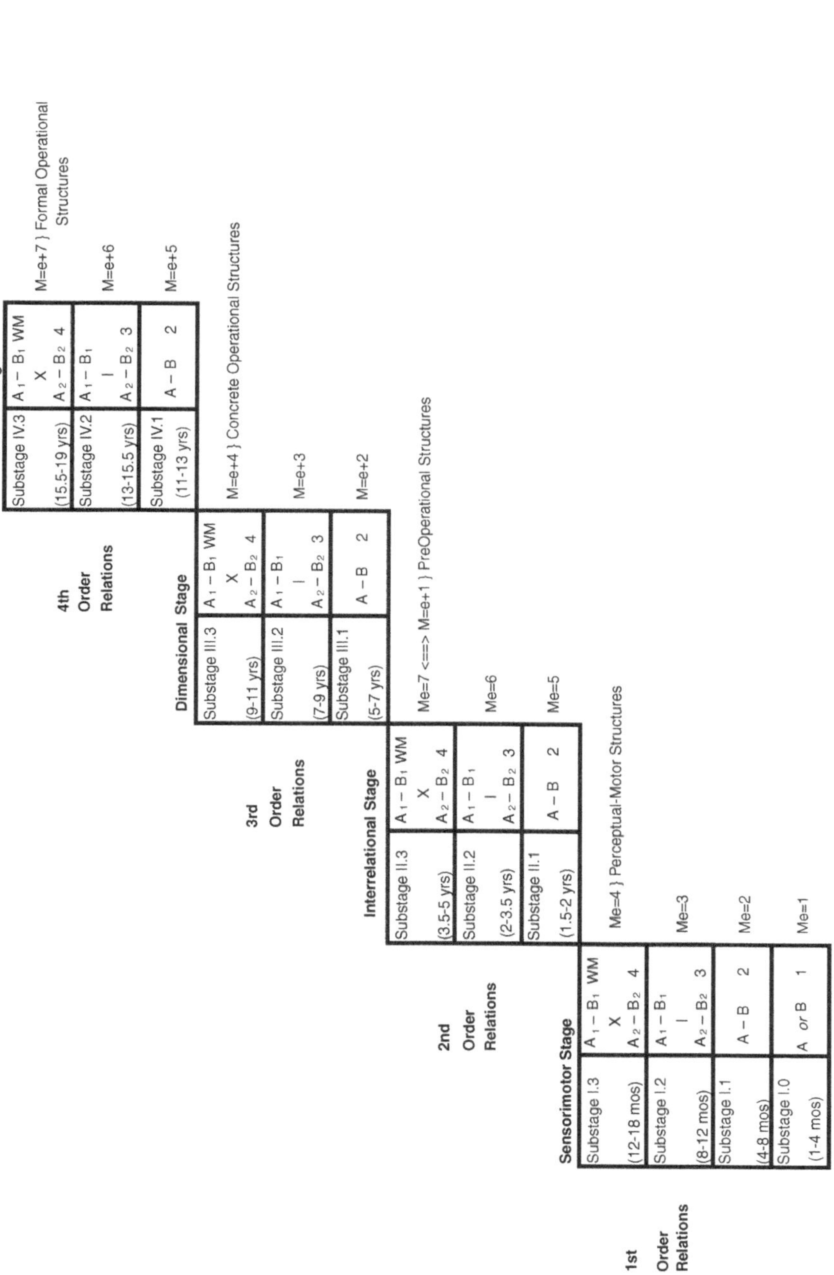

Fig. 1 Case's staircase model of developmental stages, integrated with Pascual-Leone's model of *M*-capacity growth

measurable dimensions of variation) within *M*-capacity: **e** (i.e., *Me*) and **k** (i.e., *Mk*). This distinction is needed particularly when capacity is assessed behaviorally by counting required schemes that *M* would have to boost concurrently for the task to be solved. In older children **e** functions as a constant (with the value of six sensorimotor units). **K** equals 1 at 3 years of age and increases by one unit every 2 years until it reaches $M = \mathbf{e} + \mathbf{7}$ at about 15 years of age. The e-units and the k-units cannot be combined or interchanged, because the mental (**k**) units are much larger, although the absolute magnitude of either unit is not known. We assess ("measure") both sorts of units behaviorally by counting, within suitably misleading tasks, the maximum number of distinct schemes that children have to boost simultaneously with *M*-capacity to solve the task (e.g., Pascual-Leone & Johnson, 1991, 1999).

Following Case's original model, we indicate for each stage (I, II, III, IV) and substage (0, 1, 2, 3) the age at which the substage in question normally occurs (see Fig. 1). We symbolize, using repeatedly the letters A and B with a developmentally changing meaning, the emergence of different sorts of integrative structures at the end of each stage (i.e., respectively, perceptual-motor, preoperational, concrete operational, or formal operational). This succession illustrates Piaget's process of reflective abstraction. Thus in substage I.0 (sensorimotor stage), A and B stand for two simple and separate schemes, perhaps belonging to distinct content domains such as vision, hearing, or prehension.

Case (1998) made the key assumption that relations progressively abstracted and coordinated within any given developmental stage are produced by the subject's activity in dynamic intercourse with the immediate (human and physical) environment. Such assumption is consistent with Piaget's view. From this neo-Piagetian perspective, which is also ours (Pascual-Leone, 1969, 1976, 1980, 1991, 1995), schemes and structures evolve locally, as a function of experience and prompted by the growth of mental-attentional and other hidden operators. Thus, individual differences clearly are expected throughout development and have been repeatedly found. Qualitative stages are not general but *situated* (relative to situational experience and contexts); only quantitative levels of *M*-capacity are purely organismic and general. This is in line with both Vygotsky's concept of *internalization* and a decentralized, situated construal of Piaget's *reflective abstraction* process (Kozulin, 1990; Pascual-Leone, 1995, 1996; Piaget, 1983, 1985). This content (*C*-) learning and relational or logical-structural (*L*-) learning is epistemically *reflective* of, and *internalized* from, the experiential contingencies or "causal texture" of the learner's actual environment (Pascual-Leone & Irwin, 1998; Tolman & Brunswik, 1935).

We have presented elsewhere (Pascual-Leone & Johnson, 2005), from the perspective of our theory, an interpretation of all the stages that Case described. We focus here on his Stage III or *Dimensional Stage*. This stage is well illustrated by the evolution of the concept of number, one among many *operational structures* (Case's Central Conceptual Structures – CCS) that Piaget, Case, and others have studied with similar results.

According to Case (1998), starting from two initial structures – the "global quantity" and the "counting" schemas, which 4-year-olds develop within play as they count small discrete amounts (like pebbles or beads) – a fairly complex and reversible *central numerical structure* begins to emerge in substage III.1. Case (1998, p. 765, Fig. 15.2) described it as a manifold "mental number line" constituted by the coordination of five series or sets of ordered schemes: (1) the sequence of written numerals: 1, 2, 3, etc.; (2) the sequence of number words: "one," "two," "three," etc.; (3) the sequence of operative acts assigning numbers to objects – produced by the *counting schema*; (4) the sequence of visual patterns formed by sets, collections, or numerosities of different sizes – figurative schemes that result from applying the *global-quantity schema*; and (5) the operative know-how for moving from one number to another by addition or subtraction of one unit. As Piaget and others (e.g., Bryant & Nunes, 2002) observed and Case (1992, 1998) has clarified, this number structure emerges in installments that cover the substages of Stage III.

As we construe this model, in substage III.1 children can acquire the skeleton of this number structure via coordination of schemes (3) and (4); this creates a dimensional structure of number (a "scale") that is relatively insensitive to misleading perceptual factors (this is the difference with 4-year-olds – see the Bryant & Nunes, 2002, experiments on "sharing singles and doubles"). Using this numerical structure children begin to calculate. The other three series of Case's "mental number line," that is, (1), (2), and (5), are *task-facilitated* ingredients in the ordinal or cardinal calculating practice within this number dimension, and initially they do not need to be abstracted as distinct – the child differentiates them later on.

As Case (1998) pointed out, whereas 5- and 6-year-olds build a "mental model" with one numerical dimension, 7- and 8-year-olds (i.e., substage III.2) build two dimensions (or "scales") of measurement within the same numerical structure. This structure has been shown to have wide applicability across contexts or content domains (Case, 1992; Case & Okamoto, 1996). Finally, at 9 and 10 years of age (i.e., substage III.3), children formulate and apply explicit rules for modeling the relationship between the two "scales" (Case, 1998). This full coordination demands the simultaneous entertaining of two scales and their integration by means of a calculation operative. Pascual-Leone and Johnson (2005) examined the mental complexity of the central conceptual structure for number, from the perspective of its mental-attentional (i.e., *M*) demand. Case and colleagues (Case, 1995; Case & Okamoto, 1996; Griffin & Case, 1996; Griffin, Case, & Capodilupo, 1995) found that when children were trained on the age-appropriate central conceptual structure for number, performance improved not only on the trained tasks, but also on other untrained tasks that relied on this operational structure. Griffin (1994) and Case (1996) reported that children's working memory was related to their ability to benefit from such training, suggesting that working memory capacity may be a necessary, but not sufficient, condition for development of central conceptual structures.

Our method of mental task analysis makes explicit the mental demand of tasks, in terms of the number of schemes that would have to be held in mind with effort. Because children should not be able to reliably pass tasks whose *M*-demand is beyond their *M*-capacity, our task analyses, combined with the theoretical growth of *M*-capacity (see Fig. 1), lead to clear predictions of the age at which children should be ready to benefit from training. Pascual-Leone and Johnson (2005) have given more detailed task analyses of Case's number tasks.

We summarize here an analysis of the mental demands of different types of multiplicative structures. This is followed by results from a training study, designed to test the prediction that sufficient *M*-capacity is necessary for children to benefit from conceptual training on multiplication problems.

The Mental Demand of Types of Multiplication Word Problems

Working memory (WM) has been theorized to be a source of developmental and individual differences in children's mathematical problem solving abilities (see LeFevre, DeStefano, Coleman, & Shanahan, 2005, for a review). In fact, measures of WM have been found to predict a variety of mathematical abilities, such as addition (Ashcraft, Donley, Halas, & Vakali, 1992; Lemaire, Abdi, & Fayol, 1996; McLean & Hitch, 1999), mental multiplication calculation competency (Seitz & Schumann-Hengsteler, 2000), and multiplication word problems (Geary & Widaman, 1992; Mabbott & Bisanz, 2003). Children with difficulties in math tend to score lower on WM measures (D'Amico & Guarnera, 2005; Passolunghi & Siegel, 2001, 2004; Swanson & Sachs-Lee, 2001). WM involves the process of holding information in an active state and manipulating it until a goal is reached (Mabbott & Bisanz, 2003).

Although there is much research showing that WM capacity (usually measured with span tasks) correlates with high-order cognitive ability (e.g., Wilhelm & Engle, 2005), there has been little attempt to explain precisely how WM capacity might impact on particular tasks. Our theory and task analytical methods attempt to do just this, and we illustrate for the case of types of multiplicative problems.

There are several types of situations in which multiplication is efficiently applied. These include scalar and Cartesian (e.g., array and combinatorial) problems. *Scalar multiplication* is applicable to situations in which there are a number of groups of objects having the same number in each group (e.g., Three children have four cookies each. How many cookies do they have altogether?). This sort of problem fits children's intuitive notion of multiplication as repeated addition, when at least one number is an integer (Fischbein, Deri, Nello, & Marino, 1985; Nesher, 1992).

To fully understand an *array problem* (a type of Cartesian problem) the individual must be able to visualize the two discrete values in the problem in terms of columns and rows and the display these two dimensions create. Consider the problem: "We are baking cookies. If we can fit 5 cookies along the long side of the tray and 3 cookies along the short side of the tray, how many cookies can we bake on the tray?" To conceptualize this problem as an array the individual must recognize that the number of one side (e.g., 5) is constant for each of the iterations indicated by the other number (e.g., 3). The individual must understand that array problems deal with one type of bidimensional entity that remains unchanged throughout.

Combinatorial word problems (a type of Cartesian problem) involve construction of a new composite entity (or unit) using two different, simpler entities. The new unit that the two simpler entities construct is semantically different from the original two entities used to create it. The following is an example of a combinatorial word problem: "Brian has 6 shirts and 3 pairs of pants. How many different outfits can he make with all his shirts and pants?" To solve this problem successfully an individual must be able to understand that each unit from one of the sets (e.g., each of the six shirts) can be combined with each item in the other set (e.g., each of the three different pants) to ultimately create a new unit (e.g., an outfit).

Although children are taught multiplication early in the school years, their understanding of the operation and the different types of multiplication applications appears to develop gradually over several years. Evidence for this gradual development comes from research examining children's abilities to solve/conceptualize word or story problems that require multiplication (Anghileri, 1989; Orozco, 1996; Severtson, 1993; Vergnaud, 1983). Children master scalar problems before Cartesian problems, and array problems before combinatorials (Severtson, 1993; Vergnaud, 1983, 1988). Vergnaud (1983) and Schwartz (1988) have conducted semantic analyses of the dimensions of multiplication problem types, and Nesher (1988, 1992) has examined difficulty from a textual perspective. Mental task analysis can help to explain the developmental emergence of multiplicative understanding.

Scalar Multiplication

To illustrate a predictive mental task analysis (MTA) of a scalar multiplication word problem consider the following: "Today at my store 1 candy costs 5 cents. How much will 3 candies cost?" For the purposes of this MTA we assume that the student recognizes the problem as a scalar one and chooses to solve the problem by multiplying 5 times 3. Conceptualizing the problem as scalar requires that the child understand the relationship between the two essential numerical entities in the question. He or she must recognize that one of the entities (e.g., the price of one piece of candy) can be chosen as the scale (or scalar) factor, which is the value by which each numerical unit of the other entity (e.g., the amount of candy to be purchased) is to be changed. The subject understands that this transformation changes the value of the second entity (producing the final/total cost of candy). Formula 1 is a symbolic representation denoting the conceptual understanding of scalar.

$$\textbf{SCALAR: = SCALE (}^{*}\textbf{y\_setsize, x, y)} \qquad (1)$$

We use capitals (e.g., **SCALE**) to symbolize *operative schemes* and lower case (e.g., **x** and **y**) to symbolize *figurative schemes*. Operative schemes apply on the figurative schemes, noted inside parentheses, to their right. The equation symbolizes the steps taken and the mental effort applied by the subject during the problem solving process. Starting from right to left, the symbol **y** stands for a figurative scheme corresponding to one of the entities (e.g., candy) in the problem, and **x** refers to the value of the other entity (e.g., cents). The asterisk appended to the next figurative scheme ***y_setsize** indicates that this scheme is a *parameter of the operative scheme* (Pascual-Leone & Johnson, 1999). A parameter, as already suggested, stands for a structural condition that stipulates how an operative scheme must be applied in order to achieve its goal; the parameter is a condition that the operative must satisfy in its application. The parameter ***y_setsize** carries the intuition that there is a set of objects of a given size (e.g., the amount of candies) that must be changed by scaling up the value of its numerical unit as indicated by a scale factor (e.g., the cents) – thus creating a total value that reflects the magnitude of the cost. This refers to the understanding that one of the values (e.g., **x** or **y**) will be used as the scalar factor and will be applied on the other value by the operative scheme **SCALE,** which represents the *operative concept* of the computational procedure.

Counting the schemes that must be hyperactivated by the *M*-operator, we find that the mental demand (i.e., *M*-demand) of conceptualizing the task is equal to e+4. Consequently we predict that children with *M*-capacity less than e+4 (typically, those younger than 9 years of age) likely will be unable to conceptualize SCALAR – that is, unable to see whether a given word problem fits the scalar conceptual structure. Once a child does recognize this structure in a word problem, the next step is to select an actual operative scheme (i.e., a scale procedure) to carry out the solution. With practice, the concept of scalar will become associated with one or more mathematical operations that serve as the scale procedure (e.g., multiplication, repeated addition, etc.).

Applying the scalar concept to solve the word problem in question requires simultaneously keeping the following in mind: (1) that the problem is scalar (notice that, once learned, to apply **SCALAR** in problem solving situations necessitates only one unit of *M* and not the original four units that were needed to rationally construct and learn it as formula (1) shows); (2) the number of candies to be purchased, which fits **y_setsize** in the formula; (3) the price of one candy which is the value of **x** in formula (1); (4) the fact that multiplication can be applied as a scale procedure to (2) and (3); and finally (5) multiplication number facts (e.g., a multiplication table). These are illustrated in Formula 2:

$$\mathbf{SCALAR^{L1}(\{MULT\}_{L1}\,(^{*}multi\_table,\ price{:}1,\ candy\#))} \qquad (2)$$

The operative scheme **SCALAR** has a superscripted **L1**, which symbolizes a logical-structure. A logical-structure (L-structure) refers to the overlearned associations between cofunctional and often co-activated schemes (i.e., chunking). An L-structure can be understood as a collection of concepts (schemes) that have strong associations to one another. The braces indicate that the scheme in question (i.e., **MULT**) is not being boosted by the *M*-operator, and thus, will not be counted as part of the *M*-demand of the task. The subscript **L1** outside the braces indicates that **MULT** is being boosted by **SCALAR**.

The operative of multiplication (**MULT**) is activated by the **SCALAR** operative when the subject recognizes the problem as scalar, and he or she previously has learned to solve scalar word problems using multiplication. **MULT** symbolizes this operation (multiplication) that is to be applied on the figurative schemes **candy#**

(the number of candies to be purchased) and **price:1** (the price of one candy). At the same time the individual must hold in mind a knowledge structure corresponding to multiplication number facts (the symbol ***multi_table** represents such a multiplication-table schema).

This predictive MTA indicates that the mental demand (i.e., *M*-demand) of the task is equal to *e*+4. This demand would increase to *e*+5 if the individual does not automatically associate the operative SCALAR with multiplication. Again, the prediction is that children younger than 9 years of age will not have the *M*-capacity to successfully solve **SCALAR** word problems.

Array Problems

To understand array problems fully one must visualize the two discrete entities/dimensions (i.e., the columns and the rows) and the display/space these two dimensions create. The following is an example of an array word problem: "I want to tile my bathroom floor. In my bathroom I can fit 6 tiles along the long side of the floor and 3 tiles along the short side of the floor. How many tiles will I need to cover the *whole* bathroom floor?" To conceptualize this problem as an array the individual must recognize that the number of one side (e.g., 6) is the same for each of the iterations indicated by the other number (e.g., 3). The following formula symbolizes the MTA for the concept of array:

$$\textbf{ARRAY:} = \textbf{SPACE}\,(^{*}\textbf{each-x-to-each-y, x, y}) \tag{3}$$

Beginning from the right, the symbol **y** corresponds to the value of one dimension and the symbol **x** to the value of the other dimension (both are figurative schemes). The symbol ***each-x-to-each-y** is a parameter that stipulates the **x** by **y** Cartesian product or relationship of correspondence among values between the two discrete dimensions. The individual must understand that one of the values (**x** or **y**) will need to be repeated by the amount of the other value; **SPACE** refers to the operative scheme of spatial structuring that underlies the concept of array. Counting all the schemes that are hyperactivated by *M*-operator we obtain a mental demand (i.e., *M*-demand) of *e*+4 for grasping the concept of an array.

Formula 4 symbolizes the MTA for solving an array problem using multiplication:

$$\textbf{ARRAY(MULT(}^{*}\textbf{multi\_table, val\_row, val\_col)} \tag{4}$$

Here the subject recognizes that the word problem is an **ARRAY** type and decides to solve it using multiplication. Recall that the symbol **MULT** refers to the operation multiplication. The operative scheme **ARRAY** (given in formula 3) applies on **MULT** and determines the schemes on which **MULT** applies to solve the problem. The symbol **val_row** corresponds to the numeric value of one of the numbers in the question (i.e., the value visualized as the rows); and **val_col** corresponds to the value of the column. Again, ***multi_table** refers to multiplication number facts. The *M*-demand of this task is *e*+5, therefore, children younger than 11 should have difficulties solving array word problems using multiplication.

M-demand can be reduced to *e*+4, however, if the child has had experience solving these types of problems using multiplication. In this case, the array concept may be chunked with (i.e., L-structured) and automatically activate the multiplication operative, as shown in formula 5.

$$\mathbf{ARRAY^{L1}(\{MULT\}_{L1}(^{*}multi\_table,\ val\_col,\ val\_row)} \tag{5}$$

We, therefore, predict that children with an *M*-capacity of *e*+4 (i.e., 9- to 10-year-olds) could readily benefit from training on use of multiplication for array problems, but that younger children would not.

Combinatorial

A combinatorial word problem involves construction of a new entity (or unit) using two different categories of entities. The new unit is different from the original two types of entities used to create it. The following is an example: "Brian has 6 shirts and 3 pairs of pants. How many different outfits can he make with all his shirts and pants?" To solve this problem successfully the child must be able to understand that each unit from one of the sets (e.g., each of the six shirts) can be combined with each item in the other set (e.g., each of the three different pants) to ultimately create a new unit (e.g., an outfit). The following formula symbolizes the MTA for the concept of combinatorial:

$$\mathbf{COMB:=PAIR(^{*}exhaust\_pairingx\&y,\ x,\ y)} \tag{6}$$

Starting from right, the symbol **y** corresponds to one set of entities, and **x** refers to the other set of entities. The word string ***exhaust_pairingx&y** symbolizes the parameter for the relationship between the two sets of items (pair each member of set **x** with each member of set **y**). The symbol **PAIR** refers to the operative scheme for the concept of combinatorial. To attain the notion of a combinatorial an *M*-capacity of *e*+4 is needed.

As predicted by the MTA in formula 7, the *M*-demand of actually solving a combinatorial problem using multiplication is *e*+5. Similar to the case of array problems, however, this could be reduced to *e*+4 with sufficient practice in solving combinatorial problems using multiplication.

$$\mathbf{COMB(MULT(^{*}multi\_table,\ \#shirts,\ \#pants))} \tag{7}$$

Testing M-Capacity Limits on Understanding Multiplicative Structures

M-capacity and previous experience with different types of multiplication word problems will jointly determine children's performance. To control, to some degree, for prior learning factors, we designed a multiplication intervention (Agostino, 2002). We predicted that a child's *M*-capacity would constrain the effectiveness of the intervention for various types of problems. The *theoretical hypothesis* behind this prediction can be formulated as follows: *Rapid learning (i.e., LM-learning) should be possible only when the task's M-demand is equal to or lower than the child's M-capacity*. Therefore, in a brief training intervention, children will learn only if their *M*-capacity is equal to or greater than the task's *M*-demand. This training experiment will serve to test our claim that *M-capacity and learning are intertwined* (i.e., are a dialectical pair that maintains a relation of complementarity): The effect on performance of growth in learning may depend on the growth level attained by the other member of the pair.

Children with an *M*-capacity of *e*+3 (7- to 8-year-olds) should not be able to benefit from brief training, because their capacity is below the predicted *M*-demand of the most basic sort of multiplication word problem (i.e., scalar). Children with *M*-capacity of *e*+4 should understand scalar problems, but have initial difficulty with solving arrays and combinatorials (which have a predicted *M*-demand of *e*+5). However, because an *M*-capacity of *e*+4 should be sufficient for grasping the concepts of array and combinatorial, it should be rather easy to train them to solve such problems using multiplication (or another operative procedure, such as count-by or repeated addition). Children with *M*-capacity of *e*+5 (11- to 12-year-olds) should have good initial understanding of the three types of multiplication problems. We thus predicted maximal effects of training for children with *M*-capacity of *e*+4.

Participants

Participants were 160 children, in grade 2 ($n = 52$), 4 ($n = 58$), and 6 ($n = 50$). They were recruited from two schools that had scored below average in Provincial math testing the previous year. Children received a written pretest with multiplication word problems. They also received the figural intersection task (FIT), a visuo-spatial measure of *M*-capacity (Pascual-Leone & Baillargeon, 1994; Pascual-Leone & Ijaz, 1989; Pascual-Leone & Johnson, 2001). Children within the same grade and school who obtained similar or equal pretest and FIT scores were paired, and one child from each pair was randomly assigned to a *multiplication intervention group* and the other to a *control group*. Students subsequently received a second measure of *M*, the mental attention memory (MAM) task (Pascual-Leone & Johnson, 2005). This is a modified span task, in which children recall consonants under varying degrees of interference. Their obtained *M*-capacity score was calculated as the average of FIT and MAM performance.

For the analyses reported here, we placed children into one of three *M*-capacity groups ($M = 3$, 4, or 5) based on their obtained *M*-capacity score. Seven students with an average *M*-score of 2 were dropped from the analysis, leaving a sample of $N = 153$. Three children with an *M*-score of 6 were combined with the $M = 5$ group. Because the average *M*-score was obtained after subject selection, the number of students at each *M*-level was not equal.

Training Procedures and Measures

Children in the training condition received a guided mediated-learning intervention designed to induce conceptual strategies and methods to solve multiplication word problems. The intervention aimed at developing the child's *intuitive understanding* of scalar, array, and combinatorial concepts ("concept" used here in a general sense, as Case used the term). The intervention required participation in two 45-minute individual sessions. For each problem type there were questions tapping at least two content areas (e.g., for array problems, questions about tiling a floor and questions about arranging cookies on a baking tray), so that generalization of training could be assessed. In general, intervention was provided only in the first three problems of each type, and involved a graded series of prompts that inevitably led the child to the correct answer. Children were given multiplication and addition tables, as well as concrete materials that could be used to represent and solve the problems.

In general, a child's initial answer to each question fell into one of three categories. (a) If the child answered correctly and used multiplication to obtain the answer, then the tester would reinforce use of multiplication and demonstrate why the child was correct. (b) If the child answered correctly, but did not use multiplication to obtain the answer, then the tester would reinforce the child's procedure and also demonstrate how multiplication could be used. (c) If the child's initial answer was incorrect, the tester began a series of graded prompts that would continue until the correct answer was reached. The final prompt inevitably ended with a display of the problem using concrete materials and such that the child could count items to obtain the answer, if needed. After the child provided the correct response, the tester would reinforce multiplication use to solve the problem. Several addition problems were interspersed among the multiplication problems, in order to discourage development of a set to simply multiply.

Children in the control condition received the same word problems and materials as the intervention group; however, they were not given feedback on their answers or shown any methods for solving the word problems. In order to introduce and demonstrate the multiplication and addition tables, control children did receive feedback (i.e., graded prompts) on the first scalar multiplication and the first addition word problem. The control condition was covered in one individual session that was approximately 1 hour in length.

Results

We focus here on children's initial responses to multiplication items in the individual sessions. Responses were coded in terms of correct or incorrect strategy use. If the child indicated a correct strategy yet failed to give the correct numeric response, the strategy was coded as correct (1). For instance, if the correct strategy was to multiply $4 \times 6=24$, and the child responded, "$4 \times 6=23$," the child received credit for providing the correct strategy, although the numeric response was incorrect. If the child's explanation indicated an incorrect strategy but provided a correct numeric response, the strategy was coded as incorrect (0). Note that additive strategies that would lead to a correct solution were scored as correct. We present descriptive data on an item-by-item basis within multiplication type, to trace the effects of training at different *M*-capacity levels.

Scalars. Table 2 presents the scalar problems posed to the children, and Fig. 2 shows the percent correct strategy use to solve the problems (listed in order of presentation) as a function of the children's obtained *M*-capacity scores. Word problem scores reflect the students' initial answers in the training condition and their only answers (unless they self-corrected) in the control condition. Two of the scalar problems concerned buying candies. The remaining problems were in the context of a snake game. In the snake game, children were shown four snakes that varied in length (10 cm, 20 cm, 30 cm, and 40 cm) and were told that how much these snakes eat depends on how long they are. The relationship between food and length was explained in the context of two learning problems presented to all

Table 2 Scalar items presented during individual sessions

Candy	Today at my store 1 candy costs 5 cents. How much will 3 candies cost?
Candy	Today at my store 1 candy costs 4 cents. How much will 6 candies cost?
Snakes	If the blue snake needs 6 grams of snake food each day, how many grams of food should I give to the brown snake for 1 day?
Snakes	If the blue snake needs 7 grams of snake food each day, how many grams should I give the green snake for 1 day?
Multidimensional snakes	If 1 blue snake needs 5 grams of snake food for 1 day, how much food should I give 2 red snakes for 3 days?

Note:

• Bolded items indicate that Training condition received a series of graded prompts if their initial answer was incorrect.

• For snakes items, the blue snake was 10 cm long, brown snake 20 cm, green 30 cm, and red 40 cm. The child was trained to understand that the amount of food eaten was relative to the length.

• The final scalar question was presented to all children in grades 4 and 6. Only grade 2 children who answered at least one simple scalar snake question correctly were presented the final, multidimensional scalar snake question.

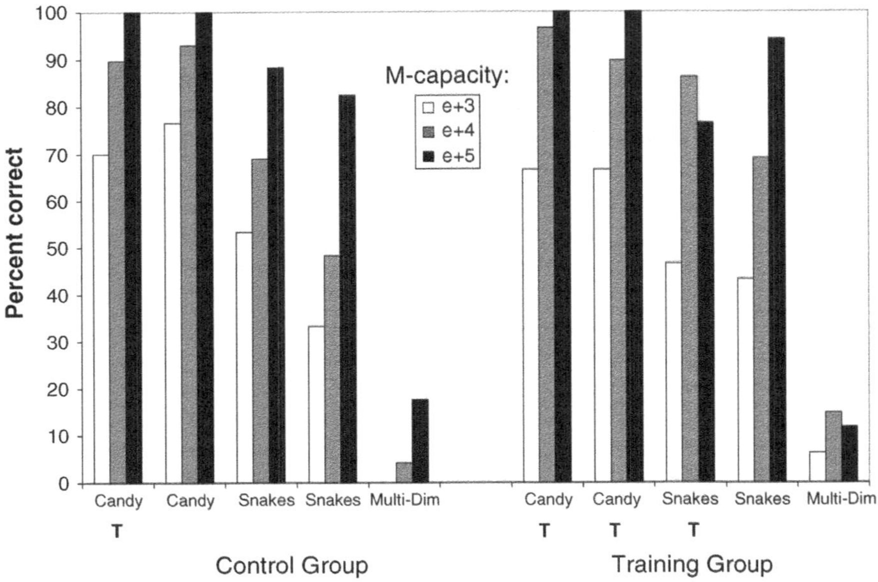

Fig. 2 Percentage correct strategy use on scalar problems as a function of item, training condition, and measured *M*-capacity. "T" indicates that intervention followed an incorrect response

children. The last scalar snake problem was a multidimensional word problem. Task analysis (Agostino, 2002) indicated that the *M*-demand of the simple scalar snake problems was *e*+4. Although the *M*-demand of the simple scalar snake problems was the same as for the candy problems, executive demand was higher in the snakes items, because they required an extra solution step to discern the relative-size relationship between the blue and the target (e.g., brown) snake (e.g., a factor of 2). For the multidimensional item, both *M*-demand and executive demand were increased, putting the problem beyond the theoretical *M*-capacity of the oldest participants. Note that the snakes game also presents an unfamiliar context, which can serve to test the limits in understanding of scalars.

We take about 70% correct as criterion for good understanding and 50% or below as evidence of poor understanding. All children received training on the first candy item, so possible differential effects of training on scalars first becomes evident only in the first snakes problem (see Fig. 2). Children with a measured *M*-capacity of *e*+3, in both conditions, show some understanding of scalars in the context of the candy problems. However, performance level falls when the simple scalar snakes problem is introduced, and training in this context does not improve the performance of children with *M*-capacity of *e*+3.

Children with *M*-capacity of *e*+4 show good understanding of scalars in the candy context. At this *M*-level, training serves to maintain good performance on the simple snakes scalars. In contrast, performance in the control condition drops off, with correct performance below 50% on the second snakes problem. As predicted, only children with sufficient *M*-capacity benefit from training. Children with *M*-capacity *e*+5 are expected to have both sufficient capacity and experience to deal with the simple scalar problems, and both control and training groups show high levels of scalar performance at this *M*-level. When the *M*-demand is raised beyond the capacity of even the oldest children (multidimensional scalar), however, performance falls drastically in both groups.

Arrays. There were four array problems, and children in the training condition received feedback on the first three questions. We focus here only on the first three array problems (see Table 3), because the fourth was in a different format. We predicted that array problems would have an initial *M*-demand of *e*+5, which could be reduced to *e*+4 with training. Figure 3 shows percentage use of correct strategies to solve array problems. As predicted, children with *M*-capacity *e*+3 had little initial understanding of arrays, and in the control condition performance at this *M*-level remained below 30%. There was some moderate success in training the *M*=*e*+3 group within the floor tiling context. However, training did not transfer, with performance in the cookies context falling to 50%.

At the *M*=*e*+4 level, children in the control group show some understanding of arrays, averaging approximately 60% correct strategy use on the first three array word problems. At this *M*-level the training group starts off at a similar level of understanding, but as predicted, shows a strong effect of training that transfers to a new context (cookies on a baking tray). As predicted, children with *M*-capacity *e*+5 show good understanding of arrays from the start. Note that the modal incorrect strategy for children at *M*-level of *e*+3 was to add the numbers together demonstrating no understanding of array. The modal incorrect strategy for the children at *M*-level *e*+4 also was to add the numbers together, and their second most common error was to add to obtain the perimeter, demonstrating a sense of the space but not of the whole space.

Combinatorials. The combinatorial section consisted of six items (see Table 4): two items about recombining clothing to make an outfit, two items about recombining boys and girls to make dancing partners (Orozco, 1996), one item about combining paper and ribbon to wrap presents, and a multidimensional problem that involved combining three types of clothing. Children in the training condition

Table 3 Array items presented during individual sessions

Tiles	I want to tile my bathroom floor. In my bathroom I can fit 6 tiles along the long side of the floor and 3 tiles along the short side of the floor. How many tiles will I need to cover the *whole* bathroom floor?
Tiles	Now, I want to tile my kitchen floor. My kitchen can fit 7 tiles along the long side of the floor and 4 tiles along the short side of the floor. How many tiles will I need to cover the *whole* kitchen floor?
Cookies	We are baking cookies. If we can fit 5 cookies along the long side of the tray and 3 cookies along the short side of the tray: How many cookies can we bake on the tray?

Note: Bolded items indicate that training condition received a series of graded prompts if their initial answer was incorrect.

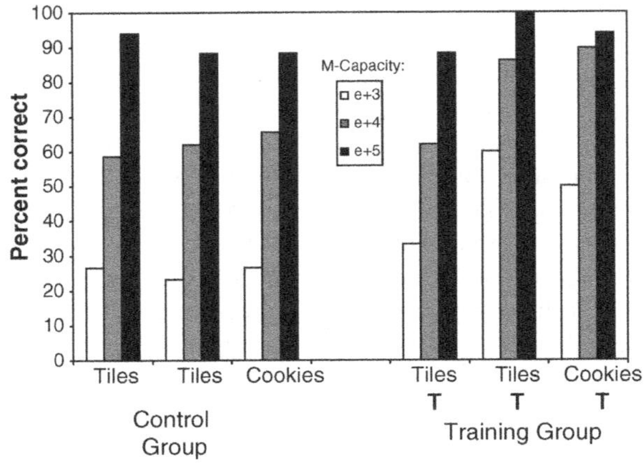

Fig. 3 Percentage correct strategy use on array problems, as a function of item, training condition, and measured *M*-capacity. "T" indicates that intervention followed an incorrect response

received feedback and prompting on the first three combinatorial items. Similar to arrays, we predicted that the basic combinatorial problems would have an initial *M*-demand of *e*+5, which could be reduced to *e*+4 with training. The multidimensional problem had greater *M*-demand (i.e., *e*+5 or *e*+6). We focus first on the basic combinatorial items (problems 1–5).

Figure 4 shows percentage correct strategy use to solve combinatorials. Children with *M*-capacity *e*+3 in the control group show little understanding of combinatorials, with correct performance hovering about 20% correct. At this *M*-level, children in the intervention group show some within-context effects of training,

Table 4 Combinatorial items presented during individual sessions

Outfits	Brian has 6 shirts and 3 pairs of pants. How many different outfits can he make with all his shirts and pants?
Outfits	Kimberley has 7 hats and 4 coats. How many different outfits can she make with all her hats and coats?
Dance	There are 4 boys and 3 girls at a dance. Each boy dances with every girl, and each girl dances with every boy. At the end of the dance, all the boys have danced with all the girls. How many different pairs of dancing partners were there?
Dance	At another dance, there are 6 boys and 5 girls. Each boy dances with every girl, and each girl dances with every boy. At the end of the dance, all the boys have danced with all the girls. How many different pairs of dancing partners were there?
Gifts	We are wrapping presents for a class party. If we have 3 colors of wrapping paper and 7 colors of ribbon, how many different ways could we wrap the presents?
Multidimensional	Jesse has 5 pairs of pants, 3 blouses, and 2 vests. How many different outfits can she make with all her pants, blouses, and vests?

Note: Bolded items indicate that training condition received a series of graded prompts if their initial answer was incorrect.

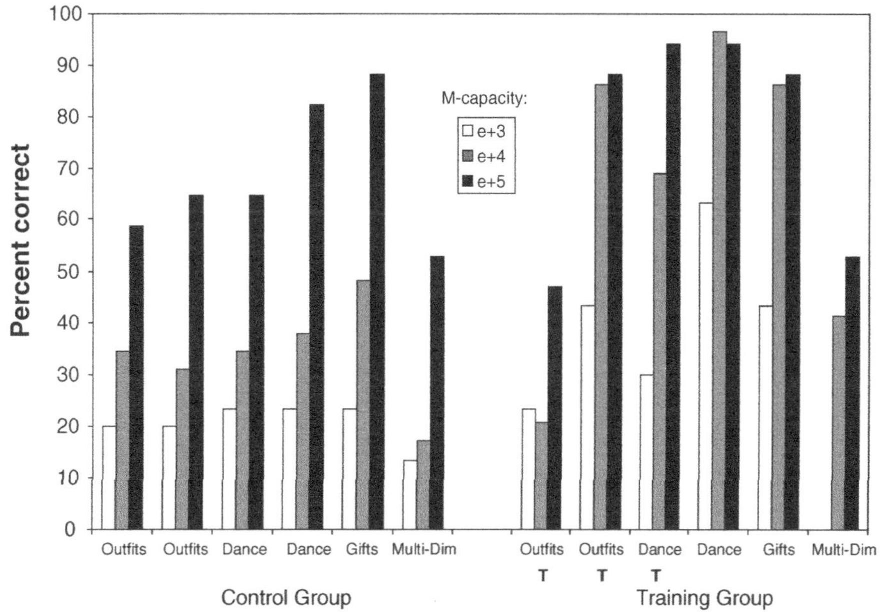

Fig. 4 Percentage correct strategy use on combinatorial problems, as a function of item, training condition, and measured *M*-capacity. "T" indicates that intervention followed an incorrect response

but this does not generalize: With change of problem context (e.g., between the second and third and between the fourth and fifth problems) performance consistently falls below 50% correct. Performance of control children at *M*-level *e*+4 also remains below 50% across problems. In contrast, as predicted, children at *M*-level *e*+4 show a strong effect of training that transfers across contexts for the basic combinatorial items.

At *M*-level *e*+5 control children start off with a moderate level of understanding and demonstrate ability to learn spontaneously from exposure to the basic combinatorial problems, reaching close to 90% correct on the fifth combinatorial item. At this *M*-level, children in the intervention group show immediate effects of training, reaching about 90% correct on the second item and sustaining that across the basic combinatorial problems. This high performance level suffers a sharp decline in both groups, however, on the more *M*-demanding multidimensional combinatorial item.

The modal incorrect strategy for children at *M*-level *e*+3 in both conditions was simply to add together the two numbers in the basic combinatorial problems – a strategy that reflects no notion of a combination. The modal incorrect strategy for children at *M*-level *e*+4 was to respond with the smaller number in the question – a strategy that implies awareness of the need to combine, but failure to recombine.

Results for the three multiplication problem types are consistent with our predictions based on an *M*-demand versus *M*-capacity trade-off (Pascual-Leone & Baillargeon, 1994). Average improvement from the first to the last item of each type (excluding multidimensional items) was correlated with *M*-capacity score in the training condition ($r = .29$, $p < .05$), but not in control ($r = .20$, ns). A structural equation model predicting improvement from the written pretest to a post-test (completed about 2 weeks after the individual sessions) showed that in the training group the effect of age on learning was fully mediated through obtained *M*-score (Pascual-Leone, Johnson, Bauer, & Agostino, 2002). These results indicate that *M*-capacity is a necessary, but not sufficient condition for performance. Relevant experience (i.e., an adequate repertoire of schemes) also is needed, but *M*-capacity places a limit on a child's conceptual learning ability.

Conclusions

In keeping with the theme of this volume, we conclude by relating our theory to the developing brain. In Fig. 1 we showed the correspondence between Case's (and Piaget's) substages and our stages of *M*-operator growth. The theories of Case and Piaget place emphasis on the qualitative stages of cognitive development, with Case describing these in terms of central conceptual structures (Piaget's operational structures) that characterize children's understanding of broad domains of experience (Case, 1998). From the perspective of cognitive-developmental neuropsychology, it may be heuristically useful to classify the many levels of processing found in different domains under four molar *levels-of-abstraction categories* relating to the classic levels of Luria (1973) and Eccles (1980). *Primary cortical areas* are where sensorial receptors or motor effectors arrive (afference) or leave (efference) the cortex. They are the fixed sites that define a particular modality of processing or *content*. Within a given restricted content domain, *secondary areas* coordinate information (schemes) that carry different aspects or attributes (visual sorting, form and depth, color, movement, etc.). *Tertiary areas* progressively coordinate schemes across content domains (vision, somatosensory, hearing, motor, etc.), so as to constitute polymodal distal objects, or action procedures, or adjunct relational information, from the world of experience. Finally, following Eccles (1980), we call *quaternary areas* (i.e., high-tertiary areas) those that are maximally polymodal, embody the highest integrations of information, and often embody localized general-purpose resources (hidden operators of the brain). The prefrontal areas within the operative ("motor") functions, and the superior temporal sulcus, and some sites in the occipital–temporal–parietal crossroad (gyrus angularis and gyrus supramarginalis, i.e., Brodmann areas 39 and 40, intraparietal sulcus), within the figurative ("sensorial") functions, are clear examples of quaternary areas. These are sites where executive processes and complex knowledge structures (such as complicated distal "objects" – for instance, model objects of universities, cities and airports) are found.

The spiral staircase model of cognitive development that Piaget, Case, and others (e.g., Lenin, Werner, Pascual-Leone, Fisher, Demetriou) put forward relates to the level-of-abstraction categories just described. As children move from one to another developmental stage (Pascual-Leone & Johnson, 2005), that is, from the Sensorimotor to the PreOperational (Case's Interrelational), to the Concrete Operational (Case's Dimensional), and the Formal Operational (Case's Vectorial), they are likely to shift their interest and main focus of cognitive growth, cumulatively, from one level of abstraction category to another: primary areas, secondary areas, tertiary areas, and quaternary areas. Concurrently with such change, children tend to shift their mind's interest from the here-and-now Present (this is Sensorial Perception and motor action); to the Inferred Present, inferred via analysis, synthesis, and interpretation (this is Intelligent Perception); to the Inferred Future (this is Intellection); to the Inferred Possible, inferred not from experience but from rational analysis of non-contradictory possibilities (this is Intellectual processing).

Pascual-Leone was the first to displace causal developmental significance from stages to substages, when he inferred the construct *M*-capacity based on task analysis of Piaget's data (Pascual-Leone, 1970; Pascual-Leone & Smith, 1969). The power of *M*-capacity grows maturationally with age up to adolescence and impacts on a child's ability to learn, as Case, ourselves, and others have demonstrated and we have illustrated here for the case of multiplicative structures.

In Fig. 1 we indicated the initial, sensorimotor *levels of M-power* as *Me* to signify that these *sensorimotor units* of *M*-capacity later are used to activate basic (well-learned) executive schemes relevant to the task at hand. We indicated the *mental-processing units* of *M*-capacity using the form $\boldsymbol{M} = \mathbf{e} + \mathbf{k}$ (Pascual-Leone, 1970). A mental-processing unit is the quantum or amount of *M*-capacity needed to hyperactivate one scheme. Hyperactivation of sensorimotor schemes should require much less capacity than the more complex mental (e.g., symbolic, representational, conceptual) schemes. It is reasonable to assume that these quanta of *M*-capacity are acquired cumulatively during development at a constant rate (so that time taken to acquire a given amount serves as indirect estimate of this amount). It is thus revealing that initially, during the first 2 years of life, transition from one *M-level* to the next occurs about every 4 (first year) or 8 (second year) months, whereas stage transitions after 3 years of age occur only every 24 months. This drastic change in rate of stage transition suggests that the sensorimotor *M*-units or quanta may be about three to six times smaller than the mental *M*-units. We, therefore, were led (Pascual-Leone, 1970) to distinguish two distinct quantitative components (or implicit measurable dimensions of variation) within *M*-capacity: **e** (i.e., *Me*) and **k** (i.e., *Mk*) – at least when this capacity is assessed behaviorally by means of counting schemes that *M* would have to boost for the task to be solved. In older children, **e** functions as a constant (with the value of six sensorimotor units). Notice that the **e**-units and the **k**-units cannot be combined or interchanged, because the mental (**k**) units are much larger, although the absolute magnitude of either unit is not known. The difference in size between **e** and **k** explains, and thus is supported by, some surprising neuroscience results obtained by Thatcher.

Figure 5 reproduces Thatcher's (1997) data showing the "sort of spiral staircase" that we have mentioned. Part A of this figure plots mean EEG coherence (correlation of neuronal firing) against age using output of left frontoparietal electrodes. In this figure there are two phases in the evolution of coherence across chronological age. In the first we see, from 1.5 to 5 years, a slow decrement in coherence with oscillations that have a high coherence point at 3 years. In the second phase there is another high jump in coherence at about 6 years followed by another slow decreasing trend of the coherence down to 16 years of age. Interestingly, the oscillations in this second phase occur about every other year. This is fully consistent with our *M*-growth model depicted in Fig. 1. Note that Thatcher credits Case's (1985) and Fischer's (1980) theories, which in fact cannot predict Thatcher's two rates of spiral change. Our *M*-model claims that there are two "hidden" rates of *M*-growth: that of the sensorimotor **e**-units and that of the mental **k**-units. *M-growth* during the former phase occurs frequently and in small amounts (when measured by the schemes being boosted by *M*). *M*-growth in the latter phase appears every 2 years and in larger amounts. Thus we expect two phases, and because this *M*-boosting leads to local differentiation of schemes, we expect in each phase the coherence to decrease as the phase proceeds.

Further, because in the first phase *M*-growth occurs often and in small increments, the rate of *M*-change with the change of time should be greater during the sensorimotor phase than during the second, mental phase of *M*-growth. This is consistent with Thatcher's results in Fig. 5 B, where the first derivative (i.e., the rate of change of coherence with the change of time) is plotted along with the mean coherence of subjects and their chronological age. Figure 5 B shows, as our model precisely predicts, that changes in the first derivative and in mean coherence are greater during the first phase. The onset of the second phase at about 6 years of age is also consistent with our model, because this is the time when the symbolic function is fully internalized and *mentation* (mental planning and thinking) becomes fully available. Consistent with this interpretation, Case (1998, Fig. 15.12) has shown

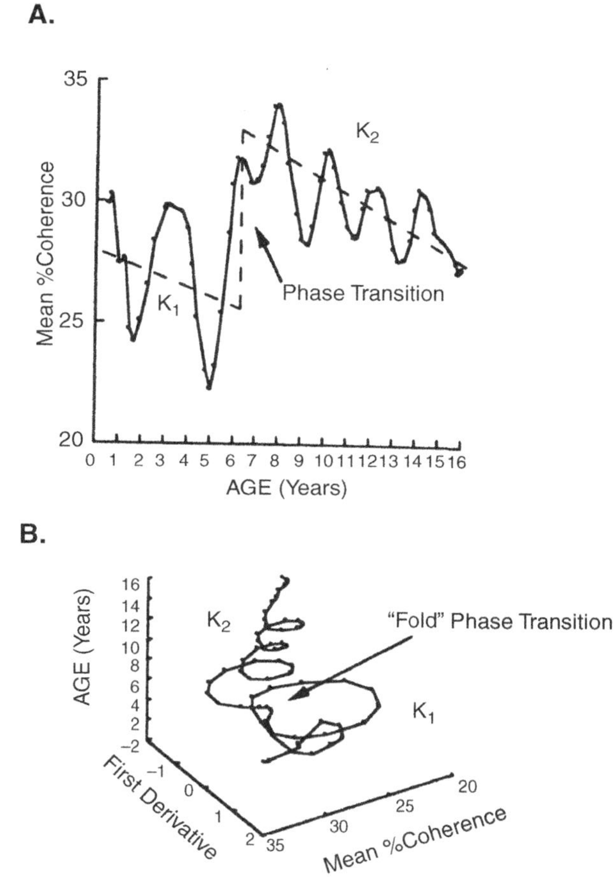

Fig. 5 (**A**) Mean percentage EEG coherence (i.e., coherence × 100) in the theta frequency band for left lateral frontal-parietal regions (i.e., F7-P3) from 6 months to 16 years. Two modes of oscillation – mode 1, from birth to approximately age 5, and mode 2, from approximately age 7 to 16 – are fit by regression lines K_1 and K_2. (**B**) A two-dimensional phase portrait represented in three dimensions by extending the phase space over age. This figure demonstrates that there are two-limit cycles or phase states of EEG coherence oscillation in the left frontal-parietal region (i.e., P3-F7) that are spirals with different radii and frequencies over the life span. (Figure and caption from Thatcher, 1997, p. 99)

suggestive curves indicating considerable cross-sectional similarity in the growth with age of EEG coherence, within Thatcher's results, and the growth of working memory (mean of counting span and spatial span) in Case's own data.

In summary, we believe to have provided evidence that mental-attentional *M-capacity* and learning are functionally intertwined (are dialectically complementary) as causal factors explaining cognitive development, something that Pascual-Leone (1970, 1976, 1980), Case (1998), and other neo-Piagetians have in various ways proposed. Further, we have intimated ways in which our theory of constructive operators can be interpreted into, and shown to explain results from, neuroscience. But a detailed account of this neuroscience story is beyond the scope of the present chapter.

Acknowledgments Preparation of this chapter was facilitated by an operating grant (#410-2001-1077) to the first two authors from the Social Sciences and Humanities Research Council of Canada (SSHRC). The reported research was funded by a SSHRC operating grant (#410-2006-2325) and a York University Faculty of Arts Research Grant. We are grateful to the following for assistance with data collection: S. Bauer, S. Cunning, D. Fisher, N. Im-Bolter, L. Hakim, and E. Polak.

References

Agostino, A. (2002). *Solving multiplication problems: The role of mental attention*. Unpublished masters thesis, York University, Toronto.

Anghileri, A. (1989). An investigation of young children's understanding of multiplication. *Educational Studies in Mathematics, 20*, 367–385.

Arbib, M. A., Érdi, P., &Szentágothai, J. (1998). *Neural organization: Structure, function, and dynamics*. Cambridge, MA: MIT Press.

Arsalidou, M. (2003). *Neural correlates of visual problem solving and complexity*. Unpublished master's thesis, York University, Toronto.

Ashcraft, M. H., Donley, R. D., Halas, M. A., & Vakali, M. (1992). Working memory, automaticity, and problem difficulty. In J. I. D. Campbell (Ed.), *The nature and origins of mathematical skills* (pp. 301–329). Amsterdam: Elsevier.

Baddeley, A. D., & Hitch, G. J. (2000). Development of working memory: Should the Pascual-Leone and the Baddeley and Hitch models be merged? *Journal of Experimental Child Psychology, 77*, 128–137.

Bohr, N. (1961). *Physique atomique et connaissance humaine*. Paris: Editions Gouthier.

Bryant, P., & Nunes, T. (2002). Children's understanding of mathematics. In U. Goswami (Ed.), *Blackwell handbook of childhood cognitive development* (pp. 412–439). Malden, MA: Blackwell.

Case, R. (1985). *Intellectual development: Birth to adulthood*. New York: Academic Press.

Case, R. (1992). *The mind's staircase*. Hillsdale, NJ: Erlbaum.

Case, R. (1995). Capacity-based explanations of working memory growth: A brief history and reevaluation. In F. Weinert & W. Schneider (Eds.), *Memory performance and competencies: Issues in growth and development* (pp. 23–44). Hillsdale, NJ: Erlbaum.

Case, R. (1996) Summary and conclusion. In R. Case & Y. Okamoto, The role of conceptual structures in the development of children's thought (pp. 189–214). *Monographs of the Society for Research in Child Development, 61* (Serial No. 246).

Case, R. (1998). The development of conceptual structures. In W. Damon (Series Ed.) & D. Kuhn & R. S. Siegler (Vol. Eds.), *Handbook of child psychology: Vol. 2. Cognition, perception, and language* (5th ed., pp. 745–800). New York: Wiley.

Case, R., & Okamoto, Y. (1996). The role of conceptual structures in the development of children's thought. *Monographs of the Society for Research in Child Development, 61* (Serial No. 246).

Cowan, N. (2005). *Working-memory capacity*. New York: Psychology Press.

D'Amico, A., & Guarnera, M. (2005). Exploring working memory in children with low arithmetical achievement. *Learning and Individual Differences, 15*, 189–202.

Demetriou, A., Christou, C., Spanoudis, G., & Platsidou, M. (2002). The development of mental processing: Efficiency, working memory, and thinking. *Monographs of the Society for Research in Child Development, 67* (Serial No. 268).

de Ribaupierre, A., & Bayeux, C. (1994). Developmental change in a spatial task of attentional capacity: An essay toward an integration of two working memory models. *International Journal of Behavioral Development, 17*, 5–35.
Eccles, J. C. (1980). *The human psyche,* Berlin: Springer-Verlag.
Edelman, G. M. (1987). *Neural Darwinism.* New York: Basic Books.
Edelman, G. M., & Tononi, G. (2000). *A universe of consciousness.* New York: Basic Books.
Fischbein, E., Deri, M., Nello, M. S., & Marino, M. S. (1985). The role of implicit models in solving verbal problems in multiplication and division. *Journal for Research in Mathematics Education, 16*, 3–17.
Fischer, K. W. (1980). A theory of cognitive development: The control and construction of hierarchies of skills. *Psychological Review, 87*, 477–531.
Fischer, K. W., & Bidell, T. R. (1998). Dynamic development of psychological structures in action and thought. In W. Damon (Series Ed.) & R. M. Lerner (Vol. Ed.), *Handbook of child psychology: Vol. 1. Theoretical models of human development* (5th ed., pp. 467–561). New York: Wiley.
Freeman, W. J. (1995). *Societies of brains.* Hillsdale, NJ: Erlbaum.
Geary, D. C., & Widaman, K. F. (1992). Numerical cognition: On the convergence of componential and psychometric models. *Intelligence, 16*, 47–80.
Griffin, S. A. (1994). *Working memory capacity and the acquisition of mathematical knowledge: Implications for learning and development.* Paper presented at the meeting of the International Society for the Study of Behavioral Development, Amsterdam.
Griffin, S. A., & Case, R. (1996). Evaluating the breadth and depth of training effects when central conceptual structures are taught. In R. Case & Y. Okamoto, The role of conceptual structures in the development of children's thought (pp. 83–102). *Monographs of the Society for Research in Child Development, 61* (Serial No. 246).
Griffin, S., Case, R., & Capodilupo, A. (1995). Teaching for understanding: The importance of the central conceptual structures in the elementary mathematics curriculum. In A. McKeough, J. Lupart, & A. Marini (Eds.), *Teaching for transfer: Fostering generalization in learning* (pp. 123–151). Hillsdale, NJ: Erlbaum.
Halford, G. S. (1993). *Children's understanding: The development of mental models.* Hillsdale, NJ: Erlbaum.
Heitz, R. P., Unsworth, N., & Engle, R. W. (2005). Working memory capacity, attention control, and fluid intelligence. In O. Wilhelm & R. W. Engle (Eds.), *Handbook of understanding and measuring intelligence* (pp. 61–77). Thousand Oaks, CA: Sage.
Hunt, J. McV. (1961). *Intelligence and experience.* New York: Ronald Press.
James, W. (1966). *Psychology: The briefer course* (G. Allport, Ed.). New York: Harper & Row.
Johnson, J., Fabian, V., & Pascual-Leone, J. (1989). Quantitative hardware-stages that constrain language development. *Human Development, 32*, 245–271.
Kozulin, A. (1990). *Vygotsky's psychology: A biography of ideas.* Cambridge, MA: Harvard University Press.
Lautrey, J. (2002). Is there a general factor of cognitive development? In R. J. Sternberg & E. L. Grigorenko (Eds.), *The general factor of intelligence: How general is it?* (pp. 117–148). Mahwah, NJ: Erlbaum.
LeFevre, J., DeStefano, D., Coleman, B., & Shanahan, T. (2005). Mathematical cognition and working memory. In J. I. D. Campbell (Ed.), *Handbook of mathematical cognition* (pp. 361–377). New York: Psychology Press.
Lemaire, P., Abdi, H., & Fayol, M. (1996). The role of working memory resources in simple cognitive arithmetic. *European Journal of Cognitive Psychology, 8*, 73–103.
Luria, A. R. (1973). *The working brain.* Middlesex, UK: Penguin Books.
Mabbott, D. J., & Bisanz, J. (2003). Developmental change and individual differences in children's multiplication. *Child Development, 74*, 1091–1107.
Marx, K., Engles, F., & Lenin, V. I. (1977). *On dialectical materialism.* Moscow: Progress Publishers.

McLean, J. F., & Hitch, G. J. (1999). Working memory impairments in children with specific arithmetic learning difficulties. *Journal of Experimental Child Psychology, 74*, 240–260.
Mounoud, P. (1986). Similarities between developmental sequences at different age periods. In I. Levin (Ed.), *Stage and structure: Reopening the debate* (pp. 119–131). Norwood, NJ: Ablex.
Morra, S. (2000). A new model of verbal short-term memory. *Journal of Experimental Child Psychology, 75*, 191–227.
Nesher, P. (1988). Multiplicative school word problems: Theoretical approaches and empirical findings. In J. Hiebert & M. Behr (Eds.), *Number concepts and operations in the middle school grades* (pp. 19–40). Reston, VA: NCIM.
Nesher, P. (1992). Solving multiplication word problems. In G. Lienhardt, R. T. Putnam, & R. A. Hattrup (Eds.), *Analysis of arithmetic for mathematics teaching* (pp. 189–219). Hillsdale, NJ: Erlbaum.
Orozco, H. M. (1996). *Analisis microgenetico y procesual de la construccion de la operacion multiplicativa*. Unpublished doctoral dissertation, Universitat de Barcelona, Barcelona.
Pascual-Leone, J. (1969). *Cognitive development and cognitive style: A general psychological integration*. Unpublished doctoral dissertation, University of Geneva, Geneva.
Pascual-Leone, J. (1970). A mathematical model for the transition rule in Piaget's developmental stages. *Acta Psychologica, 63*, 301–345.
Pascual-Leone, J. (1976). On learning and development, Piagetian style: I. A reply to Lefebvre-Pinard. *Canadian Psychological Review, 17*, 270–288.
Pascual-Leone, J. (1980). Constructive problems for constructive theories: The current relevance of Piaget's work and a critique of information-processing simulation psychology. In R. Kluwe & H. Spada (Eds.), *Developmental models of thinking* (pp. 263–296). New York: Academic Press.
Pascual-Leone, J. (1987). Organismic processes for neo-Piagetian theories: A dialectical causal account of cognitive development. *International Journal of Psychology, 22*, 531–570.
Pascual-Leone, J (1989). An organismic process model of Witkin's field-dependence-independence. In T. Globerson & T. Zelniker (Eds.), *Cognitive style and cognitive development* (pp. 36–70). Norwood, NJ: Ablex.
Pascual-Leone, J. (1991). A commentary on Boom and Juckes' on the learning paradox. *Human Development, 34*, 288–293.
Pascual-Leone, J. (1995). Learning and development as dialectical factors in cognitive growth. *Human Development, 38*, 338–348.
Pascual-Leone, J. (1996). Vygotsky, Piaget, and the problems of Plato. *Swiss Journal of Psychology, 55*, 84–92.
Pascual-Leone, J. (1998) SSSs or functionalist modes of processing? A commentary on Kargopoulos and Demetriou's paper. *New Ideas in Psychology, 16*, 89–95.
Pascual-Leone, J. (2000). Reflections on working memory: Are the two models complementary? *Journal of Experimental Child Psychology, 77*, 138–154.
Pascual-Leone, J. (2001). If the magical number is 4, how does one account for operations within working memory? *Behavioral and Brain Sciences, 24*, 136–138.
Pascual-Leone, J., & Baillargeon, R. (1994). Developmental measure of mental attention. *International Journal of Behavioral Development, 17*, 161–200.
Pascual-Leone, J., & Goodman, D. (1979). Intelligence and experience: A neoPiagetian approach. *Instructional Science, 8*, 301–367.
Pascual-Leone, J., & Ijaz, H. (1989). Mental capacity testing as a form of intellectual-developmental assessment. In R. Samuda, S. Kong, J. Cummings, J. Pascual-Leone, & J. Lewis (Eds.), *Assessment and placement of minority students* (pp. 144–171). Toronto: Hogrefe International.
Pascual-Leone, J., & Irwin, R. (1998). Abstraction, the will, the self, and models of learning in adulthood. In M. C. Smith & T. Pourchot (Eds.), *Adult learning and development: Perspectives from educational psychology* (pp. 35–66). Hillsdale, NJ: Erlbaum.

Pascual-Leone, J., & Johnson, J. (1991). The psychological unit and its role in task analysis: A reinterpretation of object permanence. In M. Chandler & M. Chapman (Eds.), *Criteria for competence* (pp. 155–187). Hillsdale. NJ: Erlbaum.

Pascual-Leone, J., & Johnson, J. (1999). A dialectical constructivist view of representation: Role of mental attention, executives, and symbols. In I. E. Sigel (Ed.), *Development of mental representation: Theories and applications* (pp. 169–200). Mahwah, NJ: Erlbaum.

Pascual-Leone, J., & Johnson, J. (2001). *Manual for FIT: Figural Intersections Test*. Unpublished manuscript, York University, Toronto.

Pascual-Leone, J., & Johnson, J. (2005). A dialectical constructivist view of developmental intelligence. In O. Wilhelm & R. W. Engle (Eds.), *Handbook of understanding and measuring intelligence* (pp. 177–201). Thousand Oaks, CA: Sage.

Pascual-Leone, J., Johnson, J., Baskind, S., Dworsky, S., & Severtson, E. (2000). Culture-fair assessment and the processes of mental attention. In A. Kozulin & Y. Rand (Eds.), *Experience of mediated learning: An impact of Feuerstein's theory in education and psychology* (pp. 191–214). New York: Pergamon.

Pascual-Leone, J., Johnson, J., Bauer, S., & Agostino, A. (2002). *How much does arithmetic proficiency in the school years owe to mental attentional capacity?* Poster presented at the meetings of the International Society for the Study of Behavioral Development, Ottawa.

Pascual-Leone, J., & Smith, J. (1969). The encoding and decoding of symbols by children: A new experimental paradigm and a neo-Piagetian model. *Journal of Experimental Child Psychology, 8*, 328–355.

Passolunghi, M. C., & Siegel, L. S. (2001). Short-term memory, working memory, and inhibitory control in children with difficulties in arithmetic problem solving. *Journal of Experimental Child Psychology, 80*, 44–57.

Passolunghi, M. C., & Siegel, L. S. (2004). Working memory and access to numerical information in children with disability in mathematics. *Journal of Experimental Child Psychology, 88*, 348–367.

Piaget, J. (1980). *Adaptation and intelligence: Organic selection and phenocopy*. Chicago: University of Chicago Press.

Piaget, J. (1983). Piaget's theory. In P. H. Mussen (Series Ed.) & W. Kessen (Vol. Ed.), *Handbook of child psychology: Vol. 1. History, theory, and methods* (4th ed., pp. 103–128). New York: Wiley.

Piaget, J. (1985). *The equilibration of cognitive structures*. Chicago: University of Chicago Press. (Original work published 1975)

Piaget, J., & Inhelder, B. (1974). *The child's construction of quantities: Conservation and atomism*. London: Routledge & Kegan Paul.

Schwartz, J. (1988). Intensive quantity and referent transforming arithmetic operations. In J. Hiebert & M. Behr (Eds.), *Number concepts and operations in the middle grades* (pp. 41–53). Hillsdale, NJ: Erlbaum.

Seitz, K., & Schumann-Hengsteler, R. (2000). Mental multiplication and working memory. *European Journal of Cognitive Psychology, 12*, 552–570.

Severtson, E. (1993). *Development of multiplicative reasoning*. Unpublished masters thesis, York University, Toronto.

Siegler, R. S. (1996). *Emerging minds: The process of change in children's thinking*. Oxford: Oxford University Press.

Spearman, C. (1927). *The abilities of man*. London: McMillan.

Swanson, H. L., & Sachs-Lee, C. (2001). Mathematical problem solving and working memory in children with learning disabilities: Both executive and phonological processes are important. *Journal of Experimental Child Psychology, 79*, 294–321.

Thatcher, R. W. (1997). Human frontal lobe development: A theory of cyclical cortical reorganization. In N. A. Krasnegor, G. R. Lyon, & P. S. Goldman-Rakic (Eds.), *Development of prefrontal cortex* (pp. 85–113). Baltimore: Paul H. Brooks.

Tolman, E. C., & Brunswik, E. (1935). The organism and the causal texture of the environment. *Psychological Review, 42*, 43–77.

Vergnaud, G. (1983). Multiplicative structures. In R. Lesh & M. Landau (Eds.), *Acquisition of mathematics concepts and processes* (pp. 127–174). New York: Academic Press.

Vergnaud, G. (1988). Multiplicative structures. In J. Hiebert & M. Behr (Eds.), *Research agenda for mathematics education: Number concepts and operations in the middle grades* (pp. 141–161). Reston, VA: NCIM.

Vuyk, R. (1981). *Overview and critique of Piaget's genetic epistemology 1965–1980* (Vol. 1). New York: Academic Press.

Wilhelm, O., & Engle, R. (Eds.) (2005). *Handbook of understanding and measuring intelligence*. Thousand Oaks, CA: Sage.

Higher-Order Network Reworking – New Findings

Robert W. Thatcher

Introduction

I had the pleasure of knowing Robbie Case for several years as a colleague and friend. We first met in Toronto at a Child Development symposium in 1987 where I first became acquainted with Robbie's wit and charm and breadth of knowledge about child development. We spoke by telephone and corresponded for several years following this meeting. In 1992, Drs. Kurt Fischer, Paul van Geert, and I received a research fellowship to meet and study child development at the Center for Advanced Study at Stanford University. Robbie Case was a visiting faculty member at Stanford at the time and he would visit with Kurt, Paul, and I and join in our many discussions and analyses of various data and theories of child development. As always, I was impressed with Robbie's breadth of knowledge and his sharp mind, delightful smile, and humor. He had the rare talent of absorbing the essence of a discussion and then adding a light and humorous note as he contributed to the group's discussion with his perspective and facts. Robbie's unfinished chapter "Approaches to behavioral and neurological research on learning disabilities: in search of a deeper synthesis" (Case, 2007) is an excellent example of the freshness of his thoughts and the breadth of his knowledge of child development and the clinical underpinnings of childhood disorders. I personally miss Robbie and feel some solace in having known him and known the depth of his many contributions to the field of human development.

In the pages to follow, I present some recent studies that add to Robbie Case's perspectives and integration of our earlier work dealing with cyclic reorganization of the human brain (Thatcher, Walker, & Guidice, 1987; Thatcher, 1992, 1994, 1998).

R.W. Thatcher (✉)
NeuroImaging Laboratory, Applied Neuroscience Research Institute, St. Petersburg, FL, USA
e-mail: rwthatcher@yahoo.com

M. Ferrari, L. Vuletic (eds.), *The Developmental Relations among Mind, Brain and Education*, DOI 10.1007/978-90-481-3666-7_4, © Springer Science+Business Media B.V. 2010

Development of EEG Coherence and Phase Differences

Neural dynamics involves the generation of electrical currents by populations of synchronously active neurons within local regions of the brain that are coupled through axonal connections to other populations of neurons (Nunez, 1981, 1994; Braitenberg, 1978; Schuz & Braitenberg, 2002). Anatomical analyses of the cerebral white matter have shown that there are three general categories of cortico-cortical connections: (1) intra-cortical unmyelinated connections within the gray matter on the order of 1 mm to approximately 3 mm, (2) short-distance "U"-shaped fibers in the cerebral white matter located beneath the gray matter (10 mm to approximately 30 mm), and (3) long-distance fasciculi located in the deep white matter below the "U"-shaped fibers with distances from 30 mm to approximately 170 mm (Braitenberg, 1978; Schuz & Braitenberg, 2002). Measures of EEG coherence and phase delays from the scalp surface commonly detect the presence of two compartments with an approximate correspondence to the short-distance "U"-shaped and long-distance fiber systems (Nunez, 1981, 1994; Thatcher, Krause, & Hrybyk, 1986; Thatcher, Biver, McAlaster, & Salazar, 1998; Thatcher, Biver, & North, 2007; Pascual-Marqui, Valdea-Sosa, & Alvarez-Amador, 1988; Shen, Nadkarni, & Zappulla, 1999; Barry, Clarke, McCarthy, & Selikowitz, 2005; Hanlon, Thatcher, & Cline, 1999; McAlaster, 1992; Srinivasan, 1999; Van Beijsterveldt, Molenaar, de Geus, & Boomsma, 1998). These studies show that EEG coherence when measured by a single common reference decreases as a function of distance from any electrode site thus characterizing the "U"-shaped fiber compartment, and coherence increases as a function of distance beyond approximately 10–12 cm, which characterizes the long-distance fascicular compartment. Studies of changes of EEG coherence with distance are usually explained by a decrease in the number of connections as a function of distance from any given population of neurons while increased coherence with distance is explained by an increase of connections between two populations through axons and fasciculi of the deep cerebral white matter (Braitenberg, 1978; Schuz & Braitenberg, 2002, Nunez, 1981, 1994; Thatcher et al., 1986, 1998, 2007; Hanlon et al., 1999; McAlaster, 1992; Srinivasan, 1999). Understanding of the differential rates of development of the local vs. distant cortical connections has been advanced by genetic analyses of identical twins in which approximately 55% of short-distance coherence measures are determined by environmental factors and approximately 45% by genetics, whereas the greater than 75% of long-distance coherence measures are determined by genetic factors (Van Beijsterveldt et al., 1998; van Baal, Boomsma, & de Geus, 2001).

A deeper understanding of cortical coupling is possible by studying the maturation of EEG coherence and phase differences in the short- vs. the long-distance compartments. EEG phase difference is an analytical measure of the time difference between coupled oscillators (Bendat & Piersol, 1980). EEG coherence is a statistical measure of the consistency of phase differences over some sample space and is a measure of "phase synchrony" or "phase stability" between spatially distant generators (Otnes & Enochson, 1972; Bendat & Piersol, 1980; Nunez, 1981). EEG phase differences are often the opposite of coherence by systematically increasing while EEG coherence decreases as a function of inter-electrode distance (Thatcher et al., 1986, 1987). The increase in phase differences as a function of inter-electrode distance is due to many potential sources such as longer conduction delays as a function of distance or slower average synaptic rise times or longer average synaptic integration times. An important advantage of measures of spontaneous EEG phase difference is that phase delays can eliminate volume conduction because volume conduction, in the absence of a defined dipole source, is defined by phase difference = 0 everywhere in the volume while network properties are measured by large phase differences. Because myelination and synaptic growth occur during human development, a study of the maturation of both coherence and phase differences may help unravel the relative contributions of the various sources of phase differences.

In the Thatcher et al. (2007) study which is summarized in this chapter, EEG coherence and phase differences were analyzed using similar methods previously published in which the spatial heterogeneity of scalp-recorded EEG coherence and phase is measured along two parallel lines with scalp electrodes equally spaced in the anterior-to-posterior and posterior-to-anterior directions (Thatcher et al., 1986, 1998). This method of EEG coherence measurement is a normalization procedure in which all electrode reference and analysis procedures are experimentally analyzed as a function of inter-electrode direction, inter-electrode distance, hemispheric symmetry, and frequency. Inflation of EEG coherence by reference electrodes was controlled in the present study (Fein, Raz, Brown, & Merrin, 1998; Rappelsberger, 1989; Nunez et al., 1997), because a single common reference or a linked ear reference was held constant while only electrode direction, distance, hemisphere symmetry, and frequency were systematically compared. This method of EEG coherence measurement is also a direct test of a two-compartmental model of EEG coherence in which dynamic differences and interactions between short inter-electrode distances (e.g., 6 cm) vs. long inter-electrode distances (e.g., 18–24 cm) have been measured (Thatcher et al., 1986; 1987, 1998; Thatcher, 1992, 1994, 1998; Pascual-Marqui et al., 1988; Nunez, 1981, 1994; Hanlon et al., 1999; McAlaster, 1992; van Baal et al., 2001; Van Beijsterveldt et al., 1998; Srinivasan, 1999).

Finally, the studies by Thatcher et al. (1987) and Thatcher (1994, 1998) reported oscillations and cyclic reorganization in EEG coherence over the age range from birth to 16 years; however, there was no parallel study of EEG phase differences in this same population. Therefore, another purpose of the Thatcher et al. (2007) study was to explore oscillations in the maturation of both coherence and phase differences in order to further understand the development of human cortical connectivity.

Methods

A total of 458 subjects ranging in age from 2 months to 16.67 years (males = 257) were included in this study. The subjects in the study were recruited using newspaper advertisements in rural and urban Maryland (Thatcher et al., 1987, 2007;

Thatcher, Walker, Biver, North, & Curtin, 2003). The inclusion/exclusion criteria were no history of neurological disorders such as epilepsy, head injuries; reported normal development and successful school performance. None of the subjects had taken medication of any kind at least 24 hours before testing in this study. All of the school-age children were within the normal range of intelligence as measured by the WISC-R and were performing at grade level in reading, spelling, and arithmetic as measured by the WRAT and none were classified as learning disabled nor were any of the school-aged children in special education classes.

The details of the EEG recordings and the computation of coherence and phase are available in Thatcher et al. (2007).

Results

Development of EEG Coherence

Figure 1 shows the development of mean EEG coherence from 0.44 to 16.22 years of age. The top row shows the anterior-to-posterior electrode combinations and the bottom row shows the posterior-to-anterior combinations. The left column shows the left hemisphere mean EEG coherence values and the right column shows the right hemisphere values. In all instances there was higher coherence in short-distance inter-electrode combinations (6 cm) than in longer inter-electrode distances with intermediate mean coherence at intermediate inter-electrode distances. Also, all inter-electrode distances exhibit oscillations in mean EEG coherence over the age range. It can be seen that there is a large increase in coherence in all four

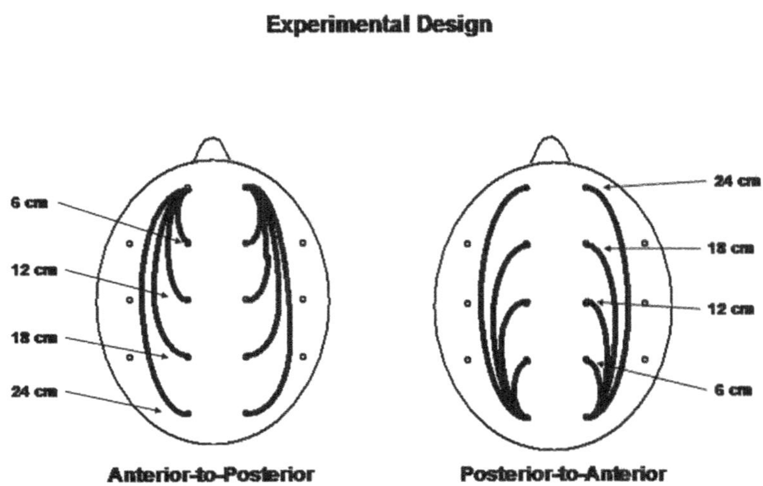

Fig. 1

inter-electrode distances from 0.44 to approximately 4 years of age. There are clear developmental trends toward higher coherence as a function of age, especially in the short inter-electrode distances and there are also differences in EEG coherence in the anterior-to-posterior vs. the posterior-to-anterior directions in both left and right hemispheres. For example, 12 cm inter-electrode distance (Fp1/2-C3/4) exhibits higher coherence in the anterior-to-posterior direction than in the posterior-to-anterior (O1/2-C3/4) direction. Mean coherence in the 24 cm long inter-electrode distance was nearly flat as a function of age and while exhibiting oscillations, nonetheless also exhibited the lowest coherence values.

Table 1 shows the results of a linear fit of the mean coherence as a function of age for all electrode pairings. It can be seen in Table 1 that 6 cm inter-electrode distances exhibited a positive slope of the linear fit to age while the 24 cm inter-electrode distances exhibited a negative slope. The only exception was in the posterior-to-anterior direction at 6 cm where the slope was essentially flat.

Table 1 Regression analyses of coherence development short-distance positive slopes and long-distance negative slopes

Left Anterior–Posterior				
	6 cm	12 cm	18 cm	24 cm
Slope	1.81	0.47	–0.34	–0.43
Intercept	22.56	13.15	9.28	6.07
Correlation	0.884	0.650	–0.617	–0.714
Significant	$P<0.0001$	$P<0.0001$	$P<0.0001$	$P<0.0001$
Left Posterior–Anterior				
	6 cm	12 cm	18 cm	24 cm
Slope	0.28	–0.71	–0.54	–0.43
Intercept	39.79	17.44	8.52	6.07
Correlation	0.343	–0.656	–0.758	–0.714
Significant	$P<0.01$	$P<0.0001$	$P<0.0001$	$P<0.0001$
Right Anterior–Posterior				
	6 cm	12 cm	18 cm	24 cm
Slope	1.75	0.44	–0.36	–0.34
Intercept	24.16	13.73	10.28	5.50
Correlation	0.908	0.604	–0.599	–0.695
Significant	$P<0.0001$	$P<0.0001$	$P<0.0001$	$P<0.0001$
Right Posterior–Anterior				
	6 cm	12 cm	18 cm	24 cm
Slope	0.08	–0.71	–0.56	–0.34
Intercept	41.50	18.01	9.12	5.50
Correlation	0.062	–0.601	–0.756	–0.695
Significant	No Sig.	$P<0.0001$	$P<0.0001$	$P<0.0001$

Note: No Sig. indicates No significance

Multivariate analyses of variance (MANOVA) were conducted with the factors being direction (anterior-to-posterior vs. posterior-to-anterior), left hemisphere vs. right hemisphere, and distance (6, 12, 18, and 24 cm). No significant left vs. right hemisphere effect was present ($F = 2.094$, $P < 0.1526$). However, there was a significant direction effect ($F = 11.598$, $P < 0.0001$) including a significant Bonferroni post hoc test ($P < 0.000686$) and a significant distance effect ($F = 2969.8$, $P < 0.0001$) including a significant Bonferroni post hoc test ($P < 0.000001$) for all pair-wise distance differences.

Development of EEG Phase Differences

Figure 2 shows the development of mean phase differences from age 0.44 to 16.22 years. The top row shows the anterior-to-posterior electrode combinations and the bottom row shows the posterior-to-anterior combinations. The left column shows the left hemisphere mean EEG phase difference values and the right column shows the right hemisphere values (see Fig. 1). In general there are higher phase differences in long-distance inter-electrode combinations (24 cm) than in short inter-electrode distances with intermediate mean phase differences at intermediate inter-electrode distances. Similar to coherence, all inter-electrode distances exhibited oscillations in mean phase differences over the age range. Unlike coherence, however, EEG

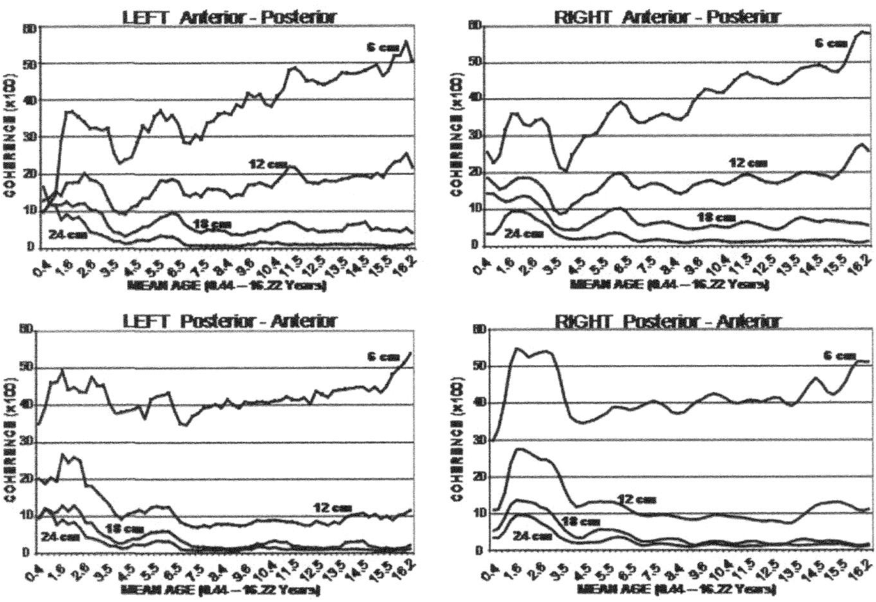

Fig. 2

phase differences in the short distance (6 cm) declined as a function of age and exhibited a negative slope, whereas the intermediate (18 cm) and long-distance (24 cm) inter-electrode combinations exhibited positive slopes and increasing phase differences as a function of age.

Table 2 shows the results of a linear fit of the mean phase differences as a function of age for all electrode pairings. It can be seen in Table 2 that 6 cm distances exhibited a negative slope of the linear fit to age while the 24 cm distances exhibited a positive slope.

There also were differences in EEG phase in the anterior-to-posterior vs. the posterior-to-anterior directions in both left and right hemispheres. For example, the 12 cm inter-electrode distance exhibited higher differences in the posterior-to-anterior direction (O1/2-C3/4) than in the anterior-to-posterior direction (Fp1/2-C3/4). The 24 cm long inter-electrode distance exhibited oscillations and a steady

Table 2 Regression analyses of phase difference development. Short-distance negative slopes and long-distance positive slopes

Left Anterior–Posterior				
	6 cm	12 cm	18 cm	24 cm
Slope	–0.98	–0.10	1.27	7.71
Intercept	18.78	6.88	3.96	3.15
Correlation	–0.613	–0.326	0.903	0.969
Significant	*P*<0.0001	*P*<0.01	*P*<0.0001	*P*<0.0001
Left Posterior–Anterior				
	6 cm	12 cm	18 cm	24 cm
Slope	0.06	0.73	3.82	7.71
Intercept	3.47	4.38	1.77	3.15
Correlation	0.309	0.905	0.933	0.969
Significant	*P*<0.05	*P*<0.0001	*P*<0.0001	*P*<0.0001
Right Anterior–Posterior				
	6 cm	12 cm	18 cm	24 cm
Slope	–1.29	–0.23	0.93	6.72
Intercept	21.45	8.15	6.24	7.30
Correlation	–0.552	–0.445	0.840	0.933
Significant	*P*<0.0001	*P*<.0001	*P*<0.0001	*P*<0.0001
Right Posterior–Anterior				
	6 cm	12 cm	18 cm	24 cm
Slope	–0.07	0.26	3.70	6.72
Intercept	5.22	8.58	5.28	7.30
Correlation	–0.168	0.239	0.918	0.933
Significant	No Sig.	No Sig.	*P*<0.0001	*P*<0.0001

Note: No Sig. indicates No significance

increase in phase difference as a function of age, especially at ages greater than approximately 4 years of age.

Multivariate analyses of variance (MANOVA) were also conducted for phase difference with the factors being direction (anterior-to-posterior vs. posterior-to-anterior), left hemisphere vs. right hemisphere, and distance (6, 12, 18, and 24 cm). No significant left vs. right hemisphere effect was present ($F = 0.2767$, $P < 0.0.599$). However, there was a significant overall direction effect ($F = 14.547$, $P < 0.0001$) including a significant Bonferroni post hoc test ($P < 0.000144$) and a significant overall distance effect ($F = 482.34$, $P < 0.0001$) including a significant Bonferroni post hoc test ($P < 0.000001$) for all pair-wise distance differences except between 6 and 12 cm.

Developmental Oscillations

Examination of Figs. 1 and 2 shows ultraslow oscillations with inter-peak intervals of approximately 2–3 years. Phase shifts between Fp1-F3 and Fp1-O1 and other pairing can be seen in Fig. 3 in which the short-distance phase differences peak at approximately 3.6 years of age while the long inter-electrode distance (24 cm) reaches a peak at approximately 4 years of age. After 4 years of age phase difference of the 6 cm inter-electrode distance declines from about 40° at age 3.6 years to

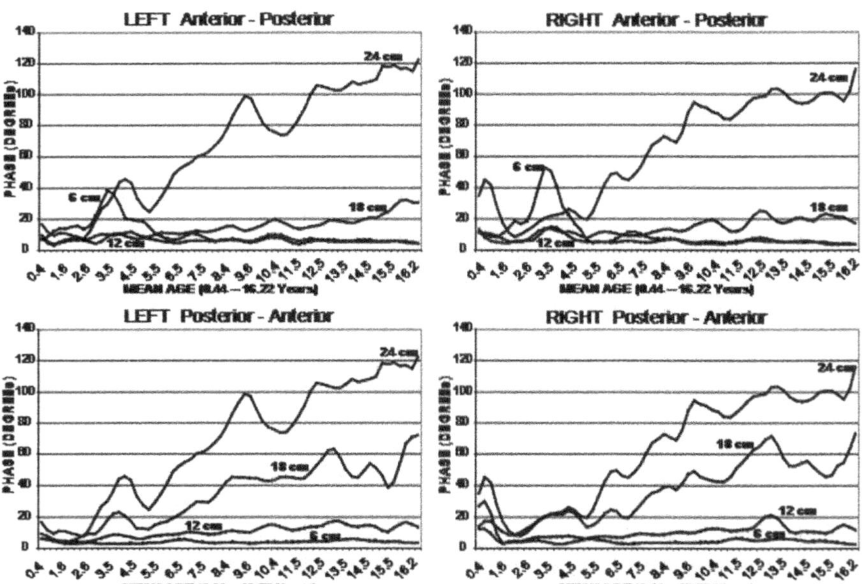

Fig. 3

about 5° at age 16.22 years, while the phase difference of the 24 cm inter-electrode distance steadily increases from about 20° at age 5 years to 120° at 16.22 years.

Figure 3 is the same as the top left chart in Fig. 3 and shows EEG phase delays in the Fp1-F3 (6 cm – dashed line) and Fp1-O1 (24 cm – solid line) from mean age of 0.44 years to the mean age of 7.04 years. It can be seen that the short- and long-distance compartments exhibit similar phase differences from 0.44 years to 3.2 years and then there is a phase shift between 3.2 and 5 years of age followed by steady divergence where phase differences increase as a function of age in the long inter-electrode distance and decrease in the short inter-electrode distances. There appears to be a competitive type of dynamic between the short and distant connections with an approximate 1 year shift between the short- and long-distance systems between approximately 3 and 4 years of age.

Oscillations in both the 6 and 24 cm inter-electrode distances were present; however, the magnitude of oscillations in phase differences was much larger in the 24 cm inter-electrode distances. A cross-correlation of the 6 vs. 24 cm time series of means showed a maximal time shift of 1.5 years with the 6 cm inter-electrode distance leading the 24 cm inter-electrode distance.

Spectral analyses of the developmental time series of coherence from 0.44 years to 16.22 years for the 6 and 24 cm inter-electrode distances are shown in Fig. 4. The top row shows the anterior-to-posterior electrode combinations and the bottom row shows the posterior-to-anterior combinations. The left column shows the left hemisphere mean FFT values and the right column shows the right hemisphere values. In

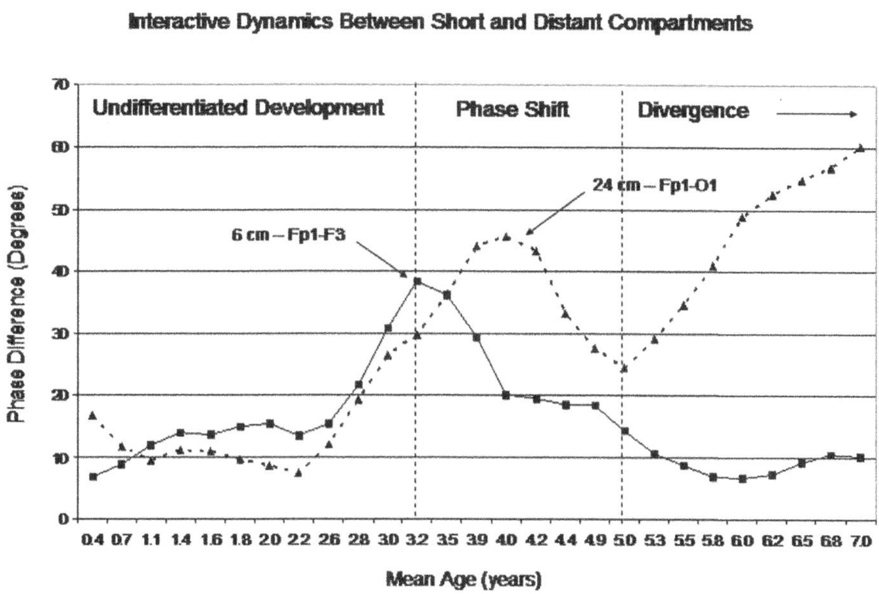

Fig. 4

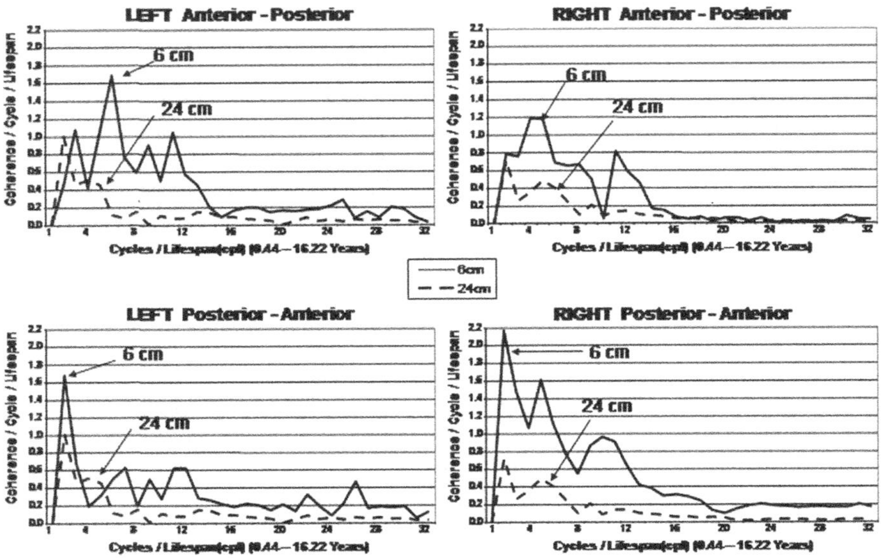
LEFT Anterior - Posterior
RIGHT Anterior - Posterior
LEFT Posterior - Anterior
RIGHT Posterior - Anterior
6 cm
24 cm
Coherence / Cycle / Lifespan
Cycles / Lifespan(cpl) (0.44—16.22 Years)
6cm
24cm

Fig. 5

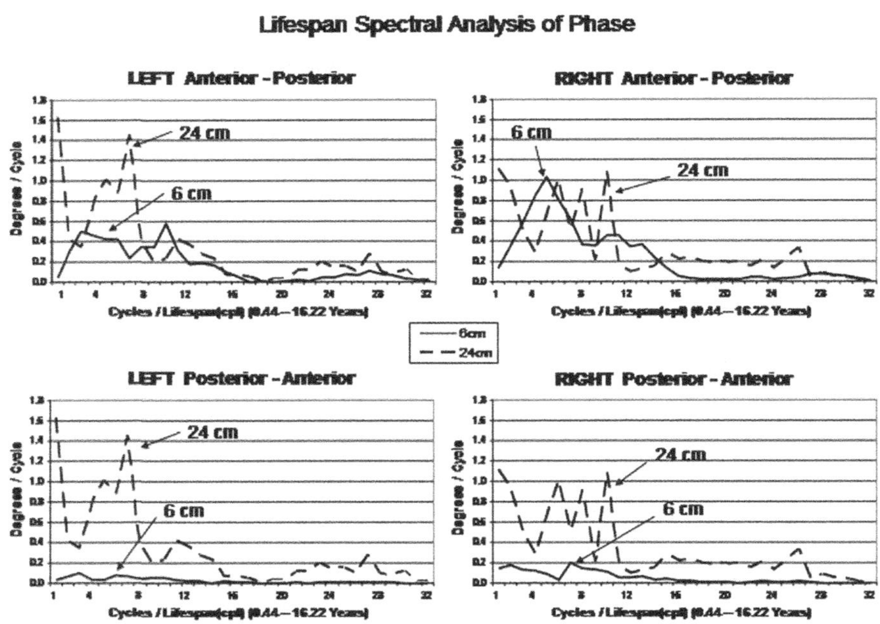
Lifespan Spectral Analysis of Phase
LEFT Anterior - Posterior
RIGHT Anterior - Posterior
LEFT Posterior - Anterior
RIGHT Posterior - Anterior
6 cm
24 cm
Degrees / Cycle
Cycles / Lifespan(cpl) (0.44—16.22 Years)
6cm
24cm

Fig. 6

general there was greater developmental spectral energy in the short inter-electrode distance (6 cm) in comparison to the long inter-electrode distance (24 cm). Most of the developmental spectral energy was in the ultraslow frequency range of 1 cycle per lifespan (i.e., a wavelength of 16 years) to approximately 12 cycles per lifespan (i.e., a wavelength of 1.33 years). The highest peak frequency was 31 cycles per lifespan (i.e., a wavelength of 0.51 years or 6.12 months).

Spectral analyses of the developmental time series of phase differences from 0.44 years to 16.22 years for the 6 and 24 cm inter-electrode distances are shown in Fig. 5. The top row of Fig. 6 shows the anterior-to-posterior electrode combinations and the bottom row shows the posterior-to-anterior combinations. The left column shows the left hemisphere FFT values and the right column shows the right hemisphere values. In comparison to coherence, a distinctly different pattern of oscillatory energies were present in phase. For example, in general there was greater spectral energy in the long inter-electrode distance (24 cm) in comparison to the short inter-electrode distance (6 cm) which is the opposite of coherence development (see Fig. 4). Similar to coherence, phase difference development exhibited most of the spectral energy in the ultraslow frequency range of 1 cycle per lifespan (i.e., a wavelength of 16

Table 3 Summary of developmental cycles and wavelengths anterior-to-posterior direction

Coherence							
Left				Right			
6 cm		24 cm		6 cm		24 cm	
CPL	λ (years)	CPL	λ (years)	CPL	λ (years)	CPL	λ (years)
2	8.00	4	4.00	2	8.00	2	8.00
3	5.33	8	2.00	4	4.00	5	3.20
5	3.20	13	1.23	8	2.00	9	1.78
8	2.00	22	0.73	11	1.45		
10	1.60			23	0.70		
25	0.64			30	0.53		
29	0.55						
Phase difference							
Left				Right			
6 cm		24 cm		6 cm		24 cm	
CPL	λ (years)	CPL	λ (years)	CPL	λ (years)	CPL	λ (years)
3	5.33	2	8.00	5	3.20	2	8.00
10	1.60	4	4.00	10	1.60	5	3.20
29	0.55	7	2.29	15	1.07	8	2.00
		11	1.45	29	0.55	10	1.60
		14	1.14			14	1.14
		16	1.00			18	0.89
		21	0.76				

years) to approximately 12 cycles per lifespan (i.e., a wavelength of 1.33 years). The highest peak frequency was 31 cycles per lifespan (i.e., a wavelength of 0.51 years or 6.12 months).

Tables 3 and 4 are summaries of the cycles per lifespan (cpl) and the wavelength (16 years/cpl) of the spectral peaks in the FFT analyses of the mean coherence and mean phase difference developmental trajectories from 0.44 to 16.22 years. Table 3 shows the FFT peak values in the anterior-to-posterior direction for both coherence (Top) and phase differences (Bottom) and Table 4 shows the values in the posterior-to-anterior direction. It can be seen that short (6 cm) and long (24 cm) are different for coherence vs. phase in both directions. In general there are more spectral peaks and greater power in the short-distance inter-electrode connections in coherence than there are in phase differences at 6 cm. The opposite is true for the development of phase differences which exhibited more spectral peaks and greater power in the long-distance inter-electrode connections than in coherence at 24 cm.

Table 4 Summary of developmental cycles and wavelengths posterior-to-anterior direction

Coherence Posterior–Anterior Left				Right			
6 cm		24 cm		6 cm		24 cm	
CPL	λ (years)	CPL	λ (years)	CPL	λ (years)	CPL	λ (years)
2	8.00	2	8.00	2	8.00	2	8.00
7	2.29	4	4.00	5	3.20	5	3.20
9	1.78	8	2.00	10	1.60	9	1.78
11	1.45	13	1.23	16	1.00	12	1.33
22	0.73			23	0.70		
26	0.62			31	0.52		
30	0.53						

Phase difference Posterior–anterior Left				Right			
6 cm		24 cm		6 cm		24 cm	
CPL	λ (years)	CPL	λ (years)	CPL	λ (years)	CPL	λ (years)
3	5.33	2	8.00	2	8.00	2	8.00
4	4.00	4	4.00	4	4.00	5	3.20
7	2.29	5	3.20	7	2.29	8	2.00
10	1.60	7	2.29	8	2.00	10	1.60
		11	1.45	13	1.23	14	1.14
		14	1.14			16	1.00
		21	0.76			18	0.89
		27	0.59				

Discussion

The results of this study are consistent with two-compartmental models of cerebral connectivity in which there is a local or short-distance compartment that is distinctly different than the long-distance compartment (Braitenberg, 1978; Schultz & Braitenberg, 2002; Nunez, 1981; Thatcher et al., 1986, 1987, 1998; Pascual-Marqui et al., 1988; Hanlon et al., 1999; McAlaster, 1992; Barry et al., 2005; Shen et al., 1999; Srinivasan, 1999; Van Beijsterveldt et al., 1998). The postnatal development of EEG coherence and EEG phase were different in both the short- and long-distance compartments. EEG coherence increased as a function of age in the short inter-electrode distance while EEG coherence in the long inter-electrode distances declined as a function of age. The opposite was observed for EEG phase differences which increased as a function of age in the long inter-electrode distances and declined in the short inter-electrode distances. Postnatal development of EEG coherence and EEG phase were also different in the anterior-to-posterior direction in comparison to the posterior-to-anterior direction even though the inter-electrode distances were the same. In addition, oscillations were prevalent in all electrode combinations in both EEG coherence and EEG phase maturation with growth spurts at specific postnatal ages. The latter finding is consistent with previous publications on the subject of cyclic reorganization using EEG coherence and phase measures (Thatcher et al. 1987; Thatcher, 1994; Hanlon et al., 1999; McAlaster, 1992; van Baal et al., 2001; Van Beijsterveldt et al., 1998; Isler, Garland, Start, & Grieve, 2005). Finally, only weak hemispheric differences in the maturation of EEG coherence and phase were found, although there were differences in the timing of growth spurts and oscillations between the two hemispheres.

Local vs. Distant Connections

An interesting finding in this study is that the development of EEG phase differences were the opposite of EEG coherence (see Figs. 2 and 3, Tables 1 and 2). Why would EEG phase differences in the long inter-electrode distances increase as a function of age? There are no published studies demonstrating delayed conduction such as reduced conduction velocities or reduced myelin concentration in cortico-cortical connections from birth to age 16. Thus, reduced conduction velocity is not a reasonable explanation of the finding of increased phase delays in long-distance connections. Increased variance of phase in distant connections also cannot explain a larger mean phase difference since the digital sample lengths used to compute the cross-spectrum were essentially the same and, in any case, random noise produces zero mean phase differences and certainly random noise cannot produce increased mean phase differences. In the absence of other explanations, the finding of phase shifts and competitive dynamics suggests an inverse relationship between the short and distant connection systems due to some type of competitive dynamic (see Fig. 3). If we assume that conduction velocity is not a critical factor to explain the findings in this study, then we can postulate a single unifying concept of an increase in the number of synaptic connections in the local systems and a reduction of synaptic connections in the distant systems as being primarily responsible for both the decrease in EEG coherence in distant connections and increased coherence in local connections. The unifying concept is that an increase in the number of connections in local domains results in an increased local processing/integration time and, therefore, longer phase delays between separated local domains. It is known that cortico-cortical connections arise primarily in layer III and terminate primarily on layers I–III and V–VI of cortical pyramidal cells and that short-distance connections primarily terminate closer to cell bodies in layer III (Jones, 1984; Barbie & Levitt, 1995; McConnel & Kaznowski, 1991; Schmahmann & Pandya, 2006). Competition for available dendritic space for synapse formation with the short distance connections "winning" the competition could reduce the number of distant connections and because the longer distant connections are located at greater distances from the cell body also result in increased local integration times and longer phase delays.

This conclusion is consistent with standard non-conduction volume models of EEG coherence (i.e., phase differences > 0) in which the magnitude of EEG coherence is mathematically modeled as equal to the average number of connections times the average strength of the connections:

$$C_{ij} = N_{ij} \times S_{ij} \tag{1}$$

where N_{ij} is a local connection matrix of the number or density of connections between neural systems i and j and S_{ij} is the synaptic strength of those connections. Phase delays can be modeled by the number of elements in a loop times the delay between elements, where delays are due to axonal conduction velocity, synaptic rise times, and dendritic integration times:

$$P_{ij} = K_{ij} \times D_{ij} \tag{2}$$

where K_{ij} is a distant connection matrix of the number or density of connections between neural systems i and j and D_{ij} is the delay between elements in a loop. A relationship between the local and distant connection systems could be combined to model competitive, cooperative, and predator/prey dynamics (Berryman, 1981; Thatcher, 1998) as

$$R_1 = N_{ij} - K_{ij}/N_{ij} \tag{3}$$

– Competition

$$R_2 = K_{ij} - N_{ij}/K_{ij} \tag{4}$$

$$R_1 = N_{ij} - K_{ij}/N_{ij} \tag{5}$$

– Predator/Prey

$$R_2 = K_{ij} + N_{ij}/K_{ij} \tag{6}$$

where R_1 is the rate of growth of connections in the local connection system and R_2 is the rate of growth of connections in the distant connection system. Further mathematical details of the effects of changing the sign and ratios of the two connection systems is described in Thatcher (1998). These generic equations are presented as models and further analyses are required to determine the best fit of the equations to the data in this study.

Due to the ultraslow frequencies and long time span from approximately 6 months of age to 16 years of age, a simple explanation of increased local coherence and increased distant phase differences is an increase in the number of local connections, which are at the expense of the number of distant connections located on the distal regions of the dendrites. That is, the average number of connections N in local domains increases in Equation (1) and K decreases in Equation (2). After the age of approximately 4 years there is a reduction in the average number of connections in the long-distance system while there is an increase in the number of connections in the short-distance compartments of the cerebral cortex. From infancy to about 3 years of age, there were relatively low levels of spatial differentiation and beyond approximately 4–5 years of age there was a steady increase in local coherence and distant phase differences (see Figs. 1, 2 and 3). The findings are generally consistent with models of coupled non-linear oscillators operating over long periods of time (Freeman, Burke, & Homes, 2003; Buzaski, 2006) as well as studies of the degree of local clustering vs. the degree of separation of clusters of connected neurons (Watts & Strogatz, 1998). According to this model, increased phase differences in long-distance connections is not due to conduction velocity changes but rather it is due to increased processing/integration time in local neural domains and/or increased dendritic distance of synaptic termination from the cell body. Similarly, the finding of reduced coherence in long inter-electrode distances is consistent with a periodic pruning in the number of connections.

Development of Complexity

The finding of an increase in short-distance coherence simultaneously with a decrease of coherence in the long-distance connections is also consistent with models of complexity in which there is a parallel increased integration in local domains and increased differentiation in long-distance connections as a function of age. Tononi, Sporns, and Edelman (1994) used quantitative models of information theory and stochastic processes to define complexity in connected neural networks. They showed that highly complex neural networks were characterized by neurons that were organized into densely linked groups, which were sparsely and reciprocally interconnected. The findings in this study are consistent with the Tononi et al. (1994) mathematical model of complexity where functional segregation and global integration are critical parameters. Specifically, increased integration due to increased number of connections within local domains of neurons is linked to increased differentiation and pruning of long-distance connections involving more precise reciprocal linkages between local and distant systems.

A neural network model is applied to the findings of this study in Fig. 7, top of which shows the standard two-compartmental model of EEG coherence for local and distant connections; the bottom of Fig. 7 is the application of the two-compartmental model to the Tononi et al. (1994) information theory of optimal neural network complexity. The distant connections are between local connection systems and are the differentiated long-association systems of the neocortex, e.g., the frontal-occipital fasciculus, uncinate fasciculus, the arcuate fasciculus, and the cingulum, which are the major long-association fibers of the human brain that terminate primarily on layers I–III and V and VI of the neocortex (Jones, 1984; Barbie & Levitt, 1995; McConnel & Kaznowski, 1991; Schmahmann & Pandya, 2006). Local synaptic connections tend to terminate closer to the cell body in layer III and are likely to be competing for dendrite membrane space for synaptogenesis (Jones, 1984). The brain development complexity curve at the bottom of Fig. 8 represents the dynamics of development that were observed in this study (see Figs. 1and 2 and Tables 1 and 2), in which there was increasing coherence in local connection

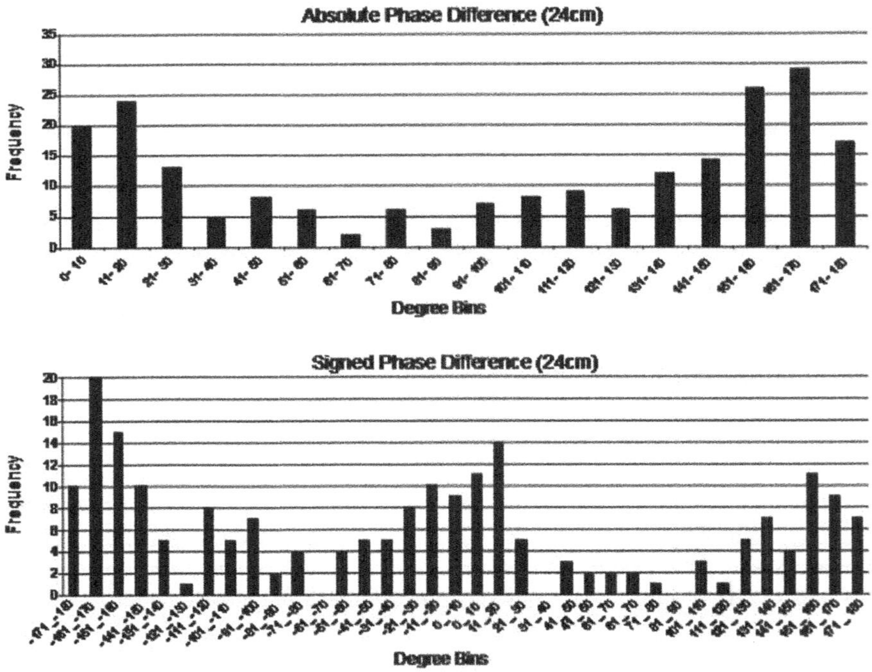

Fig. 7

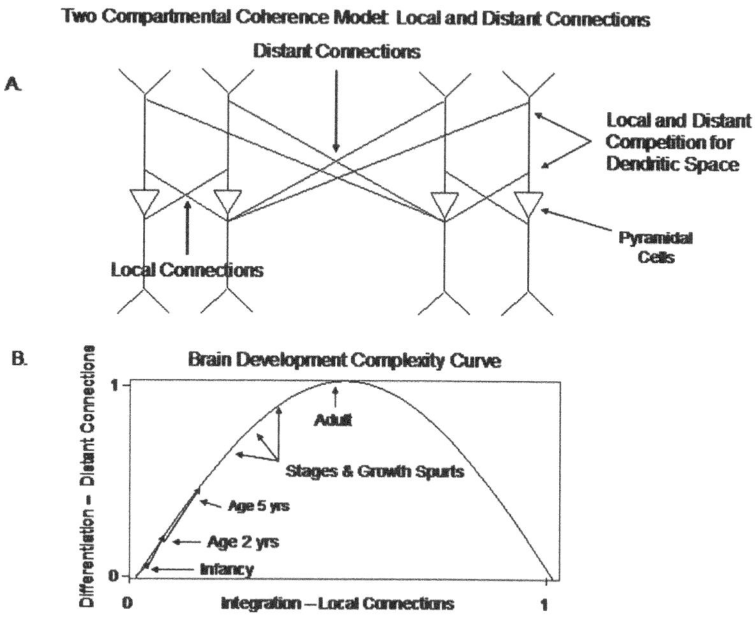

Fig. 8

systems (e.g., 6 cm) that represent increased local integration. In contrast, the distant connections (24 cm) spatially differentiate, which is consistent with selective pruning and refined connectivity during maturation. The combination of increased local integration and increased distant differentiation gives rise to increased brain complexity and increased efficiency. The arrows pointing to different ages are illustrative only and designed to indicate non-linear rates of growth at different ages which fall on the continuum of complexity as measured by Tononi et al. (1994). The right half of the brain complexity curve indicates states of declining complexity, which may occur with pathology, aging, and states of non-optimal organization.

Differences in the Anterior-to-Posterior vs. the Posterior-to-Anterior Direction

The strongest difference between the anterior-to-posterior vs. the posterior-to-anterior direction of electrode placement is the coherence and phase values of the intermediate inter-electrode distances. The development of EEG coherence in the anterior-to-posterior direction exhibits higher coherence values in intermediate inter-electrode distances (e.g., 18 cm), whereas there is little difference between the intermediate and long inter-electrode distance in the posterior-to-anterior direction. If we consider the coherence connectivity model in Equation (1), where coherence =

number of connections times the strength of connections, then the direction factor can be explained by assuming an increase in the number of connections between the frontal pole and the sensory motor cortex or between Fp1/2 and C3/4. For example, intermediate inter-electrode distances exhibited higher coherence in the anterior-to-posterior direction (i.e., Fp1/2-C3/4), because there are more connections between the frontal lobes (Fp1/2) and the sensory motor strip (C3/4) than between the occipital lobes and the sensory motor strip (i.e., the posterior-to-anterior direction). Similarly, the lower coherence in O1/2-C3/4 in contrast to Fp1/2-C3/4 is due to fewer connections between the occipital lobes and the sensory motor strip than between the frontal lobes and the sensory motor strip.

EEG phase developmental trajectories are the opposite of EEG coherence developmental trajectories in the intermediate inter-electrode distances (see Fig. 2). For example, intermediate inter-electrodes exhibited larger EEG phase differences in the posterior-to-anterior direction than in the anterior-to-posterior direction. If we assume again that increased phase delay is proportional to an increased number of connections, then the difference in direction can be explained by assuming that there are a larger number of local connections in the occipital lobes than in the frontal lobes. That is, the frontal-parietal relationship (Fp1/2- P3/4) has shorter phase delays in comparison to the occipital-frontal relationship (O1/2-F3/4) because of a larger number of connections in the local occipital cortex in comparison to the local frontal cortex. This explanation is consistent with the higher packing density in the occipital lobes compared to the frontal lobes (Carpenter & Sutin, 1983) and it is consistent with the coherence model in Equation (1) used to explain the difference in the maturational trajectories of EEG coherence and phase.

Ultraslow Oscillations and Competitive Dynamics

The Fourier transform of the EEG coherence and EEG phase developmental trajectories demonstrated significant ultraslow oscillations over the lifespan of 16 years. The mean frequency of oscillation was different in the anterior-to-posterior and posterior-to-anterior directions and for left and right hemispheres. However, common frequencies of oscillation were observed in all electrode combinations. The strongest spectral magnitudes for EEG coherence and phase development were repetitive cycles at wavelengths between 5 and 2 years using detrending in the FFT analysis. The highest frequency of oscillations was 6-month wavelengths and the higher frequency oscillations exhibited the lowest power. Cross-correlation analyses indicated a competitive relationship between short- and long-distance connections (see Fig. 3). An important fact is that there was a diversity of different environments and experiences in the lives of all of the 458 subjects in this study. In other words, the regularity of growth spurts and the strength of the repetitive cycles of coherence and phase differences cannot be explained by a common environmental factor. The most likely explanation is that a common genetic factor is responsible for the regular rhythms and slopes of change in mean coherence and mean phase over a

16-year period. The findings in this study are consistent with earlier studies demonstrating ultraslow oscillations and growth spurts in EEG coherence (Thatcher et al., 1987; Thatcher, 1992, 1994, 1998; Hanlon et al., 1999; McAlaster, 1992) as well as genetic studies of the ultraslow rates of development of local vs. distant coherence measures (Van Beijsterveldt et al., 1998; van Baal et al., 2001). The studies by Van Beijsterveldt et al. (1998) and van Baal et al. (2001) demonstrated different genetic contributions to local vs. distant connections in which there is more genetic influence on distant connections than on local connections but both compartments dynamically evolve with growth spurts at specific ages. Reduced long-distance connections in expanding neural networks often leads to increased complexity and efficiency (Buzaski, 2006). When considering efficiency and complexity models, the present findings support the view that genetics cyclically produces an excess of synaptic connections followed by pruning of the excess connections based on experience. This process is relatively slow and occurs over decades of the human lifespan.

In summary, the results are consistent with a genetic model of rhythmic long-term connection formation that occurs in cycles along a curvilinear trajectory toward adulthood. Studies of the prenatal and postnatal development of cortical synapses have shown competitive and predator-/prey-type dynamics (Edelman, 1987; Finkel & Edelman, 1989; Sporns, Tononi, & Edelman, 1991, 1994; Levay, Stryker, Shatz, 1978; Thatcher, 1996, 1998). It would be consistent with these studies to conclude that periodic increased connections and reduction of connections is linked to the cyclic genetic reshaping of cortical connectivity during postnatal development.

Educational Implications

The findings of cyclic reorganization and growth spurts in particular regions of the brain at specific ages carry several educational implications. One implication is that there may be "critical periods" associated with the rising or falling phase of the growth spurts in which educational intervention will have a greater impact than at other times during development. For example, right local frontal developmental growth spurts coincide with the development of social skills and the awareness of self and the awareness of others called the "Theory of Mind". The phase of the growth spurt (i.e., rising vs. falling phases) during which an educational intervention is applied toward better socialization may have greater benefit than at other ages or developmental periods. Similarly, the rising vs. falling phase of growth spurts in the left temporal lobes during the ages of 5–7 years may represent optimal windows of time when educational programs will have a maximal impact on language and reading development, etc.

Another educational implication is the measure of complexity that was shown in Fig. 8 in which the level of sophistication and the capacity to absorb and deal with complex information is different at different ages. A child that is behind in complexity development, as measured by EEG coherence and phase, may respond to specific educational interventions at a particular age. Also, repeated measures of the development of coherence and phase in short- and long-distance connection systems may aid in the evaluation of the efficacy of a given educational intervention.

The linkage of brain development with curriculum development is another educational implication of these studies. There are specific ages when the development of connections and synaptic efficacy are at a peak which are periods when particular educational content may have its greatest impact. For example, foreign language education during early periods of frontal and temporal lobe development may be more propitious than at other ages. Similarly, mathematical education may be accelerated for individuals with earlier or more pronounced formal operational development, e.g., right hemisphere frontal-parietal development and local bilateral frontal lobe development at ages 11–13.

References

Barbie, M. F., & Levitt, P. (1995). Age-dependent specification of the corticocortical connections of cerebral grafts. *Journal of Neuroscience*, *15*(3), 1819–1834.

Barry, R. J., Clarke, A. R., McCarthy, R., & Selikowitz, M. (2005). Adjusting EEG coherence for inter-electrode distance effects: an exploration in normal children. *International Journal of Psychophysiology*, *55*(3), 313–321.

Berryman, A. A. (1981). *Population systems: A general introduction*. New York: Plenum Press.

Bendat, J. S., & Piersol, A. G. (1980). *Engineering applications of correlation and spectral analysis*. New York: John Wiley & Sons.

Braitenberg, V. (1978). Cortical architectonics: General and areal. In M. A. B. Brazier & H. Petsche (Eds.), *Architectonics of the cerebral cortex* (pp. 443–465). New York: Raven Press.

Buzaski, G. B. (2006). *Rhythms of the Brain*. New York: Oxford University Press.

Case, R. (2007), Approaches to behavioral and neurological research on learning disabilities: in search of a deeper synthesis. In K. W. Fischer, J. H. Bernstein, & M. H. Immordino-Yang (Eds.), *Mind, brain and education in reading disorders*. Boston, MA: Cambridge University Press.

Carpenter, M. B., & Sutin, J. (1983). *Human neuroanatomy* (8th ed.). Baltimore, MD: Williams and Wilkins.

Edelman, G. M. (1987). *Neural Darwinism: The theory of neuronal group selection*. New York: Basic.

Fein, G., Raz, J., Brown, F. F., & Merrin, E. L. (1998). Common reference coherence data are confounded by power and phase effects. *Electroencephalography and Clinical Neurophysiology*, *69*, 581–584.

Finkel, L. H., & Edelman, G. M. (1989). The integration of distributed cortical systems by reentry: A computer simulation of interactive functionally segregated visual areas. *Journal of Neuroscience*, *9*, 3188–3208.

Freeman, W. J., Burke, B. C.,& Homes, M. D. (2003). Aperiodic phase-resetting in scalp EEG of beta-gamma-oscillations by state transitions at alpha-theta-rates. *Human Brain Mapping*, *19*, 248–272.

Hanlon, H. W., Thatcher, R. W., & Cline, M. J. (1999). Gender differences in the development of EEG coherence in normal children. *Developmental Neuropsychology*, *16* (3), 479–506.

Isler, J. R., Garland, M., Start, R. I., & Grieve, P. G. (2005). Local coherence oscillations in the EEG during development in the fetal baboon. *Clinical Neurophysiology*, *116*(9), 2121–2128.

Jones, E. G. (1984). History of cortical cytology. In A. Peters & E. G. Jones (Eds.), *Cerebral cortex vol 1: Cellular components of the cerebral cortex*. New York: Plenum Press.

Levay, S., Stryker, M. P., & Shatz, C. J. (1978). Ocular dominance columns and their development in layer IV of the cat's visual cortex. A quantitative study. *Journal of Comparative Neurology, 191*, 1–51.

McAlaster, R. (1992). Postnatal cerebral maturation in Down's syndrome children: a developmental EEG coherence study. *The International Journal of Neuroscience, 65*(1–4), 221–2237.

McConnel, S. K., & Kaznowski, C. E. (1991). Cell cycle dependence of laminar determination in developing cerebral cortex. *Science, 254*, 893–978.

Nunez, P. (1981). *Electrical fields of the brain*. New York: Oxford University Press.

Nunez, P. (1994). *Neocortical dynamics and human EEG rhythms*. New York: Oxford University Press.

Nunez, P. L., Srinivasan, R., Westdorp, A. F., Wijesinghe, R. S., Tucker, D. M., Silberstein, R. B., et al. (1997, November). EEG coherency. I: Statistics, reference electrode, volume conduction, Laplacians, cortical imaging, and interpretation at multiple scales. *Electroencephalography and Clinical Neurophysiology, 103*(5), 499–515.

Otnes, R. K., & Enochson, L. (1972). *Digital time series analysis*. New York: John Wiley and Sons.

Pascual-Marqui, R. D., Valdea-Sosa, S. L, & Alvarez-Amador, A. (1988). A parametric model for multichannel EEG spectra. *The International Journal of Neuroscience, 40*, 89–99.

Pascual-Marqui, R. D. (2007) Coherence and phase synchronization: generalization to pairs of multivariate time series, and removal of zero-lag contributions. arXiv:0706.1776v3 [stat.ME] 12 July 2007. (http://arxiv.org/pdf/0706.1776).

Rappelsberger, P. (1989). The reference problem and mapping of coherence: A simulation study. *Brain Topography, 2*(1/2), 63–72.

Schmahmann, J., & Pandya, D. N. (2006). *Fiber pathways of the brain*. New York: Oxford University Press

Schuz, A., & Braitenberg, V. (2002). The human cortical white matter: Quantitative aspects of cortico-cortical long-range connectivity. In A. Schultz & R. Miller (Eds.), *Cortical areas: Unity and diversity: Conceptual advances in brain research* (pp. 377–386). London: Taylor & Francis.

Shen, B., Nadkarni, M., & Zappulla, R. A. (1999). Spatial-spectral signature of human cortical synchrony, *Electroencephalography and Clinical Neurophysiology, 110*(1), 115–125.

Sporns, O., Tononi, G., & Edelman, G. M. (1991). Modeling perceptual grouping and figure-ground segregation by means of active reentrant connections. *Proceedings of the National Academy of Sciences (USA), 88*, 129–133.

Sporns, O., Tononi, G., & Edelman, G. M. (1994). Neural models of cortical integration. In R. Thatcher, M. Hallett, T. Zeffiro, E. John, & M. Huerta (Eds.), *Functional neuroimaging: Technical foundations*. New York: Academic Press.

Srinivasan, R. (1999). Spatial structure of the human alpha rhythm: Global correlation in adults and local correlation in children. *Clinical Neurophysiology, 110*, 1351–1362.

Thatcher, R. W., Krause, P, & Hrybyk, M. (1986). Corticocortical association fibers and EEG coherence: A two compartmental model. *Electroencephalography and Clinical Neurophysiology, 64*, 123–143.

Thatcher, R. W., Walker, R. A., & Guidice, S. (1987). Human cerebral hemispheres develop at different rates and ages. *Science, 236*, 1110–1113.

Thatcher, R. W. (1992). Cyclic cortical reorganization during early childhood. *Brain and Cognition, 20*, 24–50.

Thatcher, R. W. (1994). Psychopathology of early frontal lobe damage: Dependence on cycles of postnatal development. *Developmental Pathology, 6*, 565–596.

Thatcher, R. W. (1996). Neuroimaging of cyclic cortical reorganization during human development, In: R. W. Thatcher, G. R. Lyon, J. Rumsey, & N. Krasnegor (Eds.), Developmental neuroimaging: Mapping the development of brain and behavior. Florida: Academic Press.

Thatcher, R. W., Biver, C., McAlaster, R, & Salazar, A. M. (1998). Biophysical linkage between MRI and EEG coherence in traumatic brain injury. *NeuroImage*, *8*(4), 307–326.
Thatcher, R. W. (1998). A predator-prey model of human cerebral development. In K. Newell & P. Molenaar (Eds.), *Dynamical systems in development*. New Jersey: L. Erlbaum Assoc.
Thatcher, R. W., Walker, R. A., Biver, C., North, D., & Curtin, R. (2003). Quantitative EEG Normative databases: Validation and clinical correlation. *Journal of Neurotherapy, 7*(3 and 4), 87–122.
Thatcher, R. W., North, D., & Biver, C. (2007). Development of cortical connectivity as measured by EEG coherence and phase. *Human Brain Mapping, October 23*.
Thatcher, R. W., Biver, C. J., & North, D. (2007). Spatial-temporal current source correlations and cortical connectivity. *Clinical EEG and Neuroscience*, *38*(1), 35–48.
Tononi, G., Sporns, O., & Edelman, G. M. (1994). A complexity measure for selective matching of signals by the brain. *Proceedings of the National Academy of Sciences (USA)*, *93*, 3422–3427.
van Baal, G. C., Boomsma, D. I., & de Geus, E. J. (2001). Longitudinal genetic analysis of EEG coherence in young twins. *Behavior Genetics*, *31*(6), 637–651.
Van Beijsterveldt, C. E., Molenaar, P. C., de Geus, E. J., & Boomsma, D. I. (1998). Genetic and environmental influences on EEG coherence. *Behavior Genetics*, *28*(6), 443–453.
Watts, D. J., & Strogatz, S. H. (1998). Collective dynamics of "small-world" networks. *Nature*, *393*, 440–442.

Typical and Atypical Development of Basic Numerical Magnitude Representations: A Review of Behavioral and Neuroimaging Studies

Daniel Ansari, Gavin Price, and Ian Holloway

Introduction

The development of mathematical competence is a complex process, which interacts with the development of many other cognitive systems (Butterworth, 2005). International comparisons of mathematical achievement have repeatedly revealed that children in many countries lag behind their peers in countries with comparable economic success (OECD, 2004; Stevenson, Lee, & Stigler, 1986). At the same time the increasing reliance on computational devices in modern societies and the labor market put an increasing pressure on educational systems to provide children with numerical and mathematical skills that will adequately prepare them for the social and economical challenges of adult life. Against this background it is important for researchers of mathematical development to conceptualize ways in which results from their research might impact mathematics education and remediation of mathematical difficulties.

As Robbie Case's research demonstrated (for a review of this see "Children's Developing Understanding of Number: Mind, Brain and Culture"), by the time children enter the formal mathematics classroom they already have had many varied experiences with numbers and possess a set of foundational competencies that will scaffold their understanding of the material taught in primary school mathematics. In this way, much like the development of reading skills, the acquisition of numerical and mathematical skills is a highly cumulative process, in which understanding of a given concept is dependent on earlier acquired knowledge and skills. This dependence has also been referred to as the "Matthew Effect" in the reading literature (Cunningham & Stanovich, 1997). The Matthew Effect suggests that long-term difficulties may arise if foundational competencies are lacking or have not been solidified in the process of building ever more complex structures. Accordingly, there is a growing consensus that the typical and atypical developmental trajectories

D. Ansari (✉)
Numerical Cognition Laboratory, Department of Psychology and Graduate Program in Neuroscience, University of Western Ontario, London, ON, Canada N6A 5C2
e-mail: daniel.ansari@uwo.ca

M. Ferrari, L. Vuletic (eds.), *The Developmental Relations among Mind, Brain and Education*, DOI 10.1007/978-90-481-3666-7_5, © Springer Science+Business Media B.V. 2010

of reading development can be best understood by delineating those foundational competencies and how they constrain the development of higher-level reading skills (Goswami, 2003).

Against this background, some have contended that, analogous to research on typical and atypical reading development, research on the origins and development of both typical and atypical numerical and mathematical skills should adopt a focus on the most fundamental aspect of number processing, the understanding of numerical quantity or "number sense" (Gersten & Chard, 1999). A better understanding of the foundational competencies that subserve the acquisition of mathematical skills will help to design better math education programs for young children as well as intervention programs that are based on scientific results.

In this context, it is important to note that the idea that number sense is critical to the successful development of mathematical competence is not a new one. In fact the notion that an understanding of quantity lies at the core of the development of mathematical skills was central to the work of Case and his collaborators. As the Chapter "Children's Developing Understanding of Number: Mind, Brain and Culture" illustrates, much of recent research on numerical magnitude processing is consistent with many of the predictions of the models put forward by Robbie Case and his collaborators as well as more recent revisions of these. While Okamoto's chapter provides a detailed review of Case's contribution to our understanding of children's mathematical development as well as a comprehensive, modern perspective on Case's thinking and theory, the present chapter provides an in-depth review of the research on the development of numerical quantity since Robbie Case's seminal work. It is our hope that this chapter, in combination with the chapter "Children's Developing Understanding of Number: Mind, Brain and Culture" will provide an impetus for neo-Piagetian researchers and Developmental Cognitive Neuroscientists to interact with one another to advance our understanding of children's number development and develop means by which to remediate mathematical difficulties.

The last 15 years have seen substantial advances in the understanding of the evolutionary origins and brain representation of numerical magnitude (S. Dehaene, 1997). The availability of sophisticated research methodology has enabled researchers to gain insights into infants' representation of number as well as the spatial and temporal neural correlates of basic magnitude processing and their developmental trajectory.

There currently exists a gulf between the literature on the educational relevance of studying basic number processing and the empirical study of the mechanisms underlying basic numerical magnitude processing from cognitive psychology and cognitive neuroscience. The aim of this chapter is to provide a critical review of relatively recent empirical evidence on the origins, development, and brain representation of numerical magnitude in both typical and atypical populations and to critically evaluate the potential educational relevance of a cognitive neuroscience framework for the study of basic number processing. We hope that this review can provide a forum for discussion between researchers interested in the foundation of numerical cognition and mathematics educators. In a similar vein, we also hope that it will provide a basis for discussions between neo-Piagetian theorists and Developmental Cognitive Neuroscientists. The chapter closes with an outlook toward the promises and challenges that lie ahead for ongoing efforts to connect the cognitive neuroscience of numerical magnitude processing with educational practice and theory.

Typical Trajectories of Numerical Magnitude Processing

Explorations of children's numerical competency have resulted in a rich, diverse, and growing literature of research studies. In order to explore the linkages between scientific research and education, it is necessary to first characterize what children know about basic numerical magnitude and how that knowledge changes as children mature.

Basic Magnitude Understanding in Early Childhood

Developmental Changes in Numerical Quantity Comparison: Behavioral Findings

Magnitude comparison is a common method with which researchers have attempted to explore the psychophysical characteristics of representations of numerical quantity and their developmental trajectory. In studies with adults and children, individuals are asked to compare which of two numerical quantities is numerically larger or to compare the relative magnitude of a number to a target number (e.g., Is the number you see smaller or larger than 5?). The reaction time and accuracy profiles have revealed several interesting effects, which are thought to reflect the nature of numerical representation (Dehaene, Dehaene-Lambertz, & Cohen, 1998). By far, the most widely studied of these effects is the "numerical distance effect." This effect is characterized by faster reaction times and higher accuracy associated with larger numerical distance separating the numbers being compared (Banks, Fujii, & Kayra-Stuart, 1976; Buckley & Gillman, 1974; Moyer & Landauer, 1967). In other words, individuals are faster at discriminating between number pairs with large distance such as 7 (e.g., 2 vs. 9) than pairs with small distance such as 2 (e.g., 3 vs. 5).

Crucial to the context of the present discussion, the effect of numerical distance on reaction time has been shown to undergo an ontogenetic decrease (Duncan & McFarland, 1980; Sekuler & Mierkiewicz, 1977), whereby the effect of numerical distance lessens over developmental time. This developmental shift has been interpreted as reflecting changes in the underlying representations of numerical magnitudes. However, new evidence (Holloway & Ansari, 2008) suggests that the decrease may not be specific to changes in the discriminability of numerical representation, but may also reflect a change in a comparison process common to both numerical and non-numerical magnitudes (e.g., length, brightness, extent). This could either mean that the numerical distance effect reflects a common underlying representation of both numerical and non-numerical magnitude (Walsh, 2003) or that the distance effect is related to response-related components of the comparison task, rather than being an index of underlying representations. In other words, it is possible that the distance effect reflects response competition (choose left vs. right side for "larger" in a numerical comparison task), which increases with increasing distance and is common to numerical and non-numerical comparison tasks (Van Opstal, Gevers, De Moor, & Verguts, 2008; Verguts, Fias, & Stevens, 2005).

A new finding, however, relates the distance effect to higher-level mathematical performance. In a recent study, it was found that the size of the symbolic distance effect was negatively correlated with mathematics, but not reading scores, as measured by the Mathematics Fluency and Calculation subtests of Woodcock Johnson III Tests of Achievement (Holloway & Ansari, 2009).

These data suggest that higher mathematics achievement scores are related to a smaller distance effect. In essence, these data reveal an important link between reaction times associated with very low-level basic magnitude processing and educationally relevant mathematical performance. Although these data are correlational, they provide empirical support for the notion that the processing and representation of numerical magnitude is associated with the development of higher-level skills, such as mental arithmetic, which are the subject of standardized tests of children's mathematical achievement.

The mechanisms that associate the symbolic distance effect and individual differences in children's mathematical competence are currently unknown and clarifying them depends greatly on better understanding the nature of the distance effect itself. However, at the very least, this type of finding underscores the importance of understanding basic number processing for understanding mathematical development. The relationship between basic number processing and math is analogous, though not equivalent, to the relatively well-defined relationship between phonological awareness and reading skills.

Another effect that could be very relevant in linking developmental changes in numerical and mathematical processing to the domain of education is the "number-size interference effect," which, because of its similarity to the well-known Stroop effect (Stroop, 1935) is often called the "numerical Stroop effect." This effect refers to the interactive influence of font size and numerical magnitude on the ability to make relative magnitude comparisons (Duncan & McFarland, 1980; Girelli, Lucangeli, & Butterworth, 2000; Rubinsten, Henik, Berger, & Shahar-Shalev, 2002) For example, when asked to choose which of two numbers is physically larger, if the larger numerosity is presented in larger font (e.g., **3** vs. **4**), individuals are faster at choosing the physically larger number (facilitation) than when the smaller numerosity is presented in larger font (e.g., **3** vs. **4;** interference). It has been contended that this paradigm is suited to investigating the automatic activation of numerical magnitude. This is because when adults are asked to compare which of two numbers is physically, rather than numerically, larger, the irrelevant numerical magnitude both interferes and facilitates the response, suggesting the automatic activation of numerical magnitude whenever a numerical symbol is presented. In addition, these findings make it unlikely that the distance effect merely reflects response-related processing, since individual differences in the distance effect were specifically correlated with variability in children's mathematical competence and not their reading abilities.

Interestingly, developmental studies of the number-size interference or size congruity effect have revealed that automatic access to numerosity information associated with a numerical symbol does not occur until some point after the beginning of first grade (Girelli et al., 2000; Rubinsten et al., 2002). In other words, while physical size interferes with numerical size judgments when children compare relative numerical magnitude, the numerical information only starts to interfere with physical size judgments after first grade. This developmental shift is thought to reflect an increase in the fluency with which children process the numerical magnitudes associated with numerical symbols. The differential contributions of the child's age and the amount of time spent using numerical symbols to this increase in fluency have yet to be systematically examined. This issue of the development of this automatic access to numerical magnitudes upon the presentation of numerical symbols could have important implications for the understanding of children with mathematical difficulties and the use of this paradigm in the context of the study of atypical number development is discussed below.

In addition to the numerical distance and "number Stroop" (or "size congruity effect") there has been a lot of work on the development of numerical estimation abilities (see Siegler & Booth, 2005 for an in-depth review of this work). Numerical estimation is another competence that is thought to be a key index of children's understanding of numerical quantity. Below we review some of these studies.

Developmental Changes in Numerical Estimation

The ability to make estimations is another basic quantitative skill whose ontogeny yields important clues about children's developing numerical understanding. Estimation is important not only because of its potential relevance for mathematical achievement (Dowker, 2003), but also because it is an ability that requires the flexible use of quantitative knowledge. Furthermore, unlike numerical comparison tasks, which infer variability in representation from the relationship of reaction time and numerical distance, estimation provides a trial-by-trial direct measurement of response variability, which is thought to be directly reflective of variability in numerical representation.

Perhaps the most relevant type of numerical estimation to a discussion of numerical magnitude representation involves translating a number into its correct spatial position on a number line. Number lines are commonplace in elementary school classrooms and Robbie Case and his colleagues also included number lines in their study of children's number development (see "Children's Developing Understanding of Number: Mind, Brain and Culture"). The so-called number line estimation paradigm may be particularly well-suited to exploring the nature in which numerosities are internally represented. Typically, experiments exploring number line estimation will give individuals a line with zero at one end and an upper limit number, often 10, 100, or 1000, at the other end. Individuals are asked to estimate where on the line a certain number falls or estimate what number is represented by a mark on the line. If an individual's representation of number is linear, one would expect his/her estimations to be appropriately spaced. However, if his/her representation of number is logarithmic, one would expect his/her estimations to be more compressed on one side of the line. For instance, estimates of smaller number could be spaced further apart and larger numbers spaced closer together. One can then use number line estimation to see how these representations and their variability change over developmental time and analyze what functional significance, if any, is associated with these changes.

Accuracy of number line estimation increases over developmental time. This trend has been observed for number lines of different sizes like 0–10 (Petitto, 1990), 0–100 (Booth & Siegler, 2006; Petitto, 1990; Siegler & Booth, 2004), and 0–1000 (Booth & Siegler, 2006; Siegler & Opfer, 2003). In addition to overall accuracy, the nature of children's number representation has also been shown by Robert Siegler and his colleagues in a number of pioneering studies to undergo age-related changes (Please also see "Children's Developing Understanding of Number: Mind, Brain and Culture," for a discussion of how these findings may be accommodated within Robbie Case's theory of children's development of number skills). In general, changes in estimation reflect a shift in representation from logarithmic in younger children to linear in older children and adults (Booth & Siegler, 2006; Siegler & Booth, 2004; Siegler & Opfer, 2003). This shift has several salient characteristics. First, this developmental change is gradual and is punctuated by a period during which children's estimates are equally well described by both linear and logarithmic functions. Second, the shift occurs later in development for larger number lines. While the estimates of second graders are better characterized by a linear representation when making estimates on a 0–100 number line, the same age group's estimates on a 0–1,000 number line are better characterized by a logarithmic representation (Siegler & Booth, 2004). While these data clearly have great theoretical value in terms of how numbers are internally represented, what is truly exciting about these data is their practical import. Increased accuracy in number line estimation (which is thought to reflect more mature numerical representation) has been found to be associated with math achievement test scores for kindergarten through second graders making estimates on a 0–100 number line (Siegler & Booth, 2004), as well as for second through fourth graders making estimates on a line marked 0–1,000 (Booth & Siegler, 2006). Furthermore, children's performance on number line estimation tasks was predictive of their success in learning new arithmetic problems (Booth & Siegler, 2008).

A second type of numerical estimation relevant to basic number representation is numerosity estimation. This type of estimation involves determining the numerosity of a non-symbolic magnitude, for example the number of seeds in a birdfeeder or the number of chickadees that have visited the feeder today. In general, estimations of non-symbolic magnitudes become less accurate as the target numerosity increases (Whalen, Gallistel, & Gelman, 1999). Accuracy of numerosity estimation improves with age (Luwel, Verschaffel, Onghena, & DeCorte, 2000; Siegel, Goldsmith, &

Madson, 1982) and the variability of the estimations has been shown to decrease over developmental time (Huntley-Fenner, 2001). Children's accuracy in numerosity estimation has also been shown to correlate with math achievement test scores (Dowker, 2003).

In sum, studies of the development of estimation abilities have contributed to the elucidation of the developmental trajectory of children's basic representation and processing of numerical quantity. Importantly, these data have shown that there exist not merely quantitative developmental changes such as the reduction of the distance effect as a function of age, but that qualitative changes such as the shift from logarithmic to linear representations of numerical magnitude also occur as a function of age and experience.

The above review highlights the importance of using multiple measures to research the children's development of mathematical skills. In what follows, we discuss how neuroimaging methods can provide another level of analysis that can further enrich our understanding of number development.

Developmental Changes in Magnitude Comparison: Neuroimaging Findings

Over the past 10 years, neuroimaging methodologies have been increasingly used as a tool for understanding the temporal characteristics (Stanislas Dehaene, 1996; Grune, Mecklinger, & Ullsperger, 1993; Libertus, Woldorff, & Brannon, 2007; Turconi, Jemel, Rossion, & Seron, 2004), the spatial organization [for reviews see (Dehaene, Molko, Cohen, & Wilson, 2004; Stanislas Dehaene, Piazza, Pinel, & Cohen, 2003)], and the structural underpinnings (van Eimeren, Niogi, McCandliss, Holloway, & Ansari, 2008) of the neural basis of numerical magnitude processing. In brief, evidence in the neuroimaging literature has identified the inferior parietal regions, particularly in and around the bilateral intraparietal sulcus (IPS), as important brain areas for the representation of numerical magnitudes. In the domain of development, neuroimaging can help clarify whether age-related changes in performance are qualitative (i.e., a result of children utilizing different processes than adults) or quantitative (i.e., a result of children using the same processes of adults at differing rates or to different extents). A small, but growing number of studies have been conducted to explore the ontogeny of the underlying neural circuitry of basic number processing.

In addition to simply describing the nature of developmental change, characterization of the typical developmental trajectory of the functional neuroanatomy involved in number processing has the potential to be highly useful in understanding the nature of dysfunction in atypical populations (Ansari & Karmiloff-Smith, 2002). Furthermore, functional neuroimaging has been utilized to track the success of remediation programs in children with reading difficulties (Shaywitz et al., 2004; Simos et al., 2002; Temple et al., 2003).

Three studies have explored the neural underpinnings of basic number processing using a magnitude comparison task to analyze developmental differences in the numerical distance effect. Two of these studies utilized functional magnetic resonance imaging (henceforth referred to as fMRI). These studies demonstrated the existence of age-related shifts in functional activity from prefrontal to more parietal areas in response to numerical distance in symbolic (Ansari, Garcia, Lucas, Hamon, & Dhital, 2005) and non-symbolic (Ansari & Dhital, 2006) visual displays. These findings are similar to those described in a recent study using the number Stroop paradigm (discussed above) to examine developmental differences in brain activation associated with the symbolic number processing (Kaufmann et al., 2006). The differences between children and adults in these studies likely reflect children's greater recruitment of areas involved in attention and working memory in order to successfully compare the relative magnitude of numerosities. Such areas are presumably activated to compensate for under-developed representations of numerical magnitude in the parietal cortex. As children's understanding of numerical magnitude becomes more fluent, they need to rely less on auxiliary processes, such as working memory, to make magnitude comparisons.

At face value, these results conflict with those reported in an earlier study utilizing event-related potentials (ERP) to characterize differences in the number processing of children and adults. This latter study found similar activation in parietal regions for children and adults when performing both symbolic and non-symbolic numerical comparison (Temple & Posner, 1998). However, this difference could be the result of differences in methodology. The spatial resolution of ERP data is very imprecise compared with that of fMRI. Furthermore, Temple and Posner did not directly statistically contrast the waveforms for children and adults, which may also account for these divergent findings.

Interestingly, Temple and Posner reported that, though the ERP waveforms associated with the distance effect for children and adults were quite similar, children's reaction times were significantly slower than adults. These authors suggested that this reaction time difference could be caused by children's difficulty in coordinating a response rather than by differences in numerical representation. This interpretation is consistent with the fMRI findings presented above as the differences in activation measured by fMRI in part are interpreted as reflecting differences in resources necessary for activating and comparing numerical magnitudes. These results leave open the intriguing possibility that the representation of numerosity in the child is actually very similar to that of an adult, but that the meaningful use of this numerosity is what undergoes developmental changes. In this view, magnitude representation is mediated by inferior parietal regions for both children and adults. However, although the representation of numerical magnitude is mediated by inferior parietal regions in children, the representations are not as elaborated and automatically accessible as they are in the adult brain. Thus, children's use of their numerical magnitude representations for tasks such as numerical comparison must be bolstered with an increased engagement of attentional resources relative to adults.

Preliminary evidence for this can be found in a recent study that utilized an fMRI adaptation paradigm (Cantlon, Brannon, Carter, & Pelphrey, 2006). In an adaptation paradigm, participants passively view a series of stimuli that hold certain visual features (called target features) of the display constant. For example, arrays of 32 dots of different sizes could be repeatedly presented. As participants repeatedly view different examples of 32 dots, the neural response in brain regions involved in representing both the number (32) and the shape (circle) gradually decreases, or adapts. If one of the target features is suddenly changed (e.g. 16 dots or 32 squares), then the brain activation associated with representing that feature shows a significant increase in intensity. Because there is no task involved in adaptation paradigms, investigators can identify brain regions that are involved in representing different visual features and be more confident that the regions they identify are associated with representing a given feature rather than associated with completing a specific kind of task. In the study reported by Cantlon and colleagues, adults and 4-year-old children were asked to passively view the displays without specific instructions about where the focus of their attention should be. Occasionally, a "deviant" was presented that could either vary in shape (e.g., the dots change to squares for one trial) or in number (e.g., the number of dots increases from 16 to 32). The changes in brain activation in response to these deviants were compared across adults and 4-year-old children. The results suggested that areas in the IPS were activated more strongly for numerical deviants than for shape deviants in both adults and children. This was interpreted as evidence for similarity in adults and children in the areas responsible for encoding of numerical magnitude information. Interestingly, these authors also highlight a significant difference in lateralization of the activation. The activations for the adults occurred in the bilateral IPS while the activations associated with children's automatic processing of number were localized only in the right IPS. In other words, the right IPS activation shows little age-related change, but the left IPS behaves differently in children and adults. This hemispheric difference could be reflective of developmental specialization of the left parietal cortex for numerical representation, as has been suggested by two different teams of investigators (Ansari & Dhital, 2006; Rivera, Reiss, Eckert, & Menon, 2005). These findings highlight the importance of considering both developmental similarity and difference in brain activation between children and adults, rather than casting these two possibilities as being dichotomous.

In sum, the developmental neuroimaging studies of basic number processing have yielded mixed results. Some studies suggest that children have very adult-like activations associated with numerical representation. Others suggest that numerical processing changes quite substantially across development. Much more study is needed to fully characterize the developmental changes in the neural underpinnings of basic number processing. Here it will be important to compare and contrast both active and passive paradigms to assess the possibility of graded representations.

The relevance of neuroimaging to education is, as yet, unknown due to the paucity of developmental neuroimaging studies in the domain of numerical cognition. Neuroimaging studies are still far behind behavioral research in the characterization of many aspects of numerical cognition including automaticity and the mapping of numerosities to symbols. One important unanswered question regards the functional implications of the developmental shift from frontal to parietal activations during magnitude comparison. Because this shift is observed with both symbolic and non-symbolic stimuli it is likely related to increases in the automaticity associated with access to magnitude representations. However, more research is required to explore the nature of these changes in a more precise way. Unfortunately, the developmental neuroimaging studies to date have focused on contrasting children with adults. A much richer understanding of the developmental changes in the neural underpinnings of numerical processing is afforded with studies that contrast children of differing age groups. Finally, the neuroimaging studies of functional brain development must also be supplemented with studies exploring ontogenetic changes of brain structure with techniques such as diffusor tensor imaging and voxel-based morphometry or measures of cortical thickness. The combination of functional and structural data will enable us to measure the similarities, differences, and interactions between age-related functional and structural changes.

Atypical Trajectories of Numerical Magnitude Processing

Studies of basic number processing in typically developing children have afforded us an insight into which numerical competencies are manifest during particular stages of development, and which of those abilities are crucial as foundations for the development of more sophisticated and complex mathematical learning. A second line of investigation, which can both inform and be informed by the research explored above, is that of atypical development of basic number processing. The study of basic numerical processing impairments is crucial not only to better inform models of typical development and hence develop better educational practices, but is particularly important in understanding the root causes of mathematical learning disabilities. If the processing and representation of basic numerical magnitude is indeed a crucial precursor to the development of mathematical skills, then an impairment of these skills may result in atypical number development.

Impairments in mathematics performance at school are complex in behavioral profile and diverse in etiology. Attentional factors, reading ability, and even socioeconomic background may play a role.

Mathematical learning disabilities have not been as widely researched as reading disabilities, but developmental dyscalculia, which is a mathematical analog of dyslexia, (DD) is receiving ever-growing attention (B. Butterworth, 2005). Developmental dyscalculia is a disorder which is currently poorly understood but presumed to be linked to impaired development of brain function in specific areas (Shalev & Gross-Tsur, 2001), and is analogous to dyslexia in that it is thought to stem from a functional impairment of a core process essential to learning in a given area. Behavioral symptoms typically include impairments in counting (Geary, Bow-Thomas, & Yao, 1992; Geary, Hoard, & Hamson, 1999; Geary, Hamson, Hoard, 2000) and delayed use of efficient arithmetic strategies as well as the inability to encode and recall arithmetic facts (Geary et al., 2000; Geary, 1990; Geary, & Brown,

1991), with prevalence estimates around 3–6% (Shalev, 2000). Here we refer to such specific developmental disorders of mathematical abilities as developmental dyscalculia. It should be noted, however, that other researchers will sometimes refer to individuals with such cognitive profiles as children with mathematics disorder or mathematical difficulties (MD).

A limiting factor in identifying a core deficit in DD has been that most studies of developmental dyscalculia have focused on higher-level arithmetic processes, typically encountered at school level (Ansari & Karmiloff-Smith, 2002) and hence may have confounded the developmental root causes of DD with other contributing cognitive processes. It is therefore necessary to investigate the extent to which problems with mental arithmetic in children with DD can be traced back to difficulties in representing and processing basic numerical quantities.

Behavioral Studies of Atypical Basic Number Processing

It has been hypothesized that developmental dyscalculia may be the consequence of an impaired basic "number sense" or "number module." To address this hypothesis, Landerl, Bevan, and Butterworth (2004) investigated basic number processing skills in children with developmental dyscalculia, dyslexia, children with both disorders, and a group of typically developing children, using a stringent criterion for dyscalculia of three standard deviations below the control mean on a timed arithmetic test, while being within the second standard deviation in reading tests. Dyscalculic and "double deficit" (those with comorbid dyslexia and dyscalculia) children were found to be significantly impaired relative to controls on a range of "basic numerical tasks," including number naming/reading, number comparison, number sequences/counting, and dot counting. Interestingly, dyslexic children performed in the same range as control subjects on these tasks. These findings provide strong evidence of a selective deficit in basic numerical processing in severe developmental dyscalculics.

Further exploration of the relative "strength" of internal numerical magnitude representation comes from two studies by Rubinsten and Henik (2005) who found that adults with developmental dyscalculia have much smaller numerical congruity effects during size comparison in a numerical Stroop task (making physical or numerical comparison of two digits in which representing the large numerical quantity may be congruent or incongruent with its physical size; see above for a detailed description of this paradigm in the context of typical number development). Adults with DD showed less interference and facilitation from the numerical information carried in the stimuli, when making comparisons based on physical size. In other words, adults with developmental dyscalulia, like children in early first grade (see review of typical development above), do not automatically activate task-irrelevant representations of numerical magnitude. The reported absence of facilitation among participants with DD may suggest that DD subjects had a weakened internal representation of magnitude, which failed to activate automatically during the task. It is important to note that the subjects in this study were adults with DD, and hence individual differences may exist in the way numerical symbols have been mapped onto numerical magnitude referents. These differences may have arisen as a consequence of different strategies and mechanisms constructed over developmental time, and so there is a need to investigate this issue not only at an earlier stage of development, but also longitudinally.

While the above evidence points to an impairment of basic number representation and the strength of its activation in DD, it is unclear at what level this impairment occurs. In other words it is unclear whether developmental dyscalculia is related to either impaired development of internal magnitude representation, or impaired access to that representation through numerical symbols, or an inability to activate representations of numerical magnitude when presented with numerical stimuli.

To address the possibility that children with DD may suffer from deficit in accessing representations of numerical magnitude rather than impaired representations per se ("Access Deficit Hypothesis"), Rousselle and Noel (2007) compared children with developmental dyscalculia with and without comorbid reading disabilities, to normally achieving peers on symbolic and non-symbolic number comparison tasks, as well as a numerical Stroop task. Developmental dyscalculia (referred to as mathematics learning disability by the authors) was defined as being below the 15th percentile on a standardized mathematics test. The Pure DD group and the comorbid group did not differ in any of the experimental tests and so they were collapsed into one larger MD group. Rouselle and Noel found that the DD group was slower and more error prone in comparing Arabic digits, and showed a reduced distance effect for symbolic comparison. The results of this study would indicate that rather than having an impaired representation of numerical magnitude, DD children are deficient in accessing that representation through numerical symbols (i.e., Arabic digits), as evidenced by significantly slower comparison. Importantly for the authors' theory, MD children showed reduced distance effects relative to controls when comparing Arabic digits but there were no similar group differences in the non-symbolic comparison condition. Thus these data support the hypothesis that it is the process of mapping numerical symbols onto their quantitative referents that is impaired among children with mathematical difficulties.

The smaller effect of numerical distance in children with mathematical difficulties is interesting in the context of evidence suggesting that the well-replicated distance effect decreases over developmental time (Duncan & McFarland, 1980; Sekuler & Mierkiewicz, 1977) and recent evidence suggesting that large distance effects are related to relatively poorer mathematic skills (Holloway & Ansari, 2008). These findings seemingly conflict with those of Rousselle and Noel (2007) who show a weaker symbolic distance effect in dyscalculic children, and thus a more systematic appraisal of the significance of the size of the distance effect in both typical and atypical development is required.

In addition to the finding of a difference for symbolic but not non-symbolic number comparison, both groups showed equal facilitation effects (that is they were faster at comparing two numerals for their physical size when the physically larger numeral was also numerically larger as in **4** 2, compared to a neutral condition in which numerals differed in physical but not numerical size **2 2**) in a "number Stroop" task. In other words, when subjects were attending to the physical dimensions of the stimulus, the numerical dimension facilitated the responses when the physical and numerical dimensions were congruent. This is in direct contrast to the findings of Rubinsten and Henik (2005) who found reduced facilitation for dyscalculics relative to controls.

In light of these conflicting findings, it remains an open question whether the arithmetical deficits, which characterize dyscalculia, are underpinned by impaired numerical representations or impaired access to those representations through the use of learned symbols or difficulties in automatically activating internal representations of numerical magnitude when presented with numerical stimuli.

Neuroimaging Studies

As discussed in the section on typical development of basic number processing above, a wealth of adult neuroimaging literature has investigated the neural correlates of basic numerical processing in normally developed adults (Dehaene, 1996; Dehaene et al., 1998; Stanislas Dehaene et al., 2003; Dehaene, Spelke, Pinel, Stanescu, & Tsivkin, 1999; Piazza, Izard, Pinel, Le Bihan, & Dehaene, 2004; Pinel, Dehaene, Riviere, & LeBihan, 2001; Pinel et al., 1999) and more recently in comparing normally developing children and adults (Ansari & Dhital, 2006; Ansari et al., 2005; Cantlon et al., 2006). Based on findings from this literature, it is generally thought that numerical magnitude is represented in the IPS of typically developing individuals. Assuming that to be true, we can investigate the neural basis of developmental dyscalculia by examining whether atypically developing populations show the same functional and structural characteristics as their typically developing peers in intraparietal areas.

Individuals with genetic developmental disorders such as Turner syndrome (TS) have provided insights into the neural correlates of atypical development of numerical processing. Molko et al. (2003) compared fMRI activations in 14 Turner Syndrome subjects with 14 controls during exact and approximate calculation (either choosing the correct answer of an arithmetic problem or choosing which of two answers is approximately correct and therefore closest to the correct answer). The TS subjects were disproportionately slower for more difficult problems in the exact calculation condition than controls. Interestingly, while the control subjects showed increased activation in the bilateral IPS as the difficulty of exact calculations increased, the TS subjects did not show the same effect. Using a morphometric analysis that examined structural length and depth of sulci, the authors found that TS subjects also showed abnormal structural organization of the IPS in the right hemisphere, in particular reduced gray matter volume, and an unusual interruption in the horizontal segment of this sulcus, an area which is systematically activated when numbers are manipulated and which is increasingly activated as the task puts greater emphasis on quantity processing (Dehaene et al., 2003). These results are interesting for two reasons. First, they show that TS subjects with developmental difficulties in numerical processing are less able than typically developing subjects to deal with increasing numerical demands in simple calculation verification, a task that requires direct numerical comparison between a mentally calculated solution and a visually presented candidate solution. Second, they show that the brain area associated with supporting the increased level of quantity processing in controls does not respond to increased demand in TS subjects, lending strong support to the idea that the internal representation of magnitude in these subjects is significantly weaker than in typically developing peers.

Isaacs, Edmonds, Lucas, and Gadian (2001) investigated the relationship between brain structure and mathematical disabilities in children of very low birth weight. Subjects with deficits in numerical operations (NOD group), including addition, subtraction, multiplication, and division were compared to those with deficits in mathematical reasoning (MDR group), including problem solving, numeration, and number concepts. Two control groups, not exhibiting deficits in either calculation or mathematical reasoning, were matched to the experimental groups for gender, age, IQ, and other perinatal variables. The NOD group showed significantly less gray matter in the left intraparietal sulcus than matched controls, while the MDR group showed no such difference. Abnormalities in the left parietal area have been historically associated with calculation deficits since the discovery of Gerstmann's Syndrome (Gerstmann, 1940). Furthermore, Simon, Mangin, Cohen, Le Bihan, and Dehaene (2002) in a within-subjects comparison of tasks associated with parietal regions, including grasping, visual saccades, and calculation, found activation uniquely associated with calculation in the left IPS. Isaacs et al. (2001) suggest their findings may imply that the NOD group is relying heavily on memory processes to complete basic calculations, or that the reduced gray matter is sufficient for simple but not complex calculations. However, it should be noted that the relationship between gray matter volume and cognitive function is not currently well understood and much of the data (including those presented by Isaacs et al. (2001) are correlational and thus no causal claims can be made.

It should also be noted that groups with different genetic disorders or other abnormalities (such as low birth weight) have sometimes been compared as though they shared a single deficit in numerical processing. It is dangerous to equate the visuospatial and numerical impairments between these groups simply because they share similar behavioral profiles on standardized arithmetic achievement tests. Although the consequences are unknown, the fact that these groups present with mathematical impairments as part of very different genetic syndromes should not be forgotten.

Recently imaging studies have begun to investigate the neural correlates of numerical processing in pure developmental dyscalculia (i.e., not part of a wider genetic developmental syndrome). Kucian et al. (2006) conducted an fMRI experiment with developmental dyscalculics in the third and sixth grades, defined by discrepancy between scores on a battery of mathematical and reading tests and general IQ, and two groups of age-matched controls. Subjects performed approximate and exact calculation in the same paradigm used by Molko et al. (2003) and magnitude comparison task, comparing small sets of different objects (e.g., strawberries vs. nuts). fMRI showed similar activation patterns, albeit generally weaker and more diffuse, for DD and control groups in all conditions, but the only significant difference between groups was found using region of interest analysis in the IPS. In this region, DD subjects showed significantly weaker activation in response to approximate calculation in the left IPS, and a non-significant trend in the same direction in the right IPS. However, this difference was not observed in direct statistical comparison between groups using repeated measures general linear model analysis. It is important to note that in this study no behavioral differences between groups were observed for any of the experimental tasks.

In a more recent fMRI study, (Price, Holloway, Räsänen, Vesterinen, & Ansari, 2007) compared the neural correlates of the distance effect during non-symbolic number comparison between dyscalculic and typically developing children. This study found that while control children showed a classical effect of numerical distance on the right IPS (i.e., stronger activation for comparisons separated by a relatively small compared to a relatively large numerical distance), the dyscalculic children showed no such distance-related modulation of brain activity. In combination with behavioral results showing a stronger effect of distance on comparison accuracy in the dyscalculic group, these results suggest an under-developed representation of numerical magnitude, which was unable to respond to the increased numerical processing demands of the task, in the dyscalculic children. It should be noted that these data are in conflict with Rouselle and Noel's (2007) findings, showing that children with mathematical difficulties are impaired in symbolic but not non-symbolic number comparison.

The differential response of the right parietal lobe to changes in numerical distance in children with developmental dyscalculia was supported by (Soltesz, Szucs, Dekany, Markus, & Csepe, 2007) who used a symbolic number comparison ERP paradigm to show that typically developing children show a distance effect over right parietal electrodes while dyscalculic children do not. However, this difference did not reach significance in a direct statistical comparison and thus requires further replication.

The results reported by Price et al. (2007) appear to contradict those reported by Kucian et al. (2006) with regards to non-symbolic comparison; however, it should be noted that Kucian et al. did not test for the effects of numerical distance. Another possible reason for this apparent contradiction is the different tasks used in each study. Kucian et al. used sets of objects such as fruits and nuts in which continuous physical variables were not controlled. Price et al., on the other hand, employed stimuli set in which continuous physical variables were strictly controlled and could not be used to reliably predict numerosity. Therefore it is possible that the task used by Kucian et al. simply did not require access to underlying representations of numerical magnitude as it could be solved by attention to non-numerical physical parameters.

Further evidence for the role impaired development of the parietal area in developmental dyscalculia comes from a case study presented by Levy, Reis, and Grafman (1999). J.S. was an 18-year-old male with developmental acalculia in the context of above average verbal skills. J.S. was particularly impaired when the complexity of problems increased or mental computation was required. While conventional MRI showed no abnormalities, magnetic resonance spectroscopy revealed a localized defect in the left temporoparietal region, specifically in the area of the angular gyrus, including defects in metabolite amplitudes. This case is particularly interesting because it shows that conventional MRI may not detect functionally relevant impairments in atypically developing brains. Naturally, as a case study the generalizability of these findings must be taken with caution.

Neuroimaging of basic number processing in atypically developing populations has so far provided variable results. Different experimental designs and populations with highly variable cognitive profiles outside the number domain have made it difficult to apply a uniform interpretation of the findings. However some consistent findings have emerged, in that almost all of these populations, when the task is well controlled, show some abnormal functional or structural modulation of the parietal region.

Applications for Education: Diagnosis and Intervention

A major hurdle in applying research findings from the cognitive neurosciences to mathematical education has been the divergent definitions of "number sense" (Berch, 2005). While in neuropsychology the construct has been defined in terms of basic cognitive processes, which can be linked to neural substrates, educational definitions have centered on intuitive understanding of concepts related to successful arithmetic performance. Neuropsychology and cognitive psychology have focused on tasks and processes that relate to perception and manipulation of numerical magnitudes, while educational research has gone further to include understanding of the ordinal relation between discreet numbers, and basic principles of counting and calculation (Griffin, 2004).

Classifications of developmental dyscalculia from sources such as ICD-10 and the Diagnostic and Statistical Manual of Mental Disorders – Fourth Edition (DSM-IV, American Psychiatric Association, 1994) have been so vague that they lack almost any utility in practical settings, as they may identify individuals as being dyscalculic, when their deficits arise from a wide range of potential causes. Performance may be influenced positively or negatively by teaching methods, socioeconomic status relating to exposure to numerical information in everyday life, and numerous other factors, which do not relate to the actual capacity to learn mathematics.

However, improved understanding of the basic features of the disorder, through the kinds of research studies discussed above, has allowed the development of the "dyscalculia screener" (Butterworth, 2003), which aims to test "basic numerical capacities," and is a valuable tool in identifying children with problems in basic numerical processing. Further developments in the field of diagnosis should be aimed toward better characterizing the range of disorders present in a typical classroom environment. It is important for educational application that developments in research address the wide spectrum of mathematical learning disabilities present in educational settings. On the other hand, it is important that research studies apply strict criteria when selected groups of dyscalculics, so that robust interpretations of data will be possible. Thus, the apparent dichotomy of needs will limit the pace at which discovery can occur, but will ultimately ensure that robust scientific findings can be applied in the way that benefits the most individuals.

Although researchers and educators may not currently share a uniform definition of "number sense," there is a growing consensus that its teaching and development is key to successful mathematical achievement, for both typically and atypically developing populations. In other words, while "number sense" means a broad set of competencies for educators and a narrow set of skills related to the representation and processing of numerical magnitude for cognitive neuroscientists, both emphasize the critical role that an understanding of numerical quantity plays in the development of mathematical abilities. Clarifying a different conceptualization of "number sense" may be an important starting point toward finding a common language necessary to guide cross-disciplinary collaborative efforts.

More recently, the concept of "number sense" has informed the construction of intervention software specifically designed to remediate children with DD. Wilson and colleagues (Wilson, Dehaene et al., 2006; Wilson, Revkin, Cohen, Cohen, & Dehaene, 2006) have developed the "Number Race" computer game for the remediation of dyscalculia stemming from a core deficit either in number sense or in the access to it through symbolic number information. In this context "number sense" was defined as the ability to "represent and manipulate numerical quantities nonverbally." This game used number comparison as its main task and used a board game-like structure to emphasize associations between number and space. "Number Race" shared some features with "Number Worlds" in that both also attempted to improve fluency in very basic calculation. A key feature emphasized in both projects was that the programs should be relevant to child's own ability, and hence the "Number Race" game was built using a computerized, multidimensional adaptive algorithm, which assessed response patterns and adjusted task difficulty accordingly. Open trial assessments have shown some positive effects of the game in improving basic numerical skills including speed of subitizing and numerical comparison and accuracy of some simple subtraction.

The development of focused and effective teaching and remediation methods can be positively informed by cognitive neuroscience research, helping educators and scientists to understand how the brain acquires basic numerical skills and what types of developmental abnormalities can impair those processes. It is important, however, to avoid an extreme position in adapting educational practices to such an extent that children are learning only those basic processes, which are well described at the neural level, such as basic magnitude comparison. It is highly important that proficiency in processes such as simple magnitude comparison are not viewed as the learning end states, but continue to be viewed as cognitive foundations on which more sophisticated learning can be built. In this sense the findings of educational researchers are essential in developing practically applicable strategies, and a union between the two disciplines will yield maximum rewards.

Future Directions and Conclusions

Analogous to developments in the field of typical and atypical reading research, there is growing consensus that early developing skills are crucial to the development of mathematical proficiency. The above review provides an overview of the available body of investigations into the typical and atypical trajectories of basic number processing from infancy onward. This review illustrates that basic representations of numerical quantity develop from infancy onward and undergo significant changes over time. Furthermore, recent evidence suggests that children who exhibit significant mathematical difficulties in school suffer from developmental impairment of their basic numerical quantity skills.

While still lagging significantly behind behavioral research, recent brain-imaging studies are starting to reveal the neural correlates of these developmental processes, pointing to both important developmental changes and continuities in the network of brain regions activated during basic number processing in adults and children.

Although the evidence reviewed in this chapter points to significant progress in the understanding of typical and atypical development of basic numerical magnitude processing, a number of significant, outstanding questions remain. Specifically, there is now a great need for researchers using both behavioral and brain-imaging methods to be more specific about different aspects of basic numerical magnitude representation and processing. In particular, the review of atypical development illustrates that it is yet unclear whether difficulties in processing numerical magnitude result from either: (a) impairments of the representational structure of numerical magnitudes, (b) impaired mechanisms for accessing these representations, or (c) difficulties in mapping symbolic representation (e.g., Arabic numerals) onto internal representations of numerical magnitude. Future research using both behavioral and neuroimaging methods should aim to further disentangle these different components of basic numerical magnitude processing and consider their possible interactions over developmental time. Neuroimaging may be particularly useful in this context by enabling researchers to potentially dissociate as well as identify interactions between these different components of numerical magnitude representation and processing on a neural level.

The research reviewed above reveals that an increasingly large body of studies point to important relationships between basic numerical magnitude processing competencies and the development of higher-level mathematical skills. In particular, recent work with atypically developing children suggests that developmental dyscalculia may be associated with impairments of basic numerical magnitude processing. There is, however, a need to further explore the specific role played by basic numerical magnitude processing in constraining the acquisition of higher-level mathematical skills that are crucial for the child's success in format mathematics instruction. While some of the evidence reviewed above suggests that number comparison and estimation correlate with the acquisition of mental arithmetic, the precise nature of these relationships remains to be described. Such studies, preferably using longitudinal designs, are particularly important for making links between behavioral and brain-imaging studies of numerical cognition and education. This will require a shift from the currently dominant focus on studying evolutionary and developmental continuity of numerical magnitude processing toward a detailed analysis of developmental changes and their functional significance. The instructional implications of the work reviewed in this chapter will become even clearer when the mechanisms by which basic numerical magnitude processing constrains the development of abilities important for success in mathematics education are better understood.

A related issue concerns the study of individual differences in mathematical development and the role of environmental factors in constraining the development of basic numerical magnitude processing. To increase their educational relevance, future investigations need to focus both on the average as well as the individual differences in the developmental trajectories of typical and atypical numerical cognition. This will require experimenters to closely evaluate the reliability of their experimental tools in the context of predicting individual differences. Furthermore, similar to recent trends in research on children's reading development (Noble, Wolmetz, Ochs, Farah, & McCandliss, 2006), a closer consideration of the effect factors such as home environment and socio-economic status (SES) on behavioral and brain-imaging measures needs to be undertaken to understand their potentially crucial, mediating role in children's development of numerical magnitude processing.

From a broader perspective, much progress in connecting education with basic research on the behavioral and brain mechanisms of typical and atypical development of numerical cognition can be made by reciprocal interactions between, on the one hand, research from within the fields of cognitive psychology and cognitive neuroscience and, on the other hand, mathematics education researchers and practitioners. The research on basic number processing can be significantly enriched by input from educational researchers and practitioners, who often have much more experience with children than experimental psychologists or cognitive neuroscientists. Through mechanisms of funding and training, efforts need to be made to bring together these diverse communities with common interest with the eventual aim of generating hypotheses and experimental designs for the purpose of understanding how children develop number concepts and how this development can go awry (Ansari & Coch, 2006; McCandliss, Kalchman, & Bryant, 2003).

References

Ansari, D., & Coch, D. (2006). Bridges over troubled waters: Education and cognitive neuroscience. *Trends in Cognitive Sciences, 10*(4), 146–151.

Ansari, D., & Dhital, B. (2006). Age-related changes in the activation of the intraparietal sulcus during non-symbolic magnitude processing: an event-related fMRI stud. *Journal of Cognitive Neuroscience, 18*, 1820–1828.

Ansari, D., Garcia, N., Lucas, E., Hamon, K., & Dhital, B. (2005). Neural correlates of symbolic number processing in children and adults. *Neuroreport, 16*(16), 1769–1773.

Ansari, D., & Karmiloff-Smith, A. (2002). Atypical trajectories of number development: a neuroconstructivist perspective. *Trends in Cognitive Sciences, 6*(12), 511–516.

American Psychiatric Association (1994). *Diagnostic and statistical manual of mental disorders*. Washington, DC: American Psychiatric Association.

Banks, W. P., Fujii, M., & Kayra-Stuart, F. (1976). Semantic congruity effects in comparative judgments of magnitudes of digits. *Journal of Experimental Psychology: Human Perception and Performance, 2*, 435–447.

Berch, D. B. (2005). Making sense of number sense: implications for children with mathematical disabilities. *Journal of Learning Disabilities, 38*(4), 333–339.
Booth, J. L., & Siegler, R. S. (2006). Developmental and individual differences in pure numerical estimation. *Developmental Psychology, 42*(1), 189–201.
Booth, J. L., & Siegler, R. S. (2008). Numerical magnitude representations influence arithmetic learning. *Child Development, 79*, 106–1031.
Buckley, P. B., & Gillman, C. B. (1974). Comparisons of digits and dot patterns. *Journal of Experimental Psychology, 103*(6), 1131–1136.
Butterworth, B. (2003). *Dyscalculia screener*. London, UK: NFER Nelson Publishing Company Ltd.
Butterworth, B. (2005). Developmental dyscalculia. In J. I. D. Campbell (Ed.), *Handbook of mathematical cognition* (pp. 455–467). Hove: Psychology Press.
Butterworth, B. (2005). The development of arithmetical abilities. *Journal of Child Psychology and Psychiatry, 46*(1), 3–18.
Cantlon, J. F., Brannon, E. M., Carter, E. J., & Pelphrey, K. A. (2006). Functional Imaging of Numerical Processing in Adults and 4-y-Old Children. *PLoS Biology, 4*(5), e125.
Cunningham, A. E., & Stanovich, K. E. (1997). Early reading acquisition and its relation to reading experience and ability 10 years later. *Developmental Psychology, 33*(6), 934–945.
Dehaene, S. (1996). The organization of brain activations in number comparison: Event-related potentials and the additive-factors method. *Journal of Cognitive Neuroscience, 8*, 47–68.
Dehaene, S. (1997). *The Number Sense*. Oxford: Oxford University Press.
Dehaene, S., Dehaene-Lambertz, G., & Cohen, L. (1998). Abstract representations of numbers in the animal and human brain. *Trends in Neurosciences, 21*(8), 355–361.
Dehaene, S., Molko, N., Cohen, L., & Wilson, A. J. (2004). Arithmetic and the brain. *Current Opinion in Neurobiology, 14*(2), 218–224.
Dehaene, S., Piazza, M., Pinel, P., & Cohen, L. (2003). Three Parietal Circuits for Number Processing. *Cognitive Neuropsychology, 20*(3–6), 487–506.
Dehaene, S., Spelke, E., Pinel, P., Stanescu, R., & Tsivkin, S. (1999). Sources of mathematical thinking: behavioral and brain-imaging evidence. *Science, 284*(5416), 970–974.
Dowker, A. (2003). Young children's estimates for addition: The zone of partial knowledge and understanding. In A. J. Baroody & A. Dowker (Eds.), *The development of arithmetic concepts and skills: Constructing adaptive expertise* (pp. 243–265). Mahwah, NJ: Erlbaum.
Duncan, E. M., & McFarland, C. E., Jr. (1980). Isolating the effects of symbolic distance and semantic congruity in comparative judgments: An additive-factors analysis. *Memory & Cognition, 8*(6), 612–622.
Geary, D. C. (1990). A componential analysis of an early learning deficit in mathematics. *Journal of Experimental Child Psychology, 49*, 363–383.
Geary, D. C. (1993). Mathematical disabilities: cognitive, neuropsychological, and genetic components. *Psychological Bulletin, 114*(2), 345–362.
Geary, D. C., Bow-Thomas, C. C., & Yao, Y. (1992). Counting knowledge and skill in cognitive addition: a comparison of normal and mathematically disabled children. *Journal of Experimental Child Psychology, 54*(3), 372–391.
Geary, D. C., & Brown, S. C. (1991). Cognitive addition: Strategy choice and speed-of-processing differences in gifted, normal, and mathematically disabled children. *Developmental Psychology, 27*, 398–406.
Geary, D. C., Hamson, C. O., & Hoard, M. K. (2000). Numerical and arithmetical cognition: a longitudinal study of process and concept deficits in children with learning disability. *Journal of Experimental Child Psychology, 77*(3), 236–263.
Geary, D. C., Hoard, M. K., & Hamson, C. O. (1999). Numerical and arithmetical cognition: Patterns of functions and deficits in children at risk for a mathematical disability. *Journal of Experimental Child Psychology, 74*, 213–239.
Gersten, R., & Chard, D. (1999). Number Sense: Rethinking Arithmetic Instruction for Students with Mathematical Disabilities. *The Journal of Special Education, 33*(1), 18–28.

Gerstmann, J. (1940). Syndrome of finger agnosia, disorientation for right and left, agraphia and acalculia. *Archives of Neurology and Psychiatry, 44*, 398–408.

Girelli, L., Lucangeli, D., & Butterworth, B. (2000). The development of automaticity in accessing number magnitude. *Journal of Experimental Child Psychology, 76*(2), 104–122.

Goswami, U. (2003). Why theories about developmental dyslexia require developmental designs. *Trends in Cognitive Sciences, 7*(12), 534–540.

Griffin, S. (2004). Building number sense with number worlds. *Early childhood research quarterly, 19*(1), 173–180.

Grune, K., Mecklinger, A., & Ullsperger, P. (1993). Mental comparison: P300 component of the ERP reflects the symbolic distance effect. *Neuroreport, 4*(11), 1272–1274.

Holloway, I. D., & Ansari, D. (2008). Domain-specific and domain-general changes in children's development of number comparison. *Developmental Science, 11*(5), 644–649.

Huntley-Fenner, G. (2001). Children's understanding of number is similar to adults' and rats': numerical estimation by 5–7-year-olds. *Cognition, 78*(3), B27–B40.

Isaacs, E. B., Edmonds, C. J., Lucas, A. ,& Gadian, D. G. (2001) Calculation difficulties in children of very low birthweight: a neural correlate. *Brain, 124*, 1701–1707.

Kaufmann, L., Koppelstaetter, F., Siedentopf, C., Haala, I., Haberlandt, E., Zimmerhackl, L. B., et al. (2006). Neural correlates of the number-size interference task in children. *Neuroreport, 17*(6), 587–591.

Kucian, K., Loenneker, T., Dietrich, T., Dosch, M., Martin, E., & von Aster, M. (2006) Impaired neural networks for approximate calculation in dyscalculic children: a functional MRI study. *Behavioral and Brain Function : BBF, 5*(2): 31.

Landerl, K., Bevan, A., & Butterworth, B. (2004). Developmental dyscalculia and basic numerical capacities: a study of 8–9-year-old students. *Cognition, 93*(2), 99–125.

Levy, L. M., Reis, I. L. & Grafman, J. (1999) Metabolic abnormalities detected by 1H-MRS in dyscalculia and dysgraphia. *Neurology,* 11, 639–641.

Libertus, M. E., Woldorff, M. G., & Brannon, E. M. (2007). Electrophysiological evidence for notation independence in numerical processing. *Behavioral and Brain Functions: BBF, 3*, 1.

Luwel, K., Verschaffel, L., Onghena, P., & DeCorte, E. (2000). Children's strategies for numerosity judgment in square grids of different sizes. *Psychologica Belgica, 40*, 183–209.

McCandliss, B. D., Kalchman, M., & Bryant, P. (2003). Design Experiment and Laboratory Approaches to Learning: Steps Towards Collaborative Exchange. *Educational Researcher, 32*(1), 14–16.

Molko, N., Cachia, A., Riviere, D., Mangin, J. F., Bruandet, M., Le Bihan, D., et al. (2003). Functional and structural alterations of the intraparietal sulcus in a developmental dyscalculia of genetic origin. *Neuron, 40*(4), 847–858.

Moyer, R. S., & Landauer, T. K. (1967). Time required for judgements of numerical inequality. *Nature, 215*(109), 1519–1520.

Noble, K. G., Wolmetz, M. E., Ochs, L. G., Farah, M. J., & McCandliss, B. D. (2006). Brain-behavior relationships in reading acquisition are modulated by socioeconomic factors. *Developmental Science, 9*(6), 642–654.

OECD. (2004). *Learning for tomorrow's world: First results from PISA 2003. Organization for Economic Co-operation and Development.*

Petitto, A. L. (1990). Development of numberline and measurement concepts. *Cognition and Instruction, 7*, 55–78.

Piazza, M., Izard, V., Pinel, P., Le Bihan, D., & Dehaene, S. (2004). Tuning curves for approximate numerosity in the human intraparietal sulcus. *Neuron, 44*(3), 547–555.

Pinel, P., Dehaene, S., Riviere, D., & LeBihan, D. (2001). Modulation of parietal activation by semantic distance in a number comparison task. *Neuroimage, 14*(5), 1013–1026.

Pinel, P., Le Clec, H. G., van de Moortele, P. F., Naccache, L., Le Bihan, D., & Dehaene, S. (1999). Event-related fMRI analysis of the cerebral circuit for number comparison. *Neuroreport, 10*(7), 1473–1479.

Price, G. R., Holloway, I., Räsänen, P., Vesterinen, M., & Ansari, D. (2007). Impaired parietal magnitude processing in developmental dyscalculia. *Current Biology, 17*(24), 1042–1043.
Rivera, S. M., Reiss, A. L., Eckert, M. A., & Menon, V. (2005). Developmental changes in mental arithmetic: evidence for increased functional specialization in the left inferior parietal cortex. *Cerebral Cortex, 15*(11), 1779–1790.
Rousselle, L., & Noel, M. P. (2007). Basic numerical skills in children with mathematics learning disabilities: A comparison of symbolic vs non-symbolic number magnitude processing. *Cognition, 102*(3), 361–395.
Rubinsten, O., & Henik, A. (2005). Automatic activation of internal magnitudes: a study of developmental dyscalculia. *Neuropsychology, 19*(5), 641–648.
Rubinsten, O., Henik, A., Berger, A., & Shahar-Shalev, S. (2002). The development of internal representations of magnitude and their association with Arabic numerals. *Journal of Experimental Child Psychology, 81*(1), 74–92.
Sekuler, R., & Mierkiewicz, D. (1977). Children's judgments of numerical inequality. *Child Development, 48*, 630–633.
Shalev, R. (2000). Developmental Dyscalculia. *Pediatric Neurology, 24*(5), 337–342.
Shalev, R. S., & Gross-Tsur, V. (2001). Developmental dyscalculia. *Pediatric Neurology, 24*(5), 337–342.
Shaywitz, B. A., Shaywitz, S. E., Blachman, B. A., Pugh, K. R., Fulbright, R. K., Skudlarski, P., et al. (2004). Development of left occipitotemporal systems for skilled reading in children after a phonologically- based intervention. *Biological Psychiatry, 55*(9), 926–933.
Siegel, A. W., Goldsmith, L. T., & Madson, C. R. (1982). Skill in estimation problems of extent and numerosity. *Journal for Research in Mathematics Education, 13*, 211–232.
Siegler, R. S., & Booth, J. (2005). Development of Numerical Estimation: A Review. In J. Campbell (Ed.), *Handbook of Mathematical Cognition* (pp. 197–213). New York, NY: Psychology Press.
Siegler, R. S., & Booth, J. L. (2004). Development of numerical estimation in young children. *Child Development, 75*(2), 428–444.
Siegler, R. S., & Opfer, J. E. (2003). The development of numerical estimation: evidence for multiple representations of numerical quantity. *Psychological Science, 14*(3), 237–243.
Simon, O., Mangin, J. F., Cohen, L., Le Bihan, D., & Dehaene, S. (2002). Topographical layout of hand, eye, calculation, and language-related areas in the human parietal lobe. *Neuron, 33*(3), 475–487.
Simos, P. G., Fletcher, J. M., Bergman, E., Breier, J. I., Foorman, B. R., Castillo, E. M., et al. (2002). Dyslexia-specific brain activation profile becomes normal following successful remedial training. *Neurology, 58*(8), 1203–1213.
Soltesz, F., Szucs, D., Dekany, J., Markus, A., & Csepe, V. (2007). A combined event-related potential and neuropsychological investigation of developmental dyscalculia. *Neuroscience Letters, 417*(2), 181–186.
Stevenson, H. W., Lee, S. Y., & Stigler, J. W. (1986). Mathematics achievement of Chinese, Japanese, and American children. *Science, 231*(4739), 693–699.
Stroop, J. R. (1935). Studies of interference in serial verbal reactions. *Journal of Experimental Psychology, 18*(6), 643–662.
Temple, E., Deutsch, G. K., Poldrack, R. A., Miller, S. L., Tallal, P., Merzenich, M. M., et al. (2003). Neural deficits in children with dyslexia ameliorated by behavioral remediation: evidence from functional MRI. *Proceedings of the National Academy of Sciences of the United States of America, 100*(5), 2860–2865.
Temple, E., & Posner, M. I. (1998). Brain mechanisms of quantity are similar in 5-year-old children and adults. *Proceedings of the National Academy of Sciences of the United States of America, 95*(13), 7836–7841.
Turconi, E., Jemel, B., Rossion, B., & Seron, X. (2004). Electrophysiological evidence for differential processing of numerical quantity and order in humans. *Brain Research. Cognitive Brain Research, 21*(1), 22–38.

van Eimeren, L., Niogi, S. N., McCandliss, B. D., Holloway, I. D., & Ansari, D. (2008). White matter microstructures underlying mathematical abilities in children. *Neuroreport*, *19*(11), 1117–1121.

Van Opstal, F., Gevers, W., De Moor, W., & Verguts, T. (2008). Dissecting the symbolic distance effect: comparison and priming effects in numerical and nonnumerical orders. *Psychonomic Bulletin and Review*, *15*(2), 419–425.

Verguts, T., Fias, W., & Stevens, M. (2005). A model of exact small-number representation. *Psychonomic Bulletin and Review*, *12*(1), 66–80.

Walsh, V. (2003). A theory of magnitude: common cortical metrics of time, space and quantity. *Trends in Cognitive Sciences, 7*(11), 483–488.

Whalen, J., Gallistel, C. R., & Gelman, I. I. (1999). Nonverbal counting in humans: The psychophysics of number representation. *Psychological Science*, *2*, 130–137.

Wilson, A. J., Dehaene, S., Pinel, P., Revkin, S. K., Cohen, L., & Cohen, D. (2006). Principles underlying the design of "The Number Race", an adaptive computer game for remediation of dyscalculia. *Behavioral and Brain Functions*, *2*, 19.

Wilson, A. J., Revkin, S. K., Cohen, D., Cohen, L., & Dehaene, S. (2006). An open trial assessment of "The Number Race", an adaptive computer game for remediation of dyscalculia. *Behavioral and Brain Functions*, *2*, 20.

Children's Developing Understanding of Number: Mind, Brain, and Culture

Yukari Okamoto

Introduction

Robbie Case was fascinated by what children say and do. Children's words and actions provided him with a wealth of information to fuel questions such as *How do they come to know that?* He was also concerned with finding ways to help children maximize their intellectual accomplishments. He devoted tremendous energy to answering questions such as *What core knowledge do children need to have in place in order to take full advantage of formal schooling?* These questions reflected two central characteristics of Case's research – one that was a theoretical interest in intellectual development and the other that was the practical pursuit of instructional programs for disadvantaged children. What is less well known about Case's work, however, was his interest in brain research: As early as 1992, he published an article that examined the role of the frontal lobes in determining cognitive development (Case, 1992a). The current volume that examines relations among developing mind, brain, and education, therefore, is a most honorable way to celebrate Robbie Case's legacy.

The goal of this chapter is to discuss children's understanding of number in light of current thinking and the empirical evidence available to us. It is in no way a comprehensive review of the field. Rather, it is a reflection of my own view of cognitive development in the domain of whole numbers. Similar to Case's, my view of cognitive development has intellectual roots in the structural perspective of neo-Piagetian thinking, but with a stronger set of assumptions about the role of innate knowledge and cultural practices. Building upon Case's theory of intellectual development, I argue that children from birth set out on a cognitive journey guided by both innate mechanisms and cultural systems of knowledge. In a way, this chapter can be thought of as my attempt to extend Case's thinking, given advances in our understandings of mind, brain, and culture.

Y. Okamoto (✉)
Department of Education, University of California, Santa Barbara, CA, USA
e-mail: yukari@education.ucsb.edu

M. Ferrari, L. Vuletic (eds.), *The Developmental Relations among Mind, Brain and Education*, DOI 10.1007/978-90-481-3666-7_6,

Core Constituents of Case's Theory of Cognitive Development

Before discussing how I extend Case's theory, it is important to point out features of Case's theory as it went through a number of revisions. Case placed great importance to capturing the true nature of children's developing minds. This, to him, required developing a theory that integrated various schools of thought (Case, 1998). While always retaining Piaget's core ideas, he consistently updated his theory to reflect contemporary theories and empirical evidence of the time. Early on, Case knew he wanted to publish a *series* of books or monographs to work out the continuing development of his thinking. And he did.

In his first book (Case, 1985), *Intellectual Development: Birth to Adulthood*, Case proposed a model of development that consisted of four stages: the sensorimotor stage (birth to 1½ years), the interrelational stage (1½–5 years), the dimensional stage (5–11 years), and the vectorial stage (11–19 years). These stages roughly corresponded to Piaget's stages of development in age but resulted from Case's analyses of children's executive control structures. Case postulated that children's control structures go through these four stages of abstraction. Development within each stage depended upon the growth of working memory as well as mastery of more complex executive processes; in contrast, transition across stages occurred as a result of abstraction and integration of two qualitatively different structures. In formulating this theory, Case retained Piaget's notion of a general cognitive structure. He argued that most researchers abandoned this notion prematurely. Instead of rejecting it in its entirety, he thought it to be more productive to rework it, taking into account new empirical evidence as well as theoretical advancement. This model thus can be thought of as Case's recasting of Piaget's theory into the framework of classical information-processing theories.

In his second book (Case, 1992b), *The Mind's Staircase: Exploring the Conceptual Underpinnings of Children's Thought and Knowledge*, Case expanded his thinking further and postulated the notion of *central conceptual structures*. The general structure of his stage model was retained in this reformulation. Reflecting Piagetian thinking, central conceptual structures were conceived as the product of children's central processing – that is, the structures themselves reflect a set of principles and constraints that are system-wide in nature and change with age in a predictable fashion. At the same time, the proposed structures were defined within a domain as networks of semantic nodes and relations. These networks have a broad yet domain-specific application and are central to children's functioning in that domain.

Four years later, Case further elaborated on the characteristics of central conceptual structures in a monograph, *The Role of Central Conceptual Structures in the Development of Children's Thought* (Case & Okamoto, 1996). This round of reformulation incorporated ideas of innate modules as well as cultural influences on cognitive functioning. Case postulated that infants in the first few months of life parse their experience into a set of basic categories, which become well-distinguished domains of knowledge during early childhood. Central conceptual structures in each domain resulted from an integration of two essential schemas that children consolidate during this time period. From this integration emerges a conceptual structure that promotes a new way of thinking – a qualitatively different way of viewing the world. This new conceptual structure then serves as a focal hub for children's understandings of a broad range of activities and situations that are culturally defined. Upon examining cross-cultural data (see Okamoto, Case, Bleiker, & Henderson, 1996), Case and I concluded that cultural influences are more likely to be reflected in children's localized skills than in general conceptual development. That is, if a culture values a particular set of skills and invests a great deal of resources in teaching them, children in that culture are more likely to excel in those skills than children who grow up in a culture that does not. However, accelerated performance in a set of skills is unlikely to influence the rate of development of central conceptual structures: Children's development of central conceptual structures require both neurobiological maturation and varied experiences of cultural practices. In the absence of either factor, development may be delayed or inhibited. To summarize, our view of cognitive development began with innate architectures in several domains that are shaped by both physiological determinants and cultural practices.

Nature of Numerical Representations in Early Years

Over the last few decades, numerous studies of number representations in infants, adults, and non-human animals have been published. Among the various points of interest is the claim that infants are capable of representing numerosity (i.e., an abstract property of collections of objects and events). This is an important claim in that it presumes the presence of an innate architecture for the domain of number. Consistent with the nativist's position (Landau, 1998), Case postulated that the human mind is predisposed to interpret the world in terms of certain categories such as language, number, and space. For the category of number, several researchers have proposed innate capabilities that support numeracy in humans (Ansari, Price, & Holloway, this volume; Dehaene, 1997, 2007; Gallistel & Gelman, 1992; Starkey, Spelke, & Gelman, 1990). This seemingly neo-Kantian perspective sees human infants coming to the world with dedicated brain circuits to detect fundamental features of the quantitative world, with numerosity being one important property.

Evidence in support of this position comes from studies on infants' and neonates' ability to discriminate between small sets of items (Antell & Keating, 1983; Starkey & Cooper, 1980; Strauss & Curtis, 1981) as well as infants' ability to detect numerical correspondences in different sensory modalities (e.g., between visual and auditory presentations of numbers; Starkey, Spelke & Gelman, 1983, 1990). Discrimination studies are typically conducted in two phases. In the first phase, infants are shown the same number of dots repeatedly (typically up to 3 dots) until they are habituated to the same stimulus – that is, until they show little interest in the display. In the second phase, they are shown a display with a different number of dots. If infants show renewed interest, this is taken as evidence that they notice changes in numerosity. It is important to point out that, in these studies, dots are shown in different configurations. If infants are attending to how the dots are arranged on each display, then they should treat each display as new and therefore find it interesting. The results, however, demonstrated that infants showed renewed interest when the number of dots was different regardless of their configurations. Infants as early as the first week of life have been reported to behave in this manner, at least for small sets of items (Antell & Keating). In the study of infants' sensitivity to numerical correspondence across different sensory modalities, Starkey et al. (1983, 1990) reported that infants, when listening to a specific number of drumbeats, looked longer at a display of dots that matched the number of drumbeats. Furthermore, infants were shown to abstract numerosity in a puppet's jumps (Wynn, 1996) as well as to respond to numerical transformations such as addition and subtraction (Wynn, 1992). Taken together, these studies suggest that, for at least small numbers of up to three items, infants attend to numerical features of stimuli and are able to represent numerosity in some way.

Subsequent studies, however, questioned whether infants were indeed responding to numerosity as claimed in earlier studies. Mix and colleagues (Clearfield & Mix, 1999; Mix, Huttenlocher, & Levine, 2002; Mix, Levine, & Huttenlocher, 1997), for example, argued that previous studies confounded numerosity with other continuous variables (e.g., contour length, surface area, and volume). Infants therefore responded not to changes in numerosity but to changes in the total amount of "stuff" in the display. In one study, Clearfield and Mix presented infants with a set of displays of squares that differed in either number or in total perimeter (i.e., contour length). Infants were first habituated to either two or three squares. They were then shown a series of displays that alternated between changes in numerosity or in contour length. Looking times between the last habituation trial and the first test trial were compared. The results indicated that infants looked longer at the test display that differed in contour length than in numerosity. Other experiments also confirmed that infants were more responsive to continuous variables than to numerosity when numerosity is contrasted against continuous variables (Feigenson, Carey, & Spelke, 2002). These findings suggest that infants are able to discriminate between two small sets of items, but that this understanding is overridden when numerosity is pitted against continuous variables.

In yet another set of complicating findings, 6-month-old infants were successful in discriminating between two larger sets of items that differ in ratio of 1:2.[1] Xu and colleagues found that 6-month-olds discriminated between 8 versus 16 dots (Xu & Spelke, 2000) and 16 versus 32 dots (Xu, Spelke, & Goddard, 2005). In these studies, other continuous variables such as total array size, volume of dots, and density of dots were controlled for. Furthermore, infants at 6 months were found to successfully discriminate between two sequences of a puppet's jumps such as 4 and 8 jumps (Wood & Spelke, 2005). Infants' representations, however, are imprecise. Six-month-old infants failed to discriminate between 2 and 4 dots (Xu, 2003); 2 and

[1] This is in accord with Weber's Law that states that discriminability of two quantities is a function of their ratio.

4 jump sequences (Wood & Spelke); and two sets of dots whose ratio is smaller than 1:2 (Xu, Spelke, & Goddard). In sum, these studies paint a picture of an infant who is able to represent and discriminate between (a) two small numerosities and (b) two large numerosities that differ in ratio of 1:2,[2] as long as other continuous variables are controlled for.

What kind of theory can account for these seemingly conflicting findings? Some have argued that infants have access to two systems of numerical representations: an object-file system[3] for keeping track of a small number of up to three items and an analog-magnitude system for estimating large numbers (Feigenson & Carey, 2005; Feigenson, Carey, & Hauser, 2002; Feigenson, Carey, & Spelke, 2002). Using the object-file system, human infants are hypothesized to represent items as distinct symbols (or files) and do so competently for up to three object files at a time.[4] Object files that correspond to one set of items or events are represented and stored in working memory. Numerical equivalence is determined by comparing this representation to a visible set or another set in working memory in a one-to-one fashion (Simon, 1997; Uller, Huntley-Fenner, Carey, & Klatt, 1999; Vogel, Woodman, & Luck, 2001). That is, a set of items is represented as symbols to stand for individual items or events in the world, not as a numerical cardinality (Le Corre & Carey, 2007). The object-file system can explain why infants are able to represent up to three items or events and compare two sets. It can also explain why they fail to compare sets of two and four items, because the object-file system does not keep track of cardinalities. It simply creates working memory symbols corresponding to up to three individuals. Most researchers agree that this system has a hard capacity limit of three working memory symbols and therefore fails to function when more individual items are to be represented.[5] Infants' success on large-number discrimination (e.g., 4 versus 8) as well as comparisons of continuous amount is explained not in terms of their ability to represent object files, but rather by their ability to represent approximate magnitudes. These two mechanisms of representations parallel what Feigenson, Dehaene, and Spelke (2004) called the core systems of number. The core systems of number allow infants to create discrete symbols to stand for up to three individual items or events as well as to represent large, approximate numerical magnitudes.

If evolution provided human infants with a predisposition to attend to numerical attributes of the world both as object files and analog magnitudes, it is reasonable to expect neurobiological evidence in the organization of the human brain that corresponds to these two ways for conceiving of number. Brain research has long imputed the parietal cortex as a potential region responsible for a domain-specific

---

[2] Infants' precision improves. The ratio of success at 9 months is 2:3 (e.g., Lipton & Spelke, 2003).

[3] Carey and colleagues refer to this system of representation as "parallel individuation."

[4] Macaque monkeys are able to track up to four items (e.g., Hauser, Carey, & Hauser, 2000).

[5] Ross-Sheehy, Oakes, and Luck (2003) reported that infants were able to hold four units.

representation of numbers (Dehaene & Cohen, 1995). The parietal lobes, however, respond to verbal, spatial, and attentional stimuli as well as numbers. Just pointing to the parietal area as a whole is far too broad to locate the tangible substrate of the brain that may be responsible for the two core systems of number. Recent studies of neuroimaging are beginning to identify subregions within the parietal area that are associated with number-related processes (Dehaene, Piazza, Pine, & Cohen, 2003). Based on the review of neuroimaging studies, Dehaene et al. proposed that three circuits in the parietal area may be responsible for different types of numerical processing: the horizontal segment of the bilateral intraparietal sulcus (HIPS) for quantity processing; the left angular gyrus region for verbal processing of number; and the posterior superior parietal region for spatial and attentional orientation of number processing.

Of the three circuits, the HIPS is a major site of activation in neuroimaging studies of number processing and appears to hold an amodal and language-independent semantic representation of symbolic and non-symoblic quantity (Brannon, 2006; Dehaene, Molko, Cohen, & Wilson, 2004). For example, Dehaene, Spelke, Stanescu, Pinel, and Tsivkin (1999) found that the HIPS area was more active when participants tended to approximate numerical calculations than when they computed exact arithmetic operations. This area was also found to be more active when comparing numerical magnitudes than reading numbers (Chochon, Cohen, van de Moortele, & Dehaene, 1999). More recently, Ansari, Dhital, and Siong (2006) found evidence that this region was involved in numerical magnitude discrimination, as opposed to area discrimination. Parallel findings come from the studies of other animals. Nieder, Freedman, and Miller (2002), for example, found neuronal firing in the prefrontal cortex of two macaque monkeys in which neurons were tuned to approximate numerosity. Taken together, these studies provide compelling evidence for neuronal underpinnings of one of the core systems of number, that is, the analog-magnitude system (for detailed discussion of neuroimaging studies of developmental changes in magnitude comparison, see Ansari, Price, & Holloway, this volume). Although neural bases for the object-file system are less clear (Feigenson, Dehaene, & Spelke, 2004), continued progress in behavioral and neuroimaging studies may unpack the biological bases of core systems of number and how such systems give rise to the development of numerical knowledge that enables one to interpret cultural systems of complex mathematics (e.g., Ansari, Lyons, van Eimeren, & Xu, 2007; Le Corre & Carey, 2007).

Essential Schemas of Counting and Global Quantity in Early Childhood

Because access to infants' brains is limited, the notion of the core systems of number currently stands as a hypothesis. Yet, this is an exciting idea. It not only explains seemingly conflicting empirical evidence, but also provides building blocks for explaining later development of numerical knowledge. As discussed earlier,

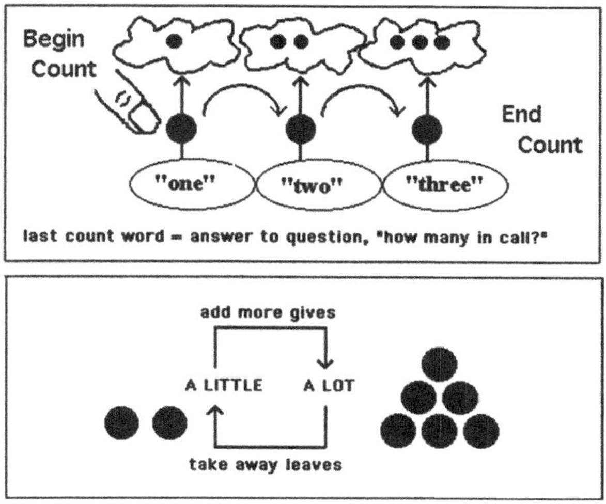

Fig. 1 Essential schemas of counting and global quantity 4-year-old children are hypothesized to develop. *Top* shows the counting schema. *Bottom* shows the global quantity schema

Case's formulation of a central conceptual structure in a domain is dependent on an integration of two essential schemas. In the domain of number, the two essential schemas are those of *counting* (e.g., Gelman & Gallistel, 1978) and *global quantity* (e.g., Starkey, 1992). Prototypes of these schemas are depicted in Fig. 1. The schemas of counting and global quantity are also described, respectively, as being "digital and sequential" and "spatial and analogic" in nature. There appears to be a parallel between the *core systems of number* – the object-file system and the analog-magnitude system – and the *essential schemas* for the domain of number – the counting schema and the global quantity schema, respectively. It is plausible that the core systems of number available to infants serve as a vehicle to shape the development of the counting and global quantity schemas. This does not necessarily imply that the core systems of number themselves evolve to become the essential schemas.[6] I argue, instead, that the core systems of number assist infants to process numerical information around them and to guide the development of the counting and global quantity schemas. Le Corre and Carey (2007) made a similar argument in that core systems of knowledge provide the cognitive primitives that support learning in childhood. They further articulate a precise mechanism in which the core systems of numerical knowledge guide the development of the verbal counting principles that are the core constitutes of the essential counting schema.

As complex as the counting and global quantity schemas may be, these schemas are yet inadequate in dealing with a cultural system of mathematics. Children

[6] There is evidence that older children and adults use an analog magnitude system to assess numerical magnitudes when prevented from counting (see, for example, Barth, Kanwisher, & Spelke, 2003).

directly or indirectly experience mathematical ideas on a daily basis. The acquisition of number words and the mapping of these words to to-be-enumerated items are some of the early cultural activities that young children in industrial nations are encouraged to master. This requires some readjustment of the way numbers and quantities are represented. At the level of neurons and synaptic connections, this means that "postnatal design-fixing" (Dennett, 1991) is taking place in order to respond to particular stimuli presented to children. That is, practices valued in a culture are transmitted into the brain repeatedly and corresponding connections become stronger. This, in turn, results in neural networks that are organized in a way to respond to cultural expectations. Cultural and environmental inputs therefore guide the development of the brain and this is particularly important in the first years of life (Nelson, Zeanah, Fox, Romer, & Walker, 2007; Scherf, Behrmann, Humphreys, & Luna, 2007; Wexler, 2006). In preparing children who can take advantage of mathematical ideas later in life, it is crucial that young children have optimal opportunities to develop number sense in everyday life. The counting and global quantity schemas are two such schemas that result from young children's attempts to make sense of the world. In a sense, these schemas can be thought of as the product of centuries of cultural development structuring the postnatal brain in the first few years of life.

Children in most industrial societies acquire the schemas of counting and global quantity typically by 4 years of age. This is by no means an automatic accomplishment. In cultures where the language of numbers is either absent or reduced, the counting schema of the sort described above does not seem to develop. For example, the Pirahã, who reside along the banks of the Maici River in the Lowland Amazonia region of Brazil, have a limited set of words to describe quantities: "hói," "hoí," and "baagi" or "aibai." These words roughly correspond to *one, two,* and *many*, respectively. When adult informants were asked to construct sets of items familiar to them that matched example sets in number, their performance was perfect for the set sizes of one and two but not for larger set sizes (Gordon, 2004).

Speakers of another language that has limited words for numbers also took part in a similar study (Pica, Lemer, Izard, & Dehaene, 2004). The Mundurukú, who live in an autonomous territory in the Parã state of Brazil, have words that roughly correspond to numerical values of 1 through 5, with no apparent verbal counting system. When Mundurukú children and adults were shown displays of 1–15 dots and asked to state the cardinal value of each set in their native language, they were not always consistent in applying the tags for particular cardinal values shown to them. Their responses tended to be more accurate for set sizes of four and fewer, but not for larger set sizes. In the absence of cultural demands for enumeration skills, the essential schemas of counting and quantity evaluation do not appear to fully develop, and enumeration is limited to the number of "files" available in the object-file system. When the Mundurukú were asked to estimate relative magnitudes of large set sizes, their success was similar to those found in other cultures (that is, accuracy increased as the ratio between the two sets increased). The core systems of number to represent up to three items as well as to compare numerical magnitudes of just-noticeable differences appear to be universal systems, whereas the essential schemas of counting and global quantity do not.

Central Numerical Understanding in Middle Childhood

In Case's theory of numerical development, a central numerical structure results from an integration of the essential schemas of counting and global quantity that takes place in the preschool years (Case & Griffin, 1989; Case & Okamoto, 1996; Case & Sandieson, 1988). During these years, children exhibit tremendous growth in many areas. They grow physically larger and stronger with development in fine and gross motor skills. Selective pruning of brain cells, which began during prenatal development, continues to take place. This process contributes to the shaping and reshaping of the soft wiring of the brain.[7] Children's vocabulary increases to about 3000 words by age 5. All these developments take place in children's social and cultural contexts. Children's developing understanding of number is not an isolated matter. As they improve their fine motor skills, for example, they are better able to coordinate the act of pointing to objects with the sequence of number words that their culture provided to them. Yet, progress in the number domain at times seems slow, especially in comparison to vocabulary development. When asked to identify which side of the balance scale would tilt, for example, preschoolers often rely on visual cues, as opposed to counting, to arrive at an answer (Case & Okamoto). This is in spite of the fact that they can count a small set of objects accurately. It appears that preschoolers have yet to understand the significance of counting in quantitative comparisons. They may not realize counting is a more reliable strategy than visual inspection when comparing two sets (Case & Okamoto; Saxe, 1977; Sophian, 1987, 1988).

Children in most industrial societies with schooling typically complete the integration of the counting and global quantity schemas by around 6 years of age. This integration results in an initial form of a central numerical structure that provides a conceptual foundation through which children interpret the numerical attributes of the world. At the same time, this structure by itself serves as a tool to create new knowledge. That is, building conceptual models is necessary for interpreting cultural concepts of telling time, currency system, and distribution of resources, as well as for taking advantage of instruction in school.

Case referred to this initial central numerical structure as a "mental number line" (Case, 1996). Although this structure implies that numerical thinking can be extended much beyond 5 on the number line, it is unlikely that children 6–7 years of age would be successful in comprehending numbers much greater than 10. Studies on numerical estimation provide support for this speculation (Pettito, 1990; Rittle-Johnson, Siegler, & Alibali, 2001; Siegler & Booth, 2004; Siegler & Opfer, 2003). Siegler and Booth, for example, asked children in kindergarten and first and second grades to indicate where a particular number would fall on a number line extending from 0 to 100. They found that kindergartners' performance was better described as logarithmic whereas second graders' performance was linear. That is, the distance between any two adjacent large numbers was much smaller than the

[7]Due to neural plasticity, neural connections may be altered reflecting life experiences.

distance between any two adjacent small numbers in younger children's responses, whereas older children's performance showed that the distance between any two adjacent numbers was similar across the range of numbers. These findings suggest that kindergartners' grasp of whole numbers has yet to become a number-line like structure.

I have argued that Case's initial central numerical structure assembled by children around 6 years of age should be better characterized as a "mental objects line" as opposed to a "mental number line" (Okamoto, 1996). In this reformulation of the central numerical structure, real world objects are represented as mental objects on a single dimension. Kindergarten and first-grade children therefore no longer need to rely on concrete objects to carry out arithmetic operations. Instead, they are able to treat mental objects as objects of manipulation – much like the way they have acted upon concrete objects. This representational system, however, is not a precise science. Mental objects are similar to mental tokens that stand for objects with no standardized size or measurement. This system also has limits in terms of a maximum number of mental objects a child is able to represent as well as a number of operations a child is capable of carrying out at any one time. A small number of mental objects is represented more accurately than a large number of mental objects; single-step addition or subtraction problems tend to result in more accurate results than multiple-step problems. Large numbers pose problems and may be represented as indeterminate "big numbers." This may be part of the reason why logarithmic functions can better account for kindergartners' and first graders' representations of whole numbers to 100.

As children gain more and varied experiences with numbers in and out of school, their central numerical structure develops from a mental objects line to a mental number line. By about 8 years of age, children's mastery of the mental number line becomes sufficiently fluent, allowing them to focus on, and tentatively begin relating, two mental number lines. As a result, new properties of numerical systems such as the base-10 system become part of their understanding (although limited to interpreting the relation between ones and tens columns). As shown in Siegler and Booth's (2004) study, second graders (close to 8 years old) have a good grasp of whole numbers that extend to nearly 100. When asked to indicate numerical magnitudes on a 0–1000 number line, however, they generated patterns fitting a logarithmic, not linear, function (Siegler & Opfer, 2003). That is, 8-year-olds understand the relation of ones to tens columns but not to hundreds column. These findings suggest that 8-year-old children's central numerical structure with two number lines does a good job of characterizing conceptual underpinnings that they possess.

It is not until about 10 years of age when an elaborate dual number-line structure develops. In this new conceptual structure, numerical relations have explicit, functional rules. That is, the numerical rules and operations developed earlier now become objects of manipulations to carry out complex arithmetic reasoning. With this new structure, 10-year-olds grasp rules of the base-10 system that extends beyond 99. The data from Opfer and Siegler's (2007) estimation study support this speculation. They found that fourth graders (10-year-olds) estimated numbers from 0 to 1000 accurately in a linear fashion. Taken together, Case's theory of central numerical structures, with a slight revision to the initial form of the structure, appears to hold good exploratory power for children's numerical thinking from about $5\frac{1}{2}$ to 10 years of age.

Having developed an elaborate dual number-line structure, children by 10 years of age have a conceptual tool to tackle many challenging mathematical problems involving whole numbers. This system, however, is far from ideal in dealing with other types of mathematical problems such as fractions and proportions. To capture the development of numerical understanding in middle childhood and beyond, Moss and Case (1999) proposed a developmental model of rational number understanding. Briefly, an in-depth and flexible understanding of rational numbers is hypothesized to develop out of two essential schemas – a schema for halving and doubling and a schema for global proportionality. Much like the essential schemas of counting and global quantity for whole numbers, Moss and Case described the halving and doubling schema as being digital and sequential, and the global proportionality schema as being spatial and analogic in nature. Another resemblance is the developmental progression of rational number understanding. They postulated that these schemas at first develop in isolation, typically by about 10 years of age, but are integrated to become the initial form of a central rational number structure. This rational number structure is presumed to go through a similar progression of differentiation and integration that completes the developmental cycle with an elaborate conceptual system to understand a full range of rational numbers (Kalchman, Moss, & Case, 2001). Although the link between central rational number development and earlier work on preschoolers' understandings of partitioning (e.g., Hunting & Sharpley, 1988) and proportional reasoning (e.g., Goswami, 1995) is unclear, this notion has proven useful in designing instructional programs to teach rational numbers for children in middle grades and beyond (Kalchman, Moss, & Case; Moss, 2005).

Central Numerical Structures, Mathematics Achievement, and Cultural Influences

In Case's theory of central conceptual structures, parallel developmental progression of central structures takes place in different domains of knowledge, such as whole numbers and rational numbers on the one hand and spatial and social/narrative knowledge on the other hand (Case & Okamoto, 1996; Kalchman, Moss, & Case, 2001). A question one might ask is how "central" a central conceptual structure is to children's thinking in each domain. In the domain of whole numbers, a central numerical structure is hypothesized to provide a foundation on which to build conceptual models to interpret cultural notions involving numbers such as telling time, money knowledge, and distribution of resources. It follows then that (1) change in central numerical understanding should result in change in performance on a broad range of specific tasks for which no training is provided and (2) mastery of a subset of specific tasks – including the content of typical school mathematics – should not result in advancement of central numerical structures.

A series of instructional studies conducted by Case and colleagues provide empirical evidence in support of the first claim. As often reported, many children encounter difficulty learning school mathematics (e.g., Jordan, Kaplan, Olah, & Locuniak, 2006). Some suspect that nearly one third of children have mathematics difficulties (e.g., Jordan, Hanich, & Kaplan, 2003). To assist kindergartners who are already behind their peers in mathematics performance, Case and colleagues designed and implemented a mathematical instructional program (Case, Griffin, & Capodilupo, 1995; Griffin & Case, 1996; Griffin, Case, & Siegler, 1994). These children were identified as not having consolidated the counting and global quantity schemas to form the initial central numerical structure. The instructional program consisted of activities that were designed to strengthen the core constituents that make up the initial central numerical structure. For example, kindergartners may play a game to figure out how many more to reach 10 when drawing a card that has one of the numbers from 1 to 9 written on it. The program was successful in helping children develop an age-appropriate central numerical structure. More important to the current thesis is that these children outperformed control children on a range of tasks, such as balance scale and money knowledge, on which they received no training. Furthermore, children's mathematics performance improved immediately following the program participation as well as 1 year later. These results support the claim that at least the acquisition of the initial central numerical structure results in improved performance on a range of specific tasks, including the content of school mathematics typical of this age group.

The second claim was that mastery of a subset of specific tasks would not result in improved central numerical structures. In support of this claim, I present cross-national comparison data on children's mathematics achievement and central numerical understanding. Children for this comparison came from middle- to upper-middle-class families in Japan and the United States (Okamoto, Case, Bleiker, & Henderson, 1996). We chose to compare these two groups of children because Japanese children in the past have fared well in mathematics among children of other high-achieving nations whereas their US counterparts performed in the middle range of achievement (Mullis, Martin, Gonzalez, & Chrostowski, 2005; Mullis, et al., 2000; Stevenson, Lee, & Stigler, 1986). We used an abbreviated version of the fifth-grade test constructed by Stevenson and his colleagues (Stevenson, Lee, & Stigler) as a measure of school mathematics achievement. Case's number knowledge and balance scale tests were used as measures of central numerical understanding. Although achievement comparison was limited to fifth graders (about 11 years old), we found a large difference in favor of Japanese children; we assumed that this difference in mathematics achievement was no coincidence and would hold up at any grade level within the same schools.

Based on this assumption, we next compared 6-, 8-, and 10-year-old children's performance on measures of central numerical understanding. The results showed only one significant group difference on the number knowledge test in favor of

Table 1 Means (standard deviations) for the number knowledge test by national group, achievement level, and age

United States						Japan		
Middle			High			High		
Age	*N*	Mean	Age	*N*	Mean	Age	*N*	Mean
6–4	22	1.82 (.31)	6–0	25	1.69 (.43)	6–5	21	2.52 (.73)
8–1	23	3.04 (.31)	8–1	26	3.12 (.53)	8–5	26	3.33 (.77)
10–5	24	4.23 (.68)	10–2	20	3.79 (.55)	10–5	20	4.05 (.76)

Note. Expected mean scores are 2, 3, and 4 for 6-, 8-, and 10-year-old groups, respectively.

Japanese 6-year-olds (see Table 1 for the US middle achievement and Japan high achievement comparison). US and Japanese children who differed in their mastery of school mathematics content did not differ in the levels of central numerical understanding. In fact, both groups of children developed age-appropriate central numerical structures. Subsequently, we collected additional data from American children who attended a school well known for its rigorous curriculum and high achievement in mathematics (Okamoto, Curtis, Chen, Kim, & Karayan, 1997). These children's development of central numerical structures was similar to that of their American counterparts in the middle achievement range as well as that of their Japanese counterparts (Table 1). These data show high-achieving American and Japanese students were not different from average-achieving American peers in central numerical development.

Findings from the instructional and cross-national studies together suggest that age-appropriate levels of central conceptual structures are necessary for the mastery of particular numerical skills and concepts emphasized in mathematics instruction. However, mastery of mathematics curriculum does not advance central numerical thinking. Instead, mathematics instruction in school provides a subset of skills to which central numerical understanding applies. An important finding from cross-national studies is that we observed cross-cultural similarities in the conceptual development of number regardless of achievement differences.

Although large-scale international comparisons of mathematics achievement report mean score differences among various nations, this does not mean that individual children cannot excel in mathematics. Our data from the second US sample showed that children attending a school that emphasized mathematics indeed performed well in mathematics. As Ericsson and colleagues (Ericsson, 2003; Ericsson, Krampe, & Tesch-Romer, 1993; Ericsson, Nandagopal, & Roring, 2005) argued, the amount of "deliberate practice" may be the key to mastery of particular skills and concepts. This is most noticeable in individual cases but could be seen at the school level (as in our second US sample) as well as at the level of cultural or national groups. With age-appropriate central numerical structures in place, the levels of expertise children reach seem to depend on the quality and quantity of practice for skills and concepts deemed important by individuals or cultural groups. Repeated experiences with a particular set of tasks in a domain are likely to result in improved performance of those tasks; repeated exposure to those tasks in and of themselves, however, is unlikely to influence the rate of development of general cognitive structures.

An Eye Toward the Future

The emerging view of numerical development identified in this chapter begins with infants whose brain organization reflects the work of human evolution, directing their attention to numerical features of the world. Recent evidence from psychological and neuropsychological research, albeit limited, suggests that this initial organization of the brain includes at least two representational systems of number – one to represent up to three objects and another to estimate numerical magnitudes. These representational systems provide a basis for developing essential schemas for counting and global quantity. I have argued that these schemas, as well as central numerical structures, do not develop as a result of maturation alone. That is, they are not part of an innate developmental sequence. Rather, the development of essential schemas and central numerical structures is a result of postnatal design-fixing, necessitated by cultural demands for numerical skills. Central numerical structures, as well as essential schemas, develop under optimal physiological and cultural circumstances. A limited emphasis on particular skills alone would not result in advanced central numerical thinking. Cross-national data presented in this chapter support this assertion. In sum, this view of numerical development is a result of my attempt to revise Case's theory, putting more emphasis on the importance of innate endowment and cultural practices.

In looking ahead, recent breakthroughs in brain research promise to enrich our current understandings of numerical development. Several clear paths have been made in neuropsychological research that monitors neural activities while performing different types of numerical tasks. For example, a synthesis of recent neuroimaging studies suggests that three specific areas of the parietal lobes are responsible for number processing (Dehaene, Piazza, Pine, & Cohen, 2003). As discussed earlier, the primary area known as the HIPS responds to processing quantity or numerical magnitudes that, depending on the types of numerical activity, may call upon resources from two other areas that process numerical information in visual or verbal form. Although more research is needed to substantiate this hypothesis, it is exciting to find neurobiological evidence in support of the analog-magnitude system. It is also intriguing to consider the relation of the "three separate circuits" hypothesis to a recent proposal that there are three representational systems of number available to preverbal infants (e.g., Le Corre & Carey, 2007). This proposal extends the earlier notion of the core systems of knowledge that attributed two systems of numerical representations – the analog-magnitude and object-file systems – available to preverbal infants. Carey and colleagues retained the analog-magnitude system as well as the object-file system (though it is termed "parallel individuation"), but included the third representational system of set-based quantification. The claim is that the verbal counting principles are acquired by mapping verbal count words onto the system that draws resources from the individuation and set-based quantification systems. How these two proposals come together to explain the postnatal design-fixing for numerical cognition is a potential direction for future research.

Another potentially interesting direction in neuropsychological research pertains to the recent discovery of "mirror neurons." Mirror neurons were first discovered to exist in the frontal lobes of macaques – more specifically in different parts of F5 (Arbib, 2006). Studies showed that the monkey responds to the experimenter's action not by overt imitation but with the neural activity in mirror neurons as if the monkey were simulating that action. Furthermore, mirror neurons respond selectively to intentional or goal-directed action. Comparable data have been gathered from humans using fMRI during action perception tasks. These data show that observing finger movements (Iacoboni, et al., 1999), hand signs (Nakamura et al., 2004), and pantomimes (Johnson-Frey, Newman-Norlund, & Grafton, 2005) all recruited a fronto-parietal network involving the posterior inferior frontal gyrus and adjacent ventral premotor cortex, as well as the inferior parietal cortex.

Although I am not aware of any work that directly links mirror neurons to numerical knowledge to date, mirror neurons have been implicated to underlie the brain mechanisms that support imitation, empathy, language, as well as musical perception (Arbib, 2006; Greenfield, 2006; Iacoboni, 2005; Molnar-Szakacs & Overy, 2006). It would be interesting if developmental theories of numerical thinking could be connected with research on mirror neurons. Most important for numerical thinking is the idea that there is a neural basis for developing shared understanding of actions. Recent research examining the neural bases of cross-cultural social communication suggests that the mirror neuron system is involved in responding to a culturally learned motor repertoire, in particular, culturally meaningful actions used in social communication (Molnar-Szakacs, Wu, Robles, & Iacoboni, 2007). Mature understanding of numbers involves mastery of culturally shared meaning and practice. Preschool children acquire numerical knowledge from participating in and observing actions of sharing, dividing, estimating, and counting. Children during snack time at preschool, for example, learn equal sharing of crackers by assisting teachers in carrying out the task. In playing a numerical board game, mothers help their children, who are trying to advance the game piece, by counting aloud and pointing to each space (Bates, Okamoto, & Romo, 2009). All of these numerical activities must be understood mutually among the participants. This may be made possible because human brains have the neurons that respond to actions of others. All of this, however, is only speculation at this point. Yet, there appears to be fertile ground for connecting what we know about the development of numerosity in behavioral, psychological, and neuroscientific research.

Acknowledgments I thank Marion Porath, Michel Ferrari, Ljiljana Vuleti, Gregory Jarrett, and John Jabagchourian for their helpful comments on earlier versions of this manuscript.

References

Ansari, D., Dhital, B., & Siong, S. C. (2006). Parametric effects of numerical distance on the intraparietal sulcus during passing viewing of rapid numerosity changes. *Bran Research, 1067*, 181–188.

Ansari, D., Lyons, I., van Eimeren, L., & Xu, F. (2007). Linking visual attention and number processing in the brain: The role of temporo-parietal junction in small and large non-symbolic number comparison. *Journal of Cognitive Neuroscience, 19*, 1845–1853.

Arbib, M. A. (2006). The mirror system hypothesis on the linkage of action and languages. In M. A. Arbib (Ed.), *Action to language via the mirror neuron system* (pp. 3–47). Cambridge, UK: Cambridge University Press.

Antell, S. E., & Keating, L. E. (1983). Perception of numerical invariance by neonates. *Child Development, 54*, 695–701.

Barth, H., Kanwisher, N., & Spelke, E. (2003). The construction of large number representations in adults. *Cognition, 86*, 201–221.

Bates, A., Okamoto, Y., & Romo, L. (2009). *Counting on mom: Maternal explanations to young children about numerical quantity comparison.* Manuscript submitted for publication.

Brannon, E. M. (2006). The representation of numerical magnitude. *Current Opinion in Neurobiology, 16*, 222–229.

Case, R. (1985). *Intellectual development: Birth to adulthood.* New York: Academic Press.

Case, R. (1992a). The role of the frontal lobes in the regulation of cognitive development. *Brain and cognition, 20*, 51–73.

Case, R. (1992b). *The mind's staircase: Exploring the conceptual underpinnings of children's thought and knowledge.* Hillsdale, NJ: Erlbaum.

Case, R. (1996).Introduction: Reconceptualizing the nature of children's conceptual structures and their development in middle childhood. In R. Case & Y. Okamoto (Eds.), *The role of central conceptual structures in the development of children's thought. Monographs of the Society for Research in Child Development, 61* (1-2, Serial No. 246), 1–26.

Case, R. (1998). The development of conceptual structures. In D. Kuhn & R. S. Siegler (Eds.), Handbook of child psychology: Volume 2: Cognition, perception, and language (pp. 745–800). Hoboken, NJ: John Wiley & Sons Inc.

Case, R., & Griffin, S. (1989). Child cognitive development: The role of central conceptual structure in the development of scientific and social thought. In C. A. Haver (Ed.), *Advances in psychology: Developmental psychology* (pp. 193–230). North Holland: Elsevier.

Case, R., Griffin, S., & Capodilupo, S. (1995). Teaching for understanding: The importance of central conceptual structures in the elementary school mathematics curriculum. In A. McKeough & J. Lupart (Eds.), *Teaching for transfer* (pp.123–152). Hillsdale, NJ: Lawrence Erlbaum Associates.

Case, R., & Okamoto, Y. (1996). The role of central conceptual structures in the development of children's thought. *Monographs of the Society for Research in Child Development, 61*(1-2, Serial No. 246).

Case, R., & Sandieson, R. (1988). A developmental approach to the identification and teaching of central conceptual structures in the middle grades. In J. Hiebert & M. Behr (Eds.), *Research agenda in mathematics education: Number concepts and operations in the middle grades* (pp. 236–270). Hillsdale, NJ: Lawrence Erlbaum Associates.

Clearfield, M. W., & Mix, K. S. (1999). Number versus contour length in infants' discrimination of small visual sets. *Psychological Science, 10*, 408–411.

Chochon, F., Cohen, L., van de Moortele, P. F., & Dehaene, S. (1999). Differential contributions of the left and right inferior parietal lobules to number processing. *Journal of Cognitive Neuroscience, 11*, 617–630.

Dehaene, S. (1997). *The number sense.* New York: Oxford University Press.

Dehaene, S., & Cohen, L. (1995). Towards an anatomical and functional model of number processing. *Mathematical Cognition, 1*, 83–120.

Dehaene, S., Molko, N., Cohen, L., & Wilson, A. J. (2004). Arithmetic and the brain. *Current Opinion in Neurobiology, 14,* 218–224.
Dehaene, S., Piazza, M., Pinel, P., & Cohen, L. (2003). Three parietal circuits for number processing. *Cognitive Neuropsychology, 20,* 487–506.
Dehaene, S., Spelke, E., Stanescu, R., Pinel, P., & Tsivkin, S. (1999). Sources of mathematical thinking: Behavioral and brain-imaging evidence. *Science, 284,* 970–974.
Dennett, D. C. (1991). *Consciousness explained.* Boston, MA: Little, Brown and Company.
Ericsson, K. A. (2003). The search for general abilities and basic capacities: Theoretical implications from the modifiability and complexity of mechanisms mediating expert performance. In R. J. Sternberg & E. L. Grigorenko (Eds.), *Perspectives on the psychology of abilities, competencies, and expertise* (pp. 93–125). Cambridge, England: Cambridge University Press.
Ericsson, K. A., Krampe, R. T., & Tesch-Romer, C. (1993). The role of deliberate practice in the acquisition of expert performance. *Psychological Review, 100,* 363–406.
Ericsson, K. A., Nandagopal, K., & Roring, R. W. (2005). Giftedness viewed from the expert performance perspective. *Journal for the Education of the Gifted, 8,* 287–311.
Feigenson, L., & Carey, S. (2005). On the limits of infants' quantification of small object arrays. *Cognition, 97,* B13–B23.
Feigenson, L., Carey, S., & Hauser, M. D. (2002). The representations underlying infants' choice of more: Object files versus analog magnitudes. *Psychological Science, 13,* 150–156.
Feigenson, L., Carey, S., & Spelke, E. (2002). Infants' discrimination of number vs. continuous extent. *Cognitive Psychology, 44,* 33–66.
Feigenson, L., Dehaene, S., & Spelke, E. (2004). Core systems of number. *Trends in Cognitive Sciences, 8,* 307–314.
Gallistel, C. R., & Gelman, R. (1992). Preverbal and verbal counting and computation. *Cognition, 44,* 43–74.
Gelman, R., & Gallistel, C. R. (1978). *The child's understanding of number.* Cambridge, MA: Harvard University Press.
Gordon, P. (2004). Numerical cognition without words: Evidence from Amazonia. *Science, 306,* 496–499.
Goswami, U. (1995). Transitive relational mappings in three-and four-year-olds: The analogy of goldilocks and the three bears. *Child Development, 66,* 877–892.
Greenfield, P. (2006). Implications of mirror neurons for the ontogeny and phylogeny of cultural processes: The examples of tools and language. In M. A. Arbib (Ed.), *Action to language via the mirror neuron system* (pp. 501–533). Cambridge, UK: Cambridge University Press.
Griffin, S., & Case, R. (1996). Evaluating the breadth and depth of training effects when central conceptual structures are taught. In R. Case & Y. Okamoto (Eds.), *The role of central conceptual structures in the development of children's thought. Monographs of the Society for Research in Child Development, 61* (1-2, Serial No. 246), 83–102.
Griffin, S., Case, R., & Siegler, R. (1994). Rightstart: Providing the central conceptual prerequisites for first formal learning of arithmetic to students at risk for school failure. In K. McGilly (Ed.), *Classroom lessons: Integrating cognitive theory and classroom practice* (pp. 25–49). Cambridge, MA: MIT Press.
Hauser, M. D., Carey, S., & Hauser, L. B. (2000). Spontaneous number representation in semifree-ranging rhesus monkeys. *Proceedings of the Royal Society of London: Biological Sciences, 267,* 829–833.
Hunting, R. P., & Sharpley, C. F. (1988). Fraction knowledge in preschool children. *Journal for Research in Mathematics Education, 19,* 175–180.
Iacoboni, M. (2005). Understanding others: Imitation, language, empathy. In S. Hurley & N. Chater (Eds.), *Perspectives on imitation: From cognitive neuroscience to social science* (pp. 77–99). Cambridge, MA: MIT Press.
Iacoboni, M., Woods, P. R., Brass, M., Bekkering, H., Mazziotta, J. C., & Rizzolatti, G. (1999). Cortical mechanisms of human imitation. *Science, 286,* 2526–2528.
Johnson-Frey, S. H., Newman-Norlund, R., & Grafton, S. T. (2005). A distributed left hemisphere network active during planning of everyday tool use skills. *Cerebral Cortex, 15,* 681–695.

Jordan, N. C., Hanich, L. B., & Kaplan, D. (2003). A longitudinal study of mathematical competencies in children with specific mathematics difficulties versus children with comorbid mathematics and reading difficulties. *Child Development, 74*, 834–850.

Jordan, N. C., Kaplan, D., Olah, L. N., & Locuniak, M. N. (2006). Number sense growth in kindergarten: A longitudinal investigation of children at risk for mathematics difficulties. *Child Development, 77*, 153–175.

Kalchman, M., Moss, J., & Case, R. (2001). Psychological models for the development of mathematical understanding: Rational numbers and functions. In S. M. Carver & D. Klahr (Eds.), *Cognition and instruction: Twenty-five years of progress* (pp. 1–38). Hillsdale, NJ: Lawrence Erlbaum Associates.

Landau, B. (1998). Innate knowledge. In W. Bechtel & G. Graham (Eds.), *A companion to cognitive science* (pp. 576–589). Malden, MA: Blackwell Publishers.

Le Corte, M., & Carey, S. (2007). One, two, three, four, nothing more: An investigation of the conceptual sources of the verbal counting principles. *Cognition, 105*, 395–438.

Lipton, J. S., & Spelke, E. S. (2003). Origins of number sense: Large-number discrimination in human infants. *Psychological Science, 14*, 396–401.

Mix, K. S., Levine, S. C., & Huttenlocher, J. (1997). Numerical abstraction in infants: Another look. *Developmental Psychology, 33*, 423–428.

Mix, K. S., Huttenlocher, J., & Levine, S. C. (2002). Multiple cues for quantification in infancy: Is number one of them? *Psychological Bulletin, 128*, 278–294.

Molnar-Szakacs, I., & Overy, K. (2006). Music and mirror neurons: From motion to 'e'motion. *Social Cognitive and Affective Neuroscience, 1*, 235–241.

Molnar-Szakacs, I., Wu, A. D., Robles, F. J., & Iacoboni, M. (2007). Do you see what I mean? Corticospinal excitability during observation of culture- specific gestures. *PLoS ONE* 2(7): e626. doi:10.1371/journal.pone. 0000626.

Moss, J. (2005) Pipes, tubes, and beakers: Teaching rational number. In J. Bransford & S. Donovan (Eds.), *How students learn: Mathematics in the classroom* (pp. 309–350). Washington, DC: National Academies Press.

Moss, J., & Case, R. (1999). Developing children's understanding of rational numbers: A new model and experimental curriculum. *Journal for Research in Mathematics Education, 330*, 122–147.

Mullis, I. V.S., Martin, M. O., Gonzalez, E. J., Gregory, K. D., Garden, R. A., O'Connor, K. M., et al. (2000). *TIMSS 1999 International Mathematics Report: Findings from IEA's Repeat of The Third International Mathematics and Science Study at the Eighth Grade*. Chestnut Hill, MA: TIMSS and PIRLS International Study Center, Boston College.

Mullis, I. V. S., Martin, M. O., Gonzalez, E. J., & Chrostowski, S. J. (2005). *TIMSS 2003 International Mathematics Report: Findings From IEA's Trends in International Mathematics and Science Study at the Fourth and Eighth Grades*. Chestnut Hill, MA: TIMSS and PIRLS International Study Center, Boston College.

Nakamura, A., Maess, B., Knösche, T. R., Gunter, T. C., Bach, P., & Friederici, A. D. (2004). Cooperation of different neuronal systems during hand sign recognition. *Neuroimage, 23*, 25–34.

Nelson, C. A., Zeanah, C. H., Fox, N. A. Romer, D., & Walker, E. F. (2007). The effects of early deprivation on brain-behavioral development: The Bucharest early Intervention project. *Adolescent psychopathology and the developing brain: Integrating brain and prevention science* (pp. 197–215). New York, NY: Oxford University Press.

Nieder, A., Freedman, D. J., & Miller, E. K. (2002). Representation of the quantity of visual items in the primate prefrontal cortex. *Science, 297*, 1708–1711.

Okamoto, Y. (1996). Developing central conceptual understandings in mathematics. *Proceedings of the International Conference on Reform Issues on Teacher Education*, 417–455.

Okamoto, Y., Case, R., Bleiker, C., & Henderson, B. (1996). Cross cultural investigations. In R. Case & Y. Okamoto (Eds.), *The role of central conceptual structures in the development*

of children's thought. Monographs of the Society for Research in Child Development, *61* (1-2, Serial No. 246), 131–155.
Okamoto, Y., Curtis, R., Chen, P. C., Kim, S., & Karayan, S. (1997). *A cross-national comparison of children's intuitive number sense: Its development and relation to formal mathematics learning: Final report.* Submitted to Spencer Foundation.
Opfer, J. E., & Siegler, R. S. (2007). Representational change and children's numerical estimation. *Cognitive Psychology, 55*, 169–195.
Pettito, A. L. (1990). Development of numberline and measurement concepts. *Cognition and Instruction, 7*, 55–78.
Pica, P., Lemer, C., Izard, V., & Dehaene, S. (2004). Exact and approximate arithmetic in an Amazonian indigene group. *Science, 306*, 499–503.
Rittle-Johnson, B., Siegler, R. S., & Alibali, M. W. (2001). Developing conceptual understanding and procedural skill in mathematics: An iterative process. *Journal of Educational Psychology, 93*, 346–362.
Ross-Sheehy, S., Oakes, L., & Luck, S. J. (2003). The development of visual short-term memory capacity in infants. *Child Development, 74*, 1807–1822.
Saxe, G. B. (1977). A developmental analysis of notational counting. *Child Development, 48*, 1512–1520.
Scherf, K. S., Behrmann, M., Humphreys, K., & Luna, B. (2007). Visual category-selectivity for faces, places and objects emerges along different developmental trajectories. *Developmental Science, 10*, F15–F30.
Siegler, R. S. & Booth, J. L. (2004). Development of numerical estimation in young children. *Child Development, 75*, 428–444.
Siegler, R. S., & Opfer, J. (2003). The development of numerical estimation: Evidence for multiple representations of numerical quantity. *Psychological Science, 14*, 237–243.
Simon, T. J. (1997). Reconceptualizing the origins of number knowledge: A non-numerical account. *Cognitive Development, 12*, 349–372.
Sophian, C. (1987). Early developments in children's use of counting to solve quantitative problems. *Cognition and Instruction, 4*, 61–90.
Sophian, C. (1988). Early development in children's understanding of number: Inferences about numerosity and one-to-one correspondence. *Child Development, 59*, 1397–1414.
Starkey, P. (1992). The early development of numerical reasoning. *Cognition, 43*, 93–126.
Starkey, P., & Cooper, R. G. (1980). Perception of numbers by human infants. *Science, 210*, 1033–1035.
Starkey, P., Spelke, E. S., & Gelman, R. (1983). Detection of intermodal numerical correspondences by human infants. *Science, 222*, 179–181.
Starkey, P., Spelke, E. S. & Gelman, R. (1990). Numerical abstraction by human infants. *Cognition, 36*, 97–128.
Stevenson, H. W., Lee, S. Y., & Stigler, J. W. (1986). Mathematics achievement of Chinese, Japanese and American children, *Science, 231*, 693–699.
Strauss, M. S., & Curtis, L. E. (1981). Infant perception of numerosity. *Child Development, 52*, 1146–1152.
Uller, C., Huntley-Fenner, G., Carey, S., & Klatt, L. (1999). What representations might underlie infant numerical knowledge? *Cognitive Development, 14*, 1–36.
Vogel, E. K., Woodman, G. F., & Luck, S. J. (2001). Storage of features, conjunctions, and objects in visual working memory. *Journal of Experimental Psychology: Human Perception and Performance, 27*, 92–114.
Wexler, B. E. (2006). Brain and culture: Neurobiology, ideology, and social change. Cambridge, MA: MIT Press.
Wood, J. N., & Spelke, E. S. (2005). Infants' enumeration of actions: Numerical discrimination and its signature limits. *Developmental Science, 8*, 173–181.
Wynn, K. (1992). Addition and subtraction by human infants. *Nature, 358*, 749–750.

Wynn, K. (1996). Infants' individuation and enumeration of actions. *Psychological Science, 7*, 164–169.
Xu, F. (2003). Numerosity discrimination in infants: Evidence for two systems of representations, *Cognition, 89*, B15–B25
Xu, F., & Spelke, E. S. (2000). Large number discrimination in 6-month-old infants. *Cognition, 74*, B1–B11.
Xu, F., Spelke, E. S., & Goddard, S. (2005). Number sense in human infants, *Developmental Science, 8*, 88–101.

Interviewing: An Insider's Insight into Learning

Marc S. Schwartz and Kurt W. Fischer

Introduction

Interviewing is often thought of as a research tool, but by shifting focus, teachers can use "interviewing" to support two important classroom goals: clarifying student understanding and in turn providing students with opportunities to organize more meaningful structures of understanding. Skill theory (Fischer, 1980; Fischer & Bidell, 2006) provides an operational definition for levels of understanding (i.e., skills) and a hierarchical framework for evaluating changes in student understanding during the interview process, and this approach has much in common with the developmental framework of Robbie Case (1985, 1991). The chapter specifically explores, through several conversations between a student and her science teacher, how the interview process can highlight and support a range of skill levels representing all or part of the student's "zone of proximal development" or ZPD (Vygotsky, 1962; Vygotsky, 1978).

From a very different perspective, the student's insights can be understood in terms of the brain's central organizational principle; brains learn about patterns in the world in order to make reliable predictions about its environment (Mountcastle, 1998). Thus, new insights are new patterns that students recognize and can test against reality within carefully constructed classroom activities or during the interview process. Furthermore, as the brain matures it follows a pattern of change in neural activity that is hypothesized to support the emergence of new stages and levels (Case, 1992; Fischer & Rose, 1998). These changes support the ability to detect richer patterns and solve more complex problems. Thus pattern recognition and changes in neural activity offer an additional dimension for understanding the dynamic interaction between the teacher/interviewer and student, which this chapter explores in detail.

M.S. Schwartz (✉)
University of Texas, Arlington, TX, USA
e-mail: SCHWARMA@uta.edu

M. Ferrari, L. Vuletic (eds.), *The Developmental Relations among Mind, Brain and Education*, DOI 10.1007/978-90-481-3666-7_7,

Overview: Change over Time

A significant challenge for educators is evaluating student understanding as they participate in classroom activities. Students also face a similar challenge as they confront or explore the depth and integrity of their knowledge. At the intersection of both tasks is one process that can help both teachers and students. The interview can help teachers recognize, represent, and evaluate student understanding. The same process can empower students to better appreciate and confront their views.

Change in Skills

How students organize and capitalize upon their observations and ideas can be thought of as a strategy or a "skill" (Fischer, 1980; Fischer & Bidell, 2006). However, an important feature of skills for researchers and educators is that they capture the organizational complexity of student understanding and action. More importantly, skills that students use to solve problems or make sense of their world are never fixed. They can vary in complexity depending on context and/or the type and degree of support they receive; thus, student abilities can vary along a range similar to what Vygotsky (1962, 1978) characterized as the zone of proximal development or ZPD. This "zone" represents the difference between how students perform when solving problems alone versus solving problems with the support of more capable individuals. "It is the distance between the actual developmental level as determined by independent problem solving and the level of potential development as determined through problem solving under adult guidance or in collaboration with more capable peers" (1978, p. 86). Because the interview can support changes in student understanding, we examine in greater detail how this process impacts one student's effort to understand a classroom problem, and how this effort impacts the skill level she uses.

Changes in Brain Activity

Changes in student understanding as measured by changes in skill level can also be viewed from the perspective of the brain. One of its key general functions is to identify patterns in the environment and compare them with stored memories of older patterns in order to detect changes and, if necessary, make predictions about future events or the success of a specific response (should one be necessary) (Hawkins & Blakeslee, 2004). When the environment changes, even in minimal ways, the challenge the brain faces is whether it will detect the difference(s) and be able to respond if necessary.

Another important change in brain activity occurs over a longer time frame as children mature. The brain's progress in its own development limits the complexity of patterns it can detect or entertain and the skill that can be coordinated. For example, changes in neural architecture underlie the initial development of coordinated action in infants, later speech in toddlers, and, in adolescents, the emergence of formal reasoning. Underlying each of these new abilities are reciprocal changes in brain activity across brain regions, which enhance brain function.

These brain-based changes will occasionally enter the main story to enhance our understanding of the dynamic relationship between skills and context as illustrated through the dialog between Eve and her science teacher. At a visible level of analysis, the interview highlights the variables Eve is considering as she looks for meaningful patterns, and re-organizes and coordinates experiences, ideas, and memories into new predictions and new skills (or in educational terms, possible solutions). Eve is 12 years old and studying electromagnets. To follow the evolution in her ideas, we first outline skill theory as a theoretical framework for analyzing with greater precision Eve's progress in integrating ideas and experiences throughout the interview. In a later section, "Exploring the Process," we focus on Eve's journey within the interview while highlighting important features of the teacher's role. The theoretical framework reappears throughout this section as a means to help the reader compare and contrast changes in the student's perspective and to consider the role that the brain plays in supporting these changes. In a later part of this section, the content of the dialog helps illustrate the scaffolding power of the interview process and its potentially important role in curriculum development.

The Site for Change – The Classroom

Educators create problems and activities for students by presenting or highlighting specific aspects of the environment they want students to consider. Students in turn discover the relevant pattern that serves as a framework to guide them in selecting and coordinating ideas and actions into a skill that serves as a response. The skill also represents the student's prediction of what best counts as an answer. Eve is about to have her first experience with electromagnets. Her ideas and questions provide not only an intimate picture of her understanding, but also reveal how students her age make sense of electricity and electromagnets (Shipstone, 1985; Schwartz, 2000; Schwartz & Fischer, 2004). Her teacher sets the stage by building a simple but functional electromagnet made of easily recognizable materials – a 12-penny nail with 20 wraps of wire (see Fig. 1). The wire is 80 cm long. Each end is stripped and attached to one end of a battery.

The teacher then demonstrates that his prototype lifts one, maybe two links of a chain. Students are offered the opportunity to inspect the teacher's design for several minutes before he presents the following challenge: "Can you improve the electromagnet so that it will pick up more links?" The challenge is carefully worded to encourage students to explore electromagnetism by providing a goal that allows them to capitalize on strategies that seem plausible and variables that seem relevant (e.g., increase the number of wraps, use a larger nail, or add layers of coils).

From the perspective of neuroscience this challenge is a natural opportunity for the brain to do what it does best – compare external patterns (i.e., observations of

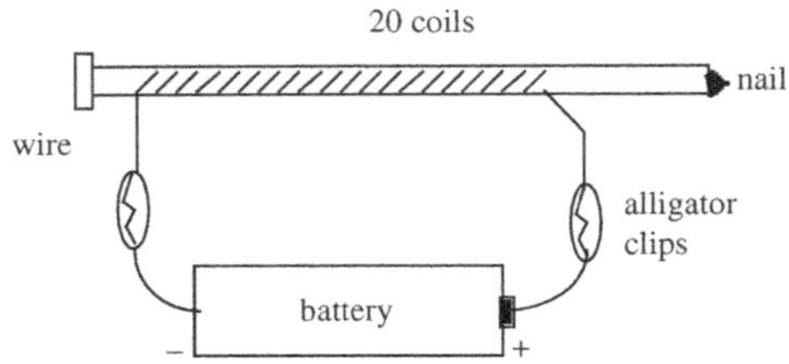

Fig. 1 Prototype electromagnet

the environment) and internal patterns (i.e., memories) of the way the world works (or is expected to work), and try to align them to reduce conflict and/or generate solutions (Hawkins & Blakeslee, 2004). The brain searches for relevant memories about the world, and tries to apply them to this new context. As it turns out, children and adults rarely refuse the opportunity to test out their predictions and will work with great intensity and focus to see if their predictions are correct (Schwartz & Sadler, 2007). They add wraps of wire around the nail; change the location of the wraps, the number of nails, or the size of the nail. After each change they measure the strength of their latest design by counting the links of chain they can lift with their electromagnet.

Within the first hour of experimenting, Eve's teacher recognizes that students can improve their electromagnets. Students quickly realize that by adding more wraps or moving the wraps closer to one of the ends of the nail, they can increase the strength of their electromagnet. But how would they explain the relationship between these changes and the results they noted? Do new patterns of understanding emerge from such an activity, and if so, are they meaningful to the student?

Theoretical Framework

When students arrive at school they also come with personal ideas about how the world works (Hugh & Novak, 1983; Driver, Guesne, & Tiberghien, 1985). These views signify important personal achievements in creating meaning out of the enormous amount of information that nature, schools, parents, friends, and the media provide. Student explanations often reflect some degree of internal consistency, account for variability in a phenomenon, and are well thought-out. Consequently these views are often highly resistant to change through instruction (Driver, Squires, Rushworth, & Wood-Robinson, 1994; Sadler, 1998).

As this chapter explores, interviews that focus on the student's experiences can help them question their ideas and support new understandings. However, recognizing the importance of these scaffolded conversations is difficult in traditional education because student achievement is often defined in terms of what students accomplish on their own. In contrast, Vygotsky (1978) offers a broader and more powerful view of achievement:

> It is generally assumed that only those things that children can do on their own are indicative of mental abilities. . . . even the profoundest thinkers never questioned the assumptions; they never entertained the notion that what children can do with the assistance of others might be in some sense even more indicative of their mental development than what they can do alone (p. 85).

This difference between what students can do alone versus what they can accomplish with support can be described with even further precision with skill theory (Fischer & Pipp, 1984). In this model of cognitive development, variability in skill performance is a function of the degree and quality of support available, and the upper limit in performance is capped by biological development.

By viewing student achievement as a function of support, teachers have an opportunity to re-evaluate as well as redefine their roles in student–teacher interactions. The interview process is one such opportunity. By focusing on the structures students use to organize their experiences and ideas, students find that they have the opportunity to better define how they are thinking about a problem or experience. When students are not sure what they understand, the student–teacher dialog allows students to construct a personal view. Students who are conscious of their structure of understanding can more easily recognize ideas they want to challenge, change, or abandon when confronting new problems and/or observations. This kind of focused dialog facilitates the student's progress toward their "potential level of development" (Vygotsky, 1978).

Teachers also benefit when shifting their focus from teaching to the purposeful attention that the interview generates. To the extent that the dialog succeeds in revealing the student's framework of understanding, the teacher can clarify the student's actual (or functional) developmental level and evaluate the student's success in moving toward his or her potential level of development. The actual level is the foundation upon which future learning is built, and a necessary insight that prepares teachers for the task of building and targeting lessons that challenge student views and in turn support growth to more sophisticated structures of understanding.

When Eve explores her ideas in an interview, so that they can make sense to both her and her teacher, Eve has the opportunity to clarify partly formed ideas and to integrate them into tentative structures for making sense of her world. Together Eve and her teacher discover or retrace paths, as necessary, to understand Eve's evolving view of electromagnetism. The teacher keeps track of and makes available to Eve her experiences and ideas when she feels lost or disoriented. This action facilitates their exploration of her structure of understanding, and indirectly supports changes in student understanding even though this is not the goal of the interview.

During such interchanges, students will often sense a growing clarity in their ideas, which motivates them to stay engaged in the dialog. However, again, the goal is not to "teach." The goal is to attain a complete picture of the student's world and the patterns they recognize as pertinent to making sense of their experiences. The work often feels satisfying to the student because the conversation is focused on their understanding; and, any change in understanding is the student's creation.

Skill Theory: Developing More Complex Structures of Understanding

As Eve's general ability to detect more nuanced patterns and coordinate ever more complex skills evolve through maturity and experience, skill theory offers a hierarchical scale of development for describing and evaluating her progress both in the short term as she navigates between her functional and optimal level and in the long term as additional and more powerful levels and tiers emerge as a result of maturation (Fischer, 1980; Case, 1992; Fischer & Bidell, 2006). Progress is measured as changes in "skill" levels. Operationally, skills highlight the complexity of understanding that emerges from the dynamic interaction between the individual's developmental progress (an outcome of maturity) and context; and thus, a skill level captures the degree of complexity in our ability to act or respond as we mature and/or as contexts change.

Skills are hierarchical in nature and, at the largest level of analysis, are grouped into four tiers that unfold during human development (reflex, action, representation, and abstraction). (This analysis has much in common with that of Case, 1991, although there are important differences also.) In each tier, the individual displays a new ability that encompasses the successes of earlier tiers. Each tier is a fundamentally new way of understanding the world. In the first-tier babies, demonstrate a set of *reflexes* that allow them to immediately respond to the world. These innate skills become the platform for the development of a set of *actions* the infant develops to allow her to interact with the world (instead of just respond in an automatic fashion). This new tier, the second, enables her to respond and interact with her world in more complex ways such as grabbing items of interest. As toddlers become children the action tier in turn become a platform that supports the emergence of a third tier, *representations*. In this new tier she can create symbolic understandings about her world that substitute for the sensorimotor experience. A striking ability that emerges in this tier is the ability to use words to represent actions (e.g., walking, drinking, laugh, cry). The pattern of encompassing and building upon earlier achievements repeats itself again in early adolescence when children become developmentally ready to use representations to create a fourth tier of understanding – *abstractions*. Figure 2 illustrates the cascade of skills growing in complexity beginning with the second tier (sometimes called the *sensorimotor* tier).

When students enter school they are developmentally ready to create and organize understandings in the third tier (i.e., representations); however, having reached this developmental milestone does not insure that they will understand the representations they encounter in school. Because skills are context specific, the transfer of representations from teachers and books to students is often a difficult and unsuccessful process (Salomon & Perkins, 1989; Pea, 1993; Nardi, 1996). "Skills are not automatically or easily generalized or integrated. Consequently, even when people have skills appropriate for a task, they frequently fail to use the skills and thereby function below the level required by the task" (Fischer, Bullock, Rotenberg, & Raya, 1993, p. 92).

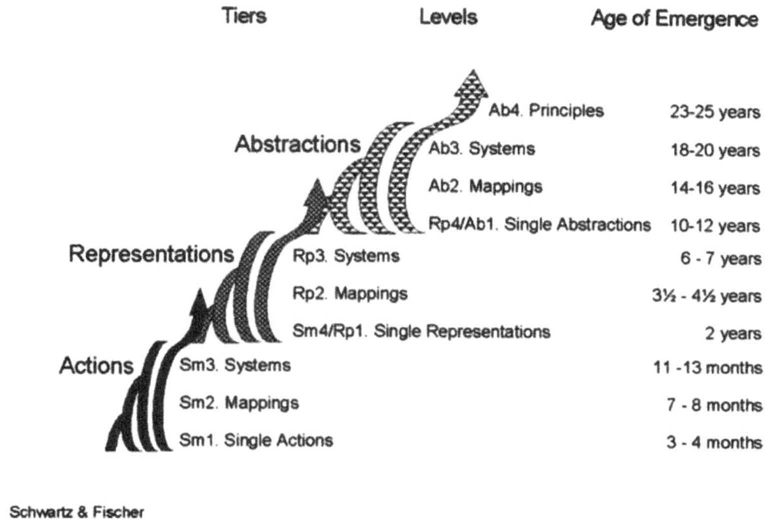

Fig. 2 Developmental scale of skill levels

In order to help students develop more complex skills, teachers not only need to recognize where students begin their learning process (i.e., their actual developmental level), but also understand that the nature and degree of support they offer plays an important role in the skills students use as contexts change. A closer inspection of the representational tier and the types of representations Eve (and students like her) creates reveals smaller incremental *levels* of development or understanding that increase in sophistication within the tier.

Within each tier there are four intermediate levels, which provide a finer grain view of development or understanding. Each level is a more complex structure (and therefore a new skill) that demonstrates further coordination and integration of earlier levels. In the representational tier the four levels are single representations, mappings of representations, systems of representations, and systems of systems. Additionally, the last level of a tier is unique in that it supports the qualitatively new way of knowing that is the beginning of the next tier and thus creates the first level of the new tier (Fischer & Bidell, 2006). Thus, by combining the four tiers and the four levels within each tier, the developmental framework can be portrayed as a 13-level developmental scale. (Note that the total number of levels is 13 instead of 16, because the last level of each tier is also the first level of the next tier. Furthermore the levels of interest in this chapter and in school learning in general begin with the first level of the action tier. See Fig. 2.)

Although the 13 levels that emerge over 30 years of maturation mark developmental milestones, they do not emerge in a continuous, uninterrupted metronomic march from one level to the next. While the metaphor of a staircase for development and its associated analogy of progress, as in climbing up the stairs, are common (Case, 1991), both are misleading. Even though the trend in development is toward increased complexity over the long term, progress is more unpredictable in the short-term (for example when confronting a new problem) and often looks more like one step forward and two steps back. This observed discontinuity in progress was previously thought to be the result of error in the tools used to measure change, but when studied through dynamic models the noticeable instability appears to be one of the prominent properties of progress (Fischer & Bidell, 2006; Van Geert, 1994; Thelen & Smith, 1998).

Ultimately maturity in the long term (and support in the short term) contributes to individuals operating at "higher" and thus more complex levels (using the stairs metaphor); however, a more nuanced view of development requires looking more closely at the discontinuities in shorter time frames such as during problem solving. At this level of analysis, the spurts and discontinuities observed in the short term highlight a prominent phenomenon when observing growth in both behavioral and neurological terms. In terms of behavior, progress is sensitive to context (to include support and/or scaffolding). In terms of brain growth, we see the same influence of a dynamic environment on the progress the brain makes in supporting the emergence of more complex skills.

A Hypothesis for How the Brain Supports the Emergence of New Skill Levels

As just highlighted, a central phenomenon when observing growth (both behaviorally and neurologically) is the presence of discontinuities. Behaviorally, discontinuities are observed in the fluctuations between optimal and functional skill levels as individuals are developing and learning to generalize optimal skill levels to new contexts. Optimal skills are at the cutting edge of a person's ability, and thus their stability and longevity is highly influenced by context (including support) and scaffolding. In a parallel fashion, discontinuities in brain activity help highlight important changes in the organization of the brain that are hypothesized to underlie the emergence of skill levels observed as individuals mature.

However, the link between brain and behavior is often not direct or obvious. Some connections are continuous while others display discontinuities over time. Dynamic modeling can help uncover order within variability when trying to understand the nature of discontinuities (Van Geert, 1994; Thelen & Smith, 1998). Just as progress in behavior can spurt forward, collapse, or halt as contexts change, discontinuities in the brain's electrical activity provide clues about how the brain is developing.

Two important metrics for evaluating changes in brain activity are coherence and relative power. Both are determined from electroencephalogram (EEG) readings of electrical brain waves. While coherence is a correlation of wave patterns in different cortical regions, power is a measure of work being done by the neurons over time (or simply, energy expended by neurons). Both measures provide clues on how changes in the neural architecture may be supporting skill development.

Relative power in brain activity measures the relative amount of power used by different regions of the brain. When looking at how the brain distributes energy over time, an important initial observation is the surge in power in the prefrontal cortex as new tiers emerge. This initial surge is also followed by peaks in power in different areas of the brain, which may mark the emergence of the intermediate levels within the tier. During the time that development within a tier is occurring, there is the opportunity for the general skill typified by the tier to diversify and grow in complexity through the four levels embedded in the tier.

In a concurrent manner the brain appears to be consolidating the robustness of each level. Nested within the power surge is an additional pattern of coordination occurring between different regions of the brain. This coordination is measured through coherence. Specifically, when regions of the brain are communicating with each other, resulting electrical wave patterns in each region are highly correlated, and thus coherence is high. In this case, the regions of importance are the prefrontal cortex and the other major lobes (parietal, temporal, occipital, and the central area of the brain). Although the pathways are numerous, the coherence between regions has been studied in a systematic way revealing a striking pattern involving the prefrontal cortex and the remaining regions (Thatcher, 1994). A compelling hypothesis is that a discontinuity in wave patterns preceding any observed increase in coherence between the prefrontal cortex and each of the remaining regions signifies the incorporation of additional networks to support a specific level (Fischer & Bidell, 2006). Furthermore, the emergence of each new level requires the coordination of existing skills at the current skill level, which the prefrontal cortex is responsible for orchestrating.

Thus, one hypothesis is that the emergence of tiers and levels follow an increase in relative power measured at specific sites. An additional hypothesis is that consolidation of each level is enhanced through communication, measured in coherence, between the prefrontal cortex and each of the other major areas of the brain. This pattern repeats itself over time as each tier develops. Thus discontinuities (as a theme) not only underscore the emergence of skill levels but of neuronal activity. While the emergence of optimal skills during problem solving depends on environmental support, support within the brain appears to build upon a redistribution of energy, which increases the power at specific sites in the brain (Fischer & Bidell, 2006; Fischer & Rose, 1998). Both coherence and relative power underscore how neuroscience is building a more complete picture of what we observe behaviorally.

A Closer Look at the Skills That Unfold for Students Like Eve

The first level of the representational tier is a one-dimensional view or understanding of the world. For example, a single representational skill for electromagnets is the name for the "wire–nail–battery ensemble" – an electromagnet (Schwartz, 2000).

When one's understanding is confined to this skill level, variations along any dimension (size of nail, number of wraps, the quality of connection between the wraps and the battery) are not obviously important unless they are extreme (i.e., more or less wraps would not matter, but wraps should be visually obvious) (Schwartz & Fischer, 2004).

Young children, 2 or 3 years old, easily demonstrate the power of this singularity. If they hold the basic view of electromagnets as a device that attracts objects, they will repeatedly try to pick up a variety of objects without noticing a pattern in what electromagnets do and do not attract. As long as the ensemble parts are present, the electromagnet should attract objects. Furthermore, if the electromagnet ceases to function, they would be unable to diagnose the problem. However, despite the obvious limitations in this level of understanding, the single representation is the foundation of the representational tier, and serves as the building block for more complex representations.

As students mature, their ability to recognize features (as potential variables) of a single representation improves. For example, they might conclude that the number of wraps influences the strength of the electromagnet. This new emergent skill, which is called a "mapping" of two representations (level Rp2), allows children to coordinate variations in a single dimension of interest such that changes in this variable lead to changes in the single representation. Metaphors often work at this level in that they reflect an understanding about relationships observed in the world (Lakoff & Johnson, 1980). For example, the metaphor "more is better" supports students concluding that more wraps would lead to a stronger electromagnet. Without failure, the first change that most students suggest in order to improve the strength of their electromagnet is to increase the number of wraps (Schwartz & Sadler, 2007). Analogies are similar to metaphors in that they offer students linear relationships that help them make sense of one specific aspect of their experiences. A limitation of representational mappings is that they only support a smaller range of predictions about the world. This skill often demonstrates a focus on the impact of only one variable as these student examples illustrate:

- Increasing the wraps will increase the strength of the electromagnet
- Moving the wraps closer to the head of the nail will increase the strength of the electromagnet
- Using a bigger nail as a core will make the electromagnet stronger

Over the longer term, as students continue to mature they become developmentally prepared to challenge metaphors or mappings. Even though students in Eve's class are developmentally ready to challenge their mappings, for many students this emerging skill is closer to their optimal level, thus they will need support. When examining more closely the connections between their explanations and their observations, they may recognize weaknesses in their metaphors and analogies. Prior to any experimentation, these simpler models provided quick explanations or predictions, but did not account for other observations or variables under inspection. To address the increased complexity needed in coordinating more variables, a more complex skill is necessary.

In skill theory, when individuals can successfully coordinate two mappings they are using a more sophisticated skill – at the level of representational systems (Rp3). Here the coordination of two mappings allows the student to consider how several observations and metaphors work at the same time. When students become more comfortable integrating new observations and ideas with their original metaphors, they are better able to entertain more sophisticated models of understanding. This skill is illustrated by the following comments or realizations:

- The strength of the electromagnet varies with both the placement of wraps and the number of wraps
- The strength of the electromagnet varies with both the number of wraps and the size of the core

As models for understanding electromagnets become more sophisticated (and approach the structures of understanding that scientists typically use to understand problems they are studying) students can account for additional variables, provide more accurate predictions, and/or extend their understanding of established mappings to additional contexts.

Sophisticated models like the field theory of electromagnetism require the coordination of multiple representational systems (Rp3) involving both electricity and magnetism. With further practice, experience, and maturity this new level of coordination can become internalized as an abstraction (Ab1). In this new tier, understanding transcends the physical, observable, concrete nature of representations. Hypothetically students could enter this tier of abstraction by recognizing the concept of "fields" as a phenomenon that both electricity and magnets create. The field's shape and density can be defined in real terms, but understanding the nature of its existence requires that one transcend the many physical variables that lead to its creation. Developmentally, Eve and her classmates have the potential of achieving this first-level abstraction, but more time, support, and practice would be necessary before their understanding in this tier emerges. Actual examples did not appear for Eve and her classmates. (Table 1 summarizes the evolution of skills concerning electromagnets from Level Rp1 through Ab1.)

Ultimately the conversation with Eve (or any student) will reveal a particular range of understanding within skill theory's 13-level scale of developmental complexity. In this case, Eve makes extensive use of skill levels within both the sensorimotor and representational tiers. Initially Eve used skills at her functional level to understand electromagnets, but the dialog with her teacher began to hint at her potential to use more sophisticated levels. These optimal levels were at the leading edge of her development, laid down through the maturation process; however as yet, Eve may not have encountered classroom contexts where this potential ability could emerge. As Vygotsky (1978) suggested, students are not bound to any one level. They can move to higher or lower levels as Eve demonstrates during the interview process.

Table 1 Levels of cognitive development from single representations to single abstractions

Level	Action	TIERS Representational	Abstract	Description and example of skill	Age of first emergence
Sm4/Rp1		Single representations **[P]** **P** = electromagnet (EM)		Relations of action systems to produce concrete representations of objects, people, or events – The name "electromagnet" as the *object* that stands for the "wire–nail–battery ensemble"	18 to 24 mos
Rp2		Representational mappings **[Q——R]** **Q** = an EM with more wraps **R** = an EM that is more powerful		Simple relations of representations (such as metaphors) – "bigger is better" – The direct relationship between increasing the number of wraps to increasing the strength of the electromagnet	3.5 to 4.5 yrs
Rp3		Representational Systems $\left[\mathbf{Q}{}^{a}_{a'} \longleftrightarrow \mathbf{S}{}^{b}_{b'}\right]$ a & a' = variations in wrappings b & b' = variations on the placement of wraps along the core		Complex relations of mappings – Two separate and coordinated relationships such as varying the number of wraps & varying the placement of those wraps along the nail and how these changes independently and in concert change the power of the electromagnet – Complete circuits is another example[1]	6 to 7 yrs

Table 1 (continued)

Level	Action	TIERS Representational	Abstract	Description and example of skill	Age of first emergence
Rp4/Ab1		$\left[\begin{matrix} \mathbf{Q}_{a'}^{a} \longleftrightarrow \mathbf{S}_{b'}^{b} \\ \Updownarrow \\ \mathbf{T}_{c'}^{c} \longleftrightarrow \mathbf{U}_{d'}^{d} \end{matrix}\right]$	Single abstractions $= [\mathcal{Y}]$	Coordination of representational systems to produce abstractions (intangible concepts) – Complete circuits and the flow of electricity through the circuit will create a magnetic "field"	10 to 12 yrs

[1] See Schwartz & Fischer (2004) for a more complete description of how complete circuits illustrate representational systems in student understanding

This process of interviewing may sound instructional, but the teacher's goal during this process is only to understand her students' views even though this particular focus can support students coordinating more complex skills. Students are most likely unable to maintain this level on their own, thus the conversation highlights the skills students will organize on their own one day, and the kind of work necessary by the teacher and curriculum to support this transition.

Exploring the Process: Eve and Her Teacher's Journey

Eve and students in her class had few problems creating single representations of electromagnets. Students recognized pictures of electromagnets as long as it included the right components: wire, battery, and a core (see Fig. 1). However students at this level of understanding (Rp1 single representations) do not yet appreciate that the number and placement of wraps matter, that opposite ends of the wire must be connected to opposite ends of the battery, that the core should be iron, etc. When students are able to coordinate these variables in order to create a richer understanding of electromagnets, they are demonstrating progress toward the next level in the representational tier (i.e., mappings at Level Rp2).

For many students, their first step toward this more sophisticated view of electromagnets takes shape around what they know about plumbing (Shipstone, 1985; Schwartz & Fischer, 2004). The plumbing model of electromagnetism is not only straightforward; it is effective. Eve sees the wires somewhat like pipes in which water or electricity flows. Pipes keep the contents within the walls just as the insulation should hold the electricity until it arrives at its destination. Her teacher, Mr. M, discovers as well as supports Eve's construction of this model early in their interchange:

M: What comes to mind when you hear the word electromagnet?

E: Well... at least something that works like a magnet but it generates electricity.

M: It works like a magnet but generates electricity...

E: Like... sort of, it could be like in (pause) ... I think it could be saying: electricity could run through...

At this point Eve is unsure what she thinks about electromagnets; however, Mr. M encourages her to develop her thoughts by prompting Eve with just one word:

M: Something... (Eve picks up the prompt and continues.)

E: Like electricity could run through it...

M: Yah...

E: ...to connect to something else.

M: Electricity could run through it to connect to something else...

E: Like in a cord.

M: So you imagine electricity passing through the cord, and then what happens?

Mr. M summarizes Eve's thinking to provide her the chance to hear what her ideas sound like, as well as offer her the opportunity to agree or change his summary.

The teacher wants Eve to know that he is attempting to follow her thoughts and that she is still free to develop or explore related ideas with him.

E: Uhm, I heard that there are electromagnets in telephones. They could be going through the cord and connecting... uhm (pause)... like when one piece of energy to another.

M: I think I see. So your idea is that electricity is passing through the cord and it's connecting one object... (Mr. M is interrupted.)

E: to another

Mr. M doesn't know what "one piece of energy" means to Eve, but recognizes her focus on "connections." He suspects that Eve is using the plumbing model, but still invites her to modify his interpretation of her ideas by restating her thought about "connecting" and by qualifying his summary with, "I think I see." Eve's growing comfort and attention in this conversation is evident at the end of the last interchange when she interrupts Mr. M and completes his sentence.

The interchange continues with a sharper focus on the details of Eve's understanding of electromagnets:

M: ok... I see. Do you think this electromagnet has any properties... things it does or doesn't do?

E: Well it is made of metal. And it probably... needs to be insulated, if you're using it. But I've never experimented with one.

The potential role of the plumbing model reappears in Eve's observation that electromagnets need to be insulated. Incidentally, this model survives well into adulthood because, for the most part, it works well in most contexts (Shipstone, 1985). Improving this model would require an understanding of complete circuits. Most adults recognize the importance of complete circuits, but they are not always successful in coordinating that understanding with their "plumbing" metaphor (Schwartz & Fischer, 2004). A representational system (Rp3) illustrates the potential coordination of these two relevant ideas: (1) electricity flows through a medium and (2) circuits of any kind only work when the circuit is complete.

Mr. M temporarily ends the interview so that Eve can continue building an electromagnet that she thinks will outperform the teacher's. When the interchange continues a few days later, Mr. M will have several questions in mind. Did experimenting help her recognize that there are problems with her plumbing model? Is she ready to look for more sophisticated strategies to account for her observations? Together Eve and her teacher will define and navigate the transition from beliefs (or simple models) toward more sophisticated models of understanding. To ensure that Eve recognizes what she believes, her teacher begins by exploring Eve's beliefs to understand them as she does. He avoids explanations or opportunities to correct mistakes to avoid disturbing Eve's focus on her beliefs. In this opening exchange Mr. M invites Eve to continue exploring with him her progress in making sense of electromagnets:

M: Do you remember what you were saying about electromagnets a few days back?

Eve: Uhm, I thought it was something that carried electricity. . . and through one object to another. . .it sort of. . . I just thought it sort of connected two things because it was magnetic and it also carried electricity through it, energy.

M: So what do you think now?

Eve: Well I thought. . .. I think. . . Well we haven't really experimented with it [the electromagnet]. We only saw how powerful it was and I'd like to try. . . while it's picking up a chain. . . I'd like to put a magnet near it. See if it will throw off the [electromagnet]. . . see if it will throw off the course.

Mr. M invites Eve to think out loud with him in order to continue their exploration in discovering the layout and boundaries of Eve's world of understanding. During their last conversation Eve mentioned that a permanent magnet might affect an electromagnet. Mr. M recognizes that the interaction between permanent magnets and electromagnets is an important issue for Eve. He takes her lead and investigates Eve's progress in making sense of her observations and experiments:

M: I remember last time you saying that if you brought a permanent magnet next to the electromagnet it might throw it off.

Eve: Yah, and I haven't tried that yet.

Eve has not yet resolved this problem; however, Mr. M does not want to discourage her from returning to the problem if she wishes. He does not judge Eve's ideas or her decision not to investigate her magnet–electromagnet hypothesis. Because there are no results to explore, Mr. M uses an open-ended question to re-launch his investigation of her progress:

M: Maybe, you'll be able to try that later. You'll have some time. So how do you think the electromagnet works?

Eve: I think. . . it probably. . . uhm, the electricity. . . the wire is carrying electricity and it is touching the nail as well and while it [the electricity] is circling really, really fast around the nail [through the wraps], the nail sort of builds up (pause) like very strong. . .. (pause) Maybe some of that electricity goes into the nail.

As Eve approaches the end of her description she senses a problem with her plumbing model. How can electricity leave the insulated wire? A few days earlier Eve observed that when the wire was hooked to the battery the nail became magnetized. How did this happen? She recognized that the wire was insulated and that insulation prevented electricity from escaping and, as she will consider later, electrocuting people. From her point of view the electricity has to leave the wire and enter the nail in order to magnetize the nail. What her plumbing model cannot explain is how the electricity can leave the wire in order to enter the nail. This understanding is deeply rooted in the sensorimotor experience of containers where liquids cannot escape unless the container has lost its integrity. Once she concedes that electricity may be entering the nail, her model of electricity is vulnerable to change. Eve recognizes the significance of this new relationship as she attempts to coordinate new ideas with older ideas, a foundation for change that Ausubel (1968) recognized as a precursor to developing new understandings. Thisre-organization process underscores how the brain looks for relevant memories to make sense of new observations in order to create a pattern that leads to reliable predictions.

Thus, the conversation not only clarifies Eve's skill level, but also supports her effort in creating more complex skills to account for her observations. Eve's teacher can later consider the kinds of follow-on lessons that would best support Eve's continued progress in working at her optimal (or potential) level of development. However, for the moment, the pair remains focused on exploring how well Eve's models work in the real world, and what options are available when they encounter problems with making reasonable or accurate predictions. Eve has not yet recognized all the problems that exist with her model. Much later she will pose the question, "How does electricity get into the nail if the wire is insulated?" Eve needs more time to clarify the problems she faces when using her mapping skill (i.e., the plumbing model) to make sense of her experiences and to explore, coordinate, and integrate observations and ideas in the face of those problems.

Mr. M maintains his attention on Eve's construction process as well as her conclusions. This attention allows her to build a picture of electromagnets where she integrates and coordinates details she might not have considered unless she was trying to articulate her picture with a partner. The interaction with Eve is analogous to how Phillips (1988) describes Winnicott's use of mirroring in psychoanalysis. The psychiatrist gives back to the client what the client brings to the relationship. In this way the client discovers feelings he does not recognize until they are reflected back to him. The process has the same effect on students. Eve discovers her thoughts and feelings about her work when her teacher gives form to her ideas. The degree to which Mr. M can accurately mirror Eve's ideas contributes to their shared understanding of electromagnets and Eve's ability to challenge the patterns she sees.

Once the image of Eve's present understanding of electromagnets takes shape, and both Mr. M and Eve can agree on the details in the pattern she sees, the teacher can accentuate the mirroring process by focusing on Eve's choice of verbs, analogies, or expressions. What are the consequences of these choices in her attempt to understand electromagnets? He focuses on those elements to explore any deeper understanding, mysteries, or confusion. To this end, he returns specifically to her use of the verb "building" when describing what happens to the nail:

M: What "builds" [up] in the nail?

Eve: Like a lot of power because there's, there's like energy and electricity running, like right around it, everywhere.

M: around it, around...

Eve: the nail, and when I tried putting the wire all the way around the nail, almost covering the entire nail, it [the electromagnet] was really powerful because like... all that... there was so much force going around that nail.

Mr. M helps Eve organize her world by keeping track of what she sees and keeping them available to her as a mirror does when you look into it. Because it is difficult to focus on all parts of the image that a mirror provides, Mr. M brings to focus elements that might be worth examining. His choice of elements can be influenced by what he knows about electromagnets, but can also be influenced by elements that seem to be important to Eve. However, again, his goal is not for Eve to guess what answers or insights he has (which would shift the focus from Eve to her teacher), but to recognize the opportunity for seeing new patterns or different aspects of an existing pattern with an experienced traveler in a new world we can call "Electromagnet Land."

Not only does the interview process help Eve recognize the consequences or implications of her views, it can also reveal places (in Electromagnet Land) where she becomes disoriented. Feeling disoriented is typical when examining a new subject from a new perspective. This is akin to being disoriented in a familiar but rarely visited part of town; you might know that you are not far from home, but not quite sure how to connect "where you are" to "where you want to go." The brain is searching for relevant patterns or a shift in focus that will allow a pattern to emerge. A bird's eye view of the terrain would help, but is only possible for the teacher at this time. So he challenges Eve to focus on those areas where the terrain is still unclear and her points of reference do not yet help. Again, this thorough investigation of Eve's understanding creates opportunities for encountering and thinking about problems they encounter. Eve and Mr. M arrive at such a problem in the following interchange:

Eve: I think that (pause)…. what I'd like to know is if you hold an electromagnet too long… uhm, it… it's going to start to burn and if… I don't know how, but if they use it [electromagnets] in telephones. I'd like to know how they use it without it getting overheated.

M: Yah, that's a good question.

Eve: And having something melt, because I saw that happening with the electromagnets. [Her team had observed that if the electromagnet remains connected to the battery for too much time, enough heat is generated to melt the insulation around the wire.[1]]

M: What do you think was happening there?

Eve: Uhm, I think the battery was… was bringing in too much power, the battery became really hot and the plastic around it starting melting and that electromagnet has to have a battery or a source. It has to sit somewhere.

M: Uh huh

Eve: And if it overheats I'd like to know how they get it [the electromagnets] in … Uh, like not overheated, because if a telephone is plugged into the wall, it has an electromagnet somewhere in it that has electricity running through it. There's if… if, I think if you unplug it, the telephone… uhm, it's going, it's going… like turn off the electromagnet and not let it overheat (pause), but the only way for a telephone to work is when it is plugged in.

[1] Even though this experience allowed Eve to encounter an interesting relationship, Mr. M decided to use C size batteries instead of D batteries in later lessons, which generates much less heat.

M: It seems odd to you that the phone is always plugged in and still it doesn't overheat?

Eve has stepped out of a familiar environment and sees a problem with an old pattern about how telephones work (i.e., they are plugged into wall sockets, they contain electromagnets, but they do not get hot). As she considers her new knowledge, which comes from building and testing electromagnets with her peers, Eve may realize that she is in an unfamiliar place in terms of her understanding of telephones. She has observed electromagnets overheating in the past. This experience creates a strong, highly organized skill within the sensorimotor tier, which is easily observed in students gingerly touching an electromagnet if they know it has been connected to a battery. Eve knows that phones contain electromagnets, and that there is a lot of electricity available at an electrical outlet. So what keeps the phone from overheating? Eve is at an impasse. She has difficulty organizing and interpreting her observations, especially when she tries to make sense of them to her teacher. She might wonder how far this new conceptual landmark (seeing electromagnets overheat) is from where she was before she embarked on this voyage (recognizing that phones use electromagnets). Is there a bridge that will close the gap she perceives here?

Naturally, a teacher would be tempted to provide an explanation to close the gap; however, explanations that come too quickly still have risks that we will explore in the next section. The interview process is still powerful enough to support the teacher and Eve in recognizing and capitalizing on opportunities to scaffold new ideas and uncover potential blind alleys, roundabouts, etc. Furthermore, the teacher's continued exploration will contribute to the lessons he designs later to challenge and support the types of problems students identify during these types of conversations. The conversation highlights the patterns of understanding students hold and what kinds of feedback might be necessary in follow-on lessons that could help direct the student's attention.

Interviewing as Scaffolding

Scaffolding, as its image might suggest, is the framework that holds an unfinished building or idea together. Scaffolding is the teacher's attempt to keep the student engaged with the problem, to limit the number of tasks needed to solve a problem in order to ensure the child can reach a solution, and to control frustration by making "problem solving less dangerous or stressful with a tutor than without" (Wood, Bruner, & Ross, 1976). The interview provides Eve the scaffolding to help her integrate the patterns that a trained eye sees in nature (like her teacher's) with the patterns that her brain is trying to detect. This effort has but one goal – to help her predict what she might see when she looks into Electromagnet Land. For example, in the following interchange Eve introduces many ideas about how to make an electromagnet stronger, but Mr. M takes only one at a time.

Eve: Because I know that sometimes the wire gets loose [the wraps around the nail], the wire goes in different directions [making for a sloppy looking electromagnet]. I think that they are probably going [to] use like, thicker wire and have it a little more powerful.... and a lot more powerful battery. Because in this case it [the telephone and the electromagnets inside] is plugged into the wall. And that has a lot more electricity going through it. So it [the phone's electromagnet] is probably more powerful.

M: Uh huh. So you think neatness is important as well, because you mentioned that...?

Eve: Yah, because every single piece of wire has to touch the nail... like I think to make a complete circuit around it.

There are a number of variables that Eve is considering: neatness, thickness of wire, the amount of electricity available, and, her latest thought, complete circuits. For example, where does neatness fit in her exploration of Electromagnet Land? This new mapping (Rp2) suggests that Eve may be trying to coordinate both neatness of wraps (which contributes to the wires ability to maintain contact with the nail) and electromagnet strength. She also seems to be trying to coordinate the "neatness–strength" mapping with another involving a second variable (i.e., thickness of wire) and its impact on the electromagnet's strength. In this case, a coordination of these two mappings would represent a new representational system (Level Rp3); however, nature's response to Eve's tentative system would be that this more complex coordination is not a pattern nature recognizes.

The interchange is also open to investigating what she means by a "complete circuit." In the last exchange, Eve was weighing the impact of neatness, thickness of wire, and complete circuits as variables; and, their importance in electromagnets do differ. The pattern is complex, and Eve needs to consider and weigh all the variables to recognize the pattern that leads to the most powerful predictions. Mr. M recognizes that some explorations will provide more insight than others, but may not be able to tell which path will be the most promising; however, he remains patient. Their investigation does not have to start or stop with neatness, but does have to begin somewhere.

By choosing to investigate any one variable with Eve, her teacher is also scaffolding the process scientists use to discover the importance of variables embedded in the patterns observed in nature. All disciplines have developed ways of knowing that teachers bring to their conversations with students. In many cases, that process is only obvious to the teacher. Even though the student is still in charge, her attention is being focused in a manner scientists would recognize. The conversation temporarily assumes the structure of a controlled experiment, where Mr. M explores the power each variable has for Eve. In follow-on conversations, Eve and Mr. M might investigate additional relationships between her ideas; discovering the dead ends in her map of Electromagnet Land, the roads that intersect, or the roads that run parallel to each other. Her teacher helps Eve keep track of her explorations, her findings, and her success in creating more sophisticated skills to coordinate her ideas and discoveries.

Given the variety of possible directions the conversation might take, Mr. M recognizes that of all the variables, one in particular resonates with the plumbing mapping, which dominated the earlier conversations. His close attention to Eve's progress allows him to recognize that an important element of neatness is Eve's concern that the wire touches the nail. The new "neatness–strength" mapping reveals her attempt to bridge what she knows about plumbing to what she has experienced with her electromagnet.

M: Oh, I see. You think the wire has to touch the nail?

Eve: Yah, touch the nail.

M: So if we wrapped the nail with paper for example... and then... wrap the paper and the nail with the wire. Do you think that would work?

Eve: Well, it depends. I think that electricity might be able to go through paper, but not like really thick surfaces.

M: All right... let's say... Oh I see, not "thick surfaces".

Eve: Yah, because I think it could [go] through paper, but not something really thick... like a piece of wood.

M: So you think the electricity leaves the wire and actually goes into the nail?

Eve: Yah

If her plumbing model of electricity holds, then the wire must touch the nail and the electricity must somehow leak into the nail. But electricity will not leak into the nail; yet, according to her mapping it must. Mr. M remains silent at this point to let Eve consider the problem she has encountered with her plumbing model. Eve is encouraged to continue her thinking, and as a result she encounters a problem that is perfectly reasonable considering her present working model. After a few seconds Eve asks, "What I would like to know is if the wire is insulated, how does it [the electricity] get into it [the nail]?"

Eve arrives at the question that began crystallizing earlier with her acknowledgment that maybe some of the electricity enters the nail. Mr. M still resists offering an explanation. More importantly, Eve is not really asking Mr. M to answer the question, so he does not. He is also conscious of the trap science educators (and possibly all educators) encounter to by assuming that their first responsibility is to offer students more sophisticated models as replacements for their ideas. Teachers find it difficult to resist the temptation to demonstrate the way they solve problems even though educators have long observed that students rarely use their teacher's models (Holt, 1964; Bredderman, 1983; Driver et al., 1985; Schneps & Sadler, 1988; Miller, 1992; Lightman & Sadler, 1993; Driver et al., 1994; Shamos, 1995; Barker, 1999).

Students more often defer to the simpler models, metaphors, or beliefs they have created when trying to make sense of a problem (Novak & Gowin, 1984). Eve demonstrates the power of the plumbing model to make sense of her question regarding insulation:

Eve: ... I think, like [the electromagnets] might be less powerful. Very little [electricity] is escaping into it [the nail] no matter how many links [of chain] we think it [our electromagnet] picks up. Because it could be uhm, that... uhm, it [our electromagnet] is less powerful, for us not to get electrocuted. But inside a telephone it's all covered and everything. So they probably do it [use wire] without the insulation. Because then they wouldn't have to worry about anyone touching it [the wire and getting electrocuted].

M: Ah, so you think if you took apart a telephone, and you saw an electromagnet, the wires wouldn't have any insulation?

Eve: Yah. Because there's no risk of anyone getting electrocuted. In this case [with the electromagnets we are making], I think that very little [electricity] is escaping into the nail.

Eve is still weighing the usefulness of the plumbing mapping. She is reasoning that the battery was not powerful enough to allow electricity to cross the wire–nail divide. She feels that this issue would not be a problem with more electricity (as an electrical outlet could provide) and wires that had no insulation (such as she suspects exists in telephones). Mr. M continues to explore with Eve the usefulness of the metaphor because it is clear that this mapping captures an important pattern that she sees in nature (i.e., in order for objects to get from one place to another, a conduit is essential). Wires do allow the electricity to travel, much in the same way that pipes transports water. This metaphor is still a useful skill for interpreting events. Accordingly, Eve concludes if the wire is not insulated, then the electricity will be able to leave the wire and move to the core. However Eve still needs to confront the limits of this pattern (characterized during much of this text as a representational mapping or, more generally, as the plumbing metaphor).

The focus on insulation and the need for contact between the nail and wire has lead to a new scenario, which Eve created. In this new context Eve is empowered to take specific action to test a specific prediction. Eve's new state of mind is also underscored by the minor theme of this chapter – the role the brain plays in this process. Its ongoing goal is to identify possible patterns in order to make more reliable predictions. Eve will find out, when she takes apart the phone, that the wire used in the electromagnets is insulated. How will Eve react to this discovery? It will not match her prediction. What will she say when she discovers that all electromagnets use insulated wire, and when all the insulation is removed, the electromagnet stops working?

Eve is at the cusp of organizing a new representational system (Level Rp3) that accounts for how insulation and conduits contribute to electromagnetism. The plumbing metaphor she uses to represent reality is an intermediate level of understanding of the world that will support more sophisticated models. Once again it is important to recognize that metaphors are important structures for making sense of reality (Lakoff & Johnson, 1980). They help bridge the gap from the known to the unknown.

This path to more sophisticated models (which in this text has often meant, "more complex skills") will be supported by her investigation of phones because this test addresses a problem Eve recognizes with the plumbing metaphor. The outcome is difficult to predict. She may ignore the evidence that electromagnets use insulated wire, and continue trying to use the plumbing model. She may modify the plumbing model by focusing on other relevant observations. There is also the risk that she may realize this model does not work and abandon electromagnetism in complete frustration. The margin between frustration and empowerment is one that the teacher must attempt to moderate. With the help of her science teacher, Eve (as well as her classmates) may be ready to consider the idea of "fields" and take a step toward an important abstraction (arising from coordinating several representational systems at Level Rp3) in electromagnetism. Eve has already noted that magnetism can impact certain objects without physically touching the object. Further consideration of this phenomenon moves her closer to a system of systems that describes both electricity and magnetism in terms of "fields."

This fields abstraction (Level Ab1) assumes that electricity passing through wires sets up an invisible field much in the same way that magnets set up an invisible field. Eve played with permanent magnets in an earlier lesson, and observed that magnets can influence certain objects as at a distance. Water, passing through pipes, cannot do this, but electricity in wires can. Recognizing this new "mapping" represents an important step in integrating it with more established mappings in order to construct a key representational system (Rp3) that coordinates ideas such as conduits, influence over space, and insulation. This coordination is a step toward the more complicated model of field theory.

Scaffolding: A Constructivist's View

Could the electricity running through a wire generate a field that affects the nail? The answer is yes, and careful lesson planning can help prepare students for this transition in understanding; however, by rushing to the answer educators risk not appreciating that the trip from "naive model" to "sophisticated model" represents critical steps in the evolution and development of more complex skills. Just offering Eve the destination does not offer her a way to find the connections between what she already understands and what science education tells her she ought to understand.

Scaffolding an exploration of electromagnets through the interview process supports the constructivist position that students must build their own meaning of concepts, and in science as in most subjects, this requires time, time, and more time. The teacher's role is to facilitate that construction with both focused questions and lessons that the student appreciates and understands. Using Eve's description of electricity is very useful from a constructivist point of view. Educators begin with what Eve knows, using the language that she uses to understand electricity. For example, Eve explains the importance of "big" (and a related metaphor) in building stronger electromagnets in the following way:

> Eve: I haven't experimented with big nails, but if it's really big like in a laboratory, scientists use really big powerful instruments. They'd probably find that if they use really thick wire and a really big nail, a lot [of electricity] will circulate through that nail. I think that's probably the second most important thing.

In Eve's comment we can still observe the importance of the plumbing model as she suggests that "really thick wire" can carry a lot of electricity. This insight makes sense if you believe that a big pipe can carry a lot of water. Here again is another opportunity for her to test her model against reality. Are there additional areas of reality for which her model does or does not account? Nature's patterns are revealed through closer and closer inspection of the world. But how far can the teacher support the student in this exploration? Without being certain of the answer for Eve or any student, the teacher offers a context that allows Eve the room to grow comfortable with her ideas so that she can begin to see where they hold and do not hold.

Eve would need to decide if she wants to invest the energy in creating a new more comprehensive model or simply ignore all the problems this investigation and conversation raises. Can the brain get tired looking for patterns? People often face this issue when confronting a problem where the old paradigm or model has been shown not to work. They know at some point they will have to expend time and energy to modify or replace the model that they have been using. It might be reasonable to expect that the resistance to changing a model is directly related to the time and energy necessary in creating a better model along with the new circuits required to support this new view. In any case, schools should serve to help Eve and her peers challenge their own views. Unfortunately too many students enter adulthood without having had the opportunity to seriously challenge any of their own models.

Conclusions

This chapter ends where most teachers want it to begin. Mr. M is satisfied that he understands Eve's construction of the world of electromagnets, and Eve is satisfied that she has made some progress in understanding through her own initiative; however, clearly there is room for improving Eve's understanding. To address this need, her teacher will need to change roles from interviewer to curriculum developer. Better informed, he is now prepared to make choices about the shape and the direction the curriculum should take for students like Eve, which skills are well established, which skills need further support, and which skills are the most sophisticated representations (or abstractions) his students will be able to coordinate.

The interview process began by focusing on how students like Eve build concepts and, while still maintaining that focus, demonstrated its potential to scaffold further inquiry. The same process highlights how students work toward more complex skills within their zone of proximal development (Vygotsky, 1978). By using skill theory to operationalize structures of understanding, teachers can evaluate a student's initial understanding as well as how changes in understanding compare with the student's original ideas (Case, 1991; Fischer & Bidell, 2006). Skill theory provides a tool for analyzing and quantifying degrees of understanding with the student's range of possible understanding. Because skill theory recognizes that changes in context will affect which skill a student will display, the interview process can be seen as a special context in which student and teacher can benefit.

Within this context, the teacher helps the student access work accomplished earlier, ideas already discussed, and/or the relationships explored between ideas and observations. Eve's teacher highlights the problems Eve needs to grapple with in order to build more sophisticated models of how electromagnets work. The world of electromagnetism is represented as a new environment where new and old patterns confront each other. The brain meets the challenge in two ways. In the short term it looks to coordinate older established patterns stored in memory with new experiences in order to make reliable predictions. In the longer term, the brain matures through the investment of energy in building networks and then coordinating those networks in different regions to establish and consolidate new levels and tiers.

The interview was portrayed as an educational tool that supports a teacher's understanding of student views, while providing students the opportunity to recognize and build upon their current structures of understanding. An outcome of the student's effort in challenging his or her ideas is temporary or fragile improvements in understanding that approach his or her optimal level, characterized more objectively through skill theory. Attaining a clearer picture of the variation in structures of understanding that students achieve can help teachers and curriculum designers plan more focused interventions as well as better evaluate the outcome of those interventions.

The goal of interviewing was to create an inviting dialog where students could experiment with their views, challenge their "actual" structure of understanding, and begin exploring structures of understanding that are closer to their optimal level. The goal was not to offer students more complex views that they somehow incorporate into their present world-view. In this environment, the student also has goals to seek a better understanding, and in this interchange with her teacher Eve is motivated to integrate new experiences, coordinate old views with new views, and build more sophisticated structures of understanding. While the conversations do offer scaffolding, they also reveal the student's potential. Curriculum planning beyond the interview would need to address the nature of ongoing support.

With greater insight into the student's world, teachers can better understand how to shape their classroom and lessons so that students can spend more time learning how to recognize and work with more complex patterns that support more powerful predictions about the world. With time and practice students can maintain their ability to perform at their full potential. However with maturity, the bar of potential development is raised, and what is today's potential level is tomorrow's actual level.

References

Ausubel, D. (1968). *Educational psychology: A cognitive view*. New York: Holt, Rinehart and Winston.

Barker, V. (1999). Students' reasoning about chemical reactions: What changes occur during a context-based post-16 chemistry course. *International Journal of Science Education, 21*(6), 645–665.

Bredderman, T. (1983). Effects of activity-based elementary science on student outcomes. *Review of Educational Research 53*(4), 499–518.

Case, R. (1985). *Intellectual development: Birth to adulthood.* New York, NY: Academic Press.

Case, R. (Ed.). (1991). *The mind's staircase: Exploring the conceptual underpinnings of children's thought and knowledge.* Hillsdale: Erlbaum.

Case, R. (1992). The role of the frontal lobes in the regulation of cognitive development. Special Issue: The role of frontal lobe maturation in cognitive and social development. *Brain & Cognition, 20*(1), 51–73.

Driver, R., Guesne E., & Tiberghien, A. (1985). Some features of children's ideas and their implications for teaching. In R. Driver, E. Guesne, & A. Tiberghien (Eds.), *Children's ideas in science* (pp. 193–201). Milton Keynes, UK: Open University Press.

Driver, R., Squires, A., Rushworth, P., & Wood-Robinson, V. (1994). *Making sense of secondary science: Research into children's ideas.* London: Routledge.

Fischer, K. W. (1980). A theory of cognitive development: The control and construction of hierarchies of skills. *Psychological Review, 87*, 477–531.

Fischer, K. W., & Bidell, T.R. (2006). Dynamic development of action and thought. Theoretical Models of Human Development. In W. Damon & R. M. Lerner (Eds.), *Handbook of child psychology* (6th ed., Vol. 1, pp. 313–339). New York, NY: Wiley.

Fischer, K. W., Bullock D., Rotenberg, E. J., & Raya, P. (1993). The dynamics of competence: How context contributes directly to skill. In R. Wozniak & K. W. Fischer (Eds.), *Development in context: Acting and thinking in specific environments* (pp. 93–117). Hillsdale, NJ: Erlbaum.

Fischer, K. W., & Pipp, S. L. (1984). Process of cognitive development: Optimal level and skill acquisition. In R. J. Sternber (Ed.), *Mechanisms of cognitive development* (pp. 45–80). New York: Freeman.

Fischer, K. W., & Rose S. P. (1998). Growth cycles of brain and mind. *Educational Leadership, 56*(3), 56–60.

Hawkins, J., & Blakeslee, S. (2004). *On intelligence.* New York: Times Books.

Holt, J. (1964). *How children fail.* New York: Dell Publishing Co.

Hugh, H., & Novak, J. D. (1983). <proc>*Proceedings of the international seminar on misconceptions in science and mathematics*</proc>. Ithaca, NY: Cornel University ED, *242*, 553.

Lakoff, G., & Johnson M. (1980). *Metaphors we live by.* Chicago, University of Chicago Press.

Lightman, A., & Sadler, P. (1993). Teacher predictions versus actual student gains. *The Physics Teacher*, 31, 162–167.

Miller, J. D. (1992). The public understanding of science and technology in the United States, 1990. Washington, DC: Report to the National Science Foundation.

Mountcastle, V. B. (1998). *Perceptual neuroscience: The cerebral cortex.* Cambridge, MA: Harvard University Press.

Nardi, B. (1996). Studying context: A comparison of activity theory, situated action models, and distributed cognition. In B. Nardi(Ed.), *Context and consciousness: Activity theory and human-computer interaction* (pp. 69–102). Cambridge, MA: MIT Press.

Novak, J. D., & Gowin D. B. (1984). *Learning how to learn.* New York: Cambridge University Press.

Pea, R. D. (1993). Practices of distributed intelligence and designs for education. In G. Salomon(Ed.), *Distributed cognitions: Psychological and educational considerations* (pp. 47–87). Cambridge, MA: Cambridge University Press.

Phillips, A. (1988). *Winnicott.* Cambridge, MA: Harvard University Press.

Sadler, P. (1998). Psychometric models of student conceptions in science: Reconciling qualitative studies and distractor-driven assessment instruments. *Journal of Research in Science Teaching, 35*(3), 265–296.

Salomon, G., & Perkins D. N. (1989). Rocky roads to transfer: Rethinking mechanisms of a neglected phenomenon. *Educational Psychologist, 24*(2), 113–142.

Schneps, M. H., & Sadler P. M. (1988). *Private universe.* Santa Monica, CA: Pyramid Films.

Schwartz, M. S. (2000). *Design challenges: A new path to understanding science concepts and skills.* Unpublished Doctoral Dissertation. Cambridge, MA: Harvard University.

Schwartz, M. S., & Fischer K. W. (2004). Building general knowledge and skill: Cognition and microdevelopment in science learning. In A. Demetriou & A. Raftopoulos(Eds.), *Emergence and transformation in the mind: Modeling and measuring cognitive change.* Cambridge, UK: Cambridge University Press.

Schwartz, M. S., & Sadler, P. S. (2007). Empowerment in science curriculum development: A microdevelopmental approach. *International Journal of Science Education, 29*(8), 987–1017.

Shamos, M. H. (1995). *The myth of scientific literacy.* New Brunswick: Rutgers University Press.

Shipstone, D. (1985). Electricity in simple circuits. In R. Driver, E. Guesne, & A. Tiberghien (Eds.), *Children's ideas in science* (pp. 33–51). Milton Keynes, UK: Open University Press.

Thatcher, R. C. (1994). Cyclic Cortical Re-Organization: Origins of Human Cognitive Development. In G. Dawson & K. Fischer (Eds.), *Human behavior and the developing brain.* New York: Guilford Press.

Thelen, E., & Smith, L. B. (1998). Dynamic systems theory. In W. Damon (Ed.), *Handbook of child psychology* (Vol. 1, pp. 563–634). New York: John Wiley & Sons.

Van Geert, P. (1994). *Dynamic systems of development: Change between complexity and chaos.* New York: Harvester Wheatsheaf.

Vygotsky, L. S. (1962). *Thought and language.* Cambridge: MIT Press.

Vygotsky, L. S. (1978). *Mind in society: The development of higher psychological processes.* Cambridge, MA: Harvard University Press.

Wood, D., Bruner J. S., & Ross, G. (1976). The role of tutoring in problem solving. *Journal of Child Psychology and Psychiatry, 17,* 89–100.

Part II
Mind and Brain in Social and Personal Development

Phases of Social–Emotional Development from Birth to School Age

Marc D. Lewis and Isabela Granic

In this chapter, we describe a series of phases of social–emotional development – the repertoire of emotional feelings, impulses, and regulatory processes that characterize children's social interactions across the period of infancy and early childhood. To help conceptualize and understand this progression, we juxtapose Robbie Case's stage model of early cognitive development with observational research on children's emotional responses to their caregivers. A great deal of information is available from researchers who have studied children and parents directly, often by videotaping them in natural and experimental environments. These researchers include Ed Tronick, Colwyn Trevarthen, Alan Fogel, Louis Sander, Margaret Mahler, Joe Campos, Michael Tomasello, Judy Dunn, and many others. Much of this literature describes behavioral phenomena that change in systematic ways with development. There is a good fit between these changes and the schedule of cognitive development proposed by Case and other neo-Piagetian theorists. Our aim is to demonstrate this fit clearly and to make sense of it by showing how children's cognitive acquisitions provide the underpinning for their social–emotional activities at each age and stage. We see that Case's model of early cognitive development explains *why* social–emotional functions appear when they appear, by specifying the cognitive tools children have (or still lack) at each age for interpreting the world in a particular way – evoking particular emotions (appraisal functions) and coping with those emotions when they arise (regulatory functions). At the same time, we see that the data on early social–emotional development put flesh on the bones of Case's timetable of cognitive stages and substages, by describing a rich behavioral domain shaped by intrinsic and extrinsic capacities and constraints.

The overall point of the chapter is to show how 11 phases of social–emotional development are nested within the first two major stages (and component substages) of cognitive development – a period from birth to 4–5 years. For the sake of

M.D. Lewis (✉)
Department of Human Development and Applied Psychology, OISE/University of Toronto, Toronto, ON, Canada
e-mail: mlewis@oise.utoronto.ca

M. Ferrari, L. Vuletic (eds.), *The Developmental Relations among Mind, Brain and Education*, DOI 10.1007/978-90-481-3666-7_8,

clarity, we denote periods of social–emotional development as "phases" and periods of cognitive development as "stages" and "substages." We also suggest some directions for educational applications of this timetable, specifically in the realm of parent education. Robbie was a great advocate of educational advances based on psychological theory and research. And parents need all the help they can get in navigating the difficult emotional terrain of infancy and toddlerhood. However, following Robbie's example, and in contrast to most attempts at parent education, we base our suggestions on research. They are thus specific, empirically based, and time-sensitive. Behind many of these suggestions is the simple logic that emotional development swings like a pendulum between periods of greater resilience, stability, and self-reliance and periods of greater vulnerability, sensitivity, and dependency. We propose that vulnerable periods correspond with substage transitions to unifocal and bifocal coordination, in both the sensorimotor and interrelational stages. These are the developmental shifts that most transform the young child's cognitive and emotional worlds. Our general message to parents is to spare children jarring life events, such as the commencement of daycare, extended parental absences, and major changes to routines such as sleeping and feeding, during these periods of vulnerability. Such challenges will be more easily negotiated during phases of development characterized by independence and security. Finally, we include a personal note here and there. Because this volume is in memory and in honor of Robbie – both the person and the scholar – we intersperse our writing with the occasional memory, image, or anecdote based on our interactions with Robbie. Both of us knew him well as a teacher and friend, particularly Marc, who was Robbie's graduate student and theoretical progeny; also Isabela Granic, who took courses with Robbie and "picked his brain" on topics from development to dinner. In fact, our last memory of Robbie, shoveling down Indian food while discussing the roller-coaster ride of his life, still resonates as an emotional blend of sadness, affection, and surprise – always surprise.

The relation between cognition and emotion has captured the attention of psychologists of many stripes. It has also captured the attention of contemporary neuroscience. Psychologists generally look at the cognitive concomitants of emotion in terms of two distinct functions: an appraisal function, by which cognitive interpretations induce or trigger particular emotions, and a regulatory function, by which cognitive capacities to shift attention, inhibit attention, or reappraise the meaning of a situation serve to alter the type or intensity of an emotional response. Conventional emotion theory, a branch of cognitive psychology, thus places some cognitive operations before emotions (appraisals) and other cognitive operations after emotions (regulation) (Frijda, 1993). As can be seen, however, there is a fair bit of overlap between these kinds of operations. Appraisal is supposed to come before emotion, but re-appraisal is supposed to come after emotion, to help regulate it. And because appraisal itself is a complex suite of operations, entailing a variety of attentional and interpretive processes, there really is no clear way to parse appraisal from regulation. They involve overlapping cognitive operations. One way out of this conundrum is to view cognition and emotion as reciprocal, iterative processes that continue to build on one another as emotional processes unfold in time (Lewis, 1995, 1996; Lewis &

Granic 1999; Scherer, 1999). A related approach is to view cognition–emotion interactions as a multi-component dynamic system that settles in different states (Lewis & Granic, 2000; Scherer, 2000). Both of these approaches lend themselves to neuroscientific investigations. A look at the brain during emotional states demonstrates activity in a variety of regions associated with attentional and interpretive cognitive processes (e.g., lateral prefrontal cortex, anterior cingulate cortex, temporal-parietal junction) as well as automatic appraisal areas that trigger emotional associations (amygdala). But the brain does not divide appraisal, emotion, and regulation in any neat or meaningful way (see Lewis, 2005, for a review and synthesis; also Pessoa, 2008).

The complexity of brain activities subserving cognition–emotion interactions makes it difficult to test age-specific cognitive operations involved in appraisal or regulation. This would seem to be a necessary condition for a neuroscientific research program relating stages of cognitive development to phases of emotional development on the basis of underlying cognitive operations. Nevertheless, specific questions have been asked by developmental neuroscientists concerning cognitive functions that may be critical for emotional appraisal and/or regulation at particular ages. Most notably, Posner and Rothbart (1998, 2000) have long postulated that maturation of the anterior cingulate cortex corresponds to children's developing capacity to apply "effortful control" to override their impulses at 3–4 years of age. Specific cognitive tasks have been used to test this hypothesis. The Eriksen flanker task, which requires subjects to avoid attention to distracting stimuli so that they can correctly identify the target stimulus, has been conducted with preschool children in conjunction with neural evaluations. However, no evidence for the maturation of the anterior cingulate at the hypothesized age has yet been reported. Studies of the neural correlates of appraisal and regulation, using emotional stimuli, have been conducted with adults (e.g., Beauregard, Lévesque, & Bourgouin, 2001; Cunningham et al., 2004; Ochsner et al., 2004; Ochsner & Gross, 2005), and much less frequently with particular age groups, including infancy (e.g., Carver & Vaccaro, 2007) and adolescence (e.g., Monk et al., 2003). Our own work has investigated age-related changes in neural activity corresponding with cognitive functions involved in emotion regulation (Lamm, Zelazo, & Lewis, 2006; Lewis et al., 2006). But none of these studies tap age differences in the content or structure of cognitive operations. In short, there is very little research relating stage-specific cognitive concomitants of emotional appraisal and emotion regulation to the developing brain, and certainly no fine-grained research program that allows us to assign an age-specific level of cognitive operations to an observed change in brain function. It should also be noted that there is very little evidence of neural changes corresponding to stages of cognitive development in general, with the exception of work by Thatcher (eg., 1991, 1998, "Higher-order network reworking: New findings"). Thus, despite the attraction of using neuroscience to study stage-specific cognition–emotion interactions in development, we presently have to overlook the brain and rely on behavioral evidence for a progression of phases of emotional development linked with neo-Piagetian stages.

Many investigators believe that children's emotional functioning depends on their level of cognitive development – how they interpret the world uniquely at each stage. A detailed model of emotional stages that parallel cognitive stages was developed by Alan Sroufe (e.g., 1979, 1995). This model was well received by Robbie, who shared it with his students enthusiastically, both in class and in casual conversation. Like Robbie, we see much merit in Sroufe's analysis, and we borrow liberally from his ideas. But how should we envision the structure of cognitive development as the foundation for children's emotional capacities and habits?

Marc remembers conversations in which Robbie referred to the stages of cognitive development as being like the floors of a house or building under construction. Each floor is constructed gradually, he said. First the vertical supports go up, then the concrete floor is laid down, then the doors and windows are framed, and finally the walls get built up around them. Moreover, this sequence of construction begins with each new floor before the floor below is completed. Robbie intended this metaphor to emphasize the gradual nature of cognitive development, within and even between stages, often in opposition to Marc's argument for rapid, global reorganizations appearing as developmental discontinuities. Robbie and Marc disagreed on a few issues concerning the nature of development, giving rise to an ongoing and incredibly fertile debate that extended from one Indian meal to the next. However, we agreed on most of the important points. A good argument with Robbie was like a duel, leaving a little blood and a lot of sweat but no major injuries. And it was always surprising to see how quickly Robbie's ideas grew, metamorphosed, and advanced, as new perspectives – e.g., from dynamic systems theory and developmental neuroscience – made themselves available. Robbie enjoyed debate and disagreement, and intellectual challenges provided him with fuel for the continual enhancement of his thinking and his theory. In any case, we see his point about the house under construction, and we use this metaphor to frame the relation of social–emotional acquisitions to cognitive-developmental stages. As shown in Fig. 1, social–emotional phases (the "windows" on each floor) are embedded within the "building" of Robbie's stages and substages.

What is responsible for the synchronization of social–emotional development with the underlying structure of cognitive development? In Robbie's view, the cognitive software for understanding the social world and for understanding the self changes in important and measurable ways from one stage or substage to the next, and it is that understanding that is responsible for generating emotions and for modifying those emotions once they appear. As noted previously, we can break this idea down into two fundamental mechanisms, one for generating emotion (often called *appraisal*) and one for regulating emotion (or *emotion regulation*). First, when the child moves from one stage to the next, and his or her mental software is upgraded accordingly, the computations that trigger emotional reactions are different, resulting in different emotions (e.g., the advent of jealousy at about 2½) and different contexts for the same emotion (e.g., the generation of anger by a threat to self-esteem by about 1½). Second, the computations used to regulate emotions (e.g., to inhibit the affective discomfort of distress or to deflect an angry impulse) also become more efficacious, sophisticated, and abstract with the progress of cognitive

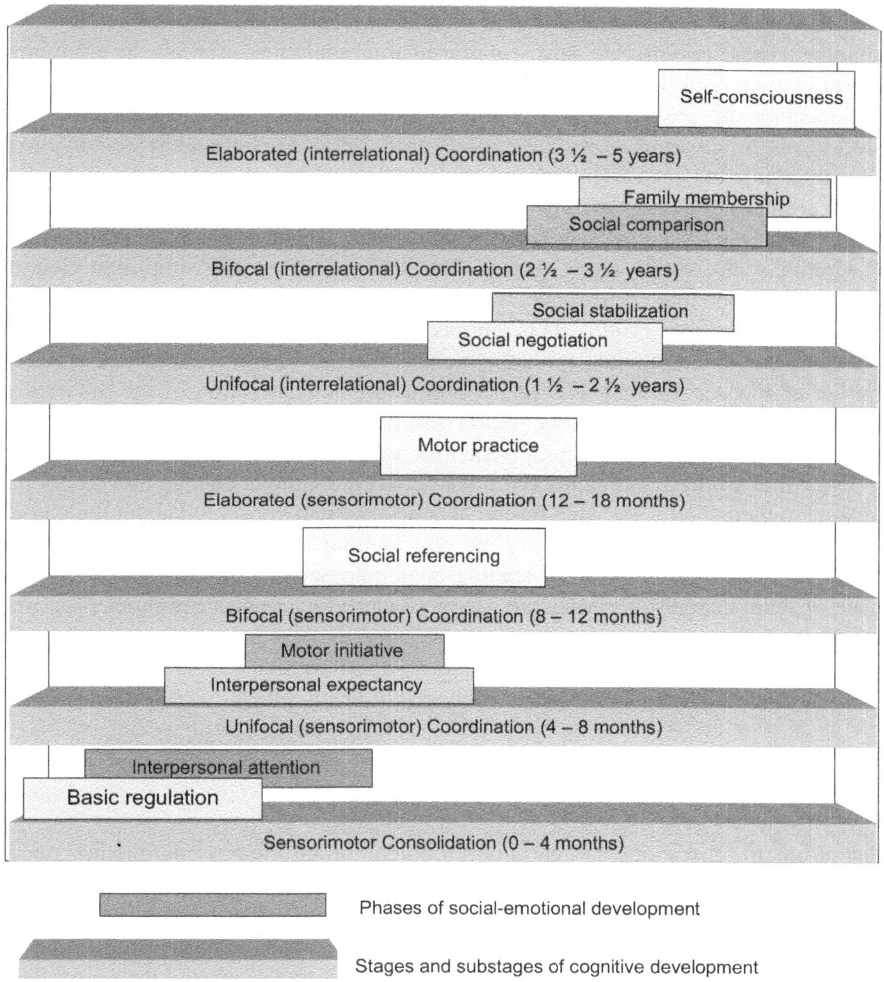

Fig. 1 Stages and substages of cognitive development as a foundation for phases of social–emotional development across the first 4–5 years of life

development. Thus, at each stage, there is a new set of *reasons* for glee, distress, excitement, or disappointment; new tools for *adjusting* thoughts and actions to minimize negative emotions (and amplify positive ones); and sometimes new emotions *themselves*. Each new stage of cognitive development brings with it a change in what the child understands, pays attention to, and finds interesting, attractive, important, and frustrating. That changes the basic cognitive appraisal that is responsible for the initial moments of an emotional response, and changes the capacities for extending and modifying that appraisal as the emotional response continues to feed back with its cognitive concomitants (in our view). For Robbie, and for us, developmental change in these two mechanisms – appraisal and regulation – retools the emotional world in sync with the milestones of cognitive development. In other words, these two mechanisms ensure that each shift in cognitive development is paralleled by a shift in emotional development (see also Sroufe, 1995). We have addressed the theoretical relation between cognitive and emotional development in great detail in other work, emphasizing our own dynamic systems perspective over the last 10 or 15 years (e.g., Case, Hayward, Lewis, & Hurst, 1988; Lewis, 1993a, 1995, 1996, 2000; Lewis & Granic, 1999, 2000). Here we leave the reader with a fairly simplified view of this relation: one that corresponds with the views we generally shared with Robbie and outlined by Case (1988). This interpretation is sufficient to map out a series of phases of social–emotional development, based on the cognitive capacities acquired by the child over the first 4–5 years. While further elaboration of the theoretical relation between cognition and emotion will be of interest to some readers, it does little to alter the basic roadmap of normative social–emotional development.

Now that we have explained the links between cognitive change and emotional change in theory, let's see what researchers have actually observed about the phases of social–emotional development. We now outline those phases, in chronological order, based on the work of leading contemporary researchers, and show how each of them depends, in large part, on the underlying cognitive abilities proposed by Case and his colleagues. That is to say, we explain *how and why* children's emotional responses to their parents' actions – routines, rules, separations, reunions, etc. – change in predictable ways at each step of development.

Phase 1: Basic Regulation

According to Case's model of early development, infants do not enter the first major stage, *sensorimotor coordination*, until 4 or 4½ months. Before then, they can't move their hands to follow their gaze. They can gaze at interesting objects continuously. They can orient to them, if they are already in their field of vision, and they can even track the movements of their mother as she moves around the room. By 3 or 4 months, babies can track more complex movements, such as those of a mobile, and they take delight in the continuous changes of shape that mobiles are famous for. Young babies can also hold onto a rattle, grasping it with their palms and fingers and feeling its texture. But they can't coordinate their gaze with their manual actions. So the grasping they do is not guided by the visual system. And their gaze at interesting objects rarely leads to reaching or grasping. Infants of this age are in the preliminary substage of sensorimotor coordination, dubbed senorimotor *consolidation,* when their capabilities are best characterized by what they *can't* do. According to Case, their limitations stem from their inability to coordinate two sensorimotor schemes. This inability makes the young infant unable to launch a two-part action, or an action intended to produce an effect. So all she can do is to continue more or less whatever she's already doing.

According to infant observers, the period of 0–3 months is the time when babies learn to regulate their basic bodily reactions, their states, and their physiology.

These little beings have spent a long time in the womb, developing all the bodily mechanisms necessary to live on this planet, to eat, to breathe, to expend energy in motion, to coordinate muscles and senses so that motion accomplishes something, and to sleep when replenishment is needed. They have also acquired the mechanisms for gaining knowledge and skill – mechanisms that will allow them to pay attention to what is most important, especially the faces, voices, and actions of other humans. Now, each of these mechanisms starts to function. And, as if that weren't enough, they have to function together, in synchrony with one another. Despite their vast complexity, bodies and brains have to start acting in a highly coordinated fashion. Systems have to be tuned to one another so that arousal, motivation, motor actions, sensory focusing, and the organs responsible for fueling them all become coordinated.

This period of developing synchrony among brain, body, and mind is referred to as the period of "basic regulation" by Louis Sander, a researcher who spent several decades observing infants and their mothers. (e.g., Sander 1975) emphasized, not just the coordination of these systems with each other, but also their coordination with the habits, states, and capabilities of the mother (or other caregiver). (When we refer to "the mother" it is out of convenience. Most primary caregivers in the vast majority of cultures are mothers. But primary caregivers can also be fathers, grandparents, elder sisters, nannies, and so forth. Our mention of "the mother" should be taken to include anyone who plays that crucial role). Sander (1975, 1983) was particularly interested in how the infant and caregiver manage to adjust to each other's needs and capacities.

The link between cognitive development and social–emotional synchronization at this age was dealt with by Case in some detail in a speculative but fascinating paper (Case, 1991). We won't summarize this work, but the main point is that the infant during this stage builds up representations of his own actions synchronized with mother's actions through a large number of recurrent associations. Because two schemes cannot be coordinated on-line, learning during this phase is gradual rather than abrupt. Rather than scheme coordination as a mechanism of learning, sensorimotor schemes are in the process of being elaborated and extended through conditioning. That is how sensory input constellations (such as the changing image of a toy as it moves through space) can be integrated with motor control representations (such as the change in muscle contractions needed to move the eye in correspondence with the toy). Similarly, shared interactions such as feeding involve component sensory and muscular processes that engage both the infant and the mother, but the representation acquired by the child does not necessarily distinguish these components. Rather, a smoothly coordinated feeding interaction becomes the object of a single sensorimotor scheme in which expected actions and outcomes are fused together in a single amalgam that is manipulated within the infant's cognitive apparatus each time feeding takes place. And Robbie was of the opinion that emotional tone was a fundamental feature of that amalgam (also see Stern, 1985). The gradual building up of such complex sensorimotor schemes sets the stage for two-scheme coordinations that arrive on the scene after 4 months. At that time learning will be fluid, but in the period prior to 4 months it is slow, gradual, and dependent on the repetition of familiar routines.

According to Sander, the success of the *basic regulation* period is marked by the smoothness, predictability, and emotional ease with which the infant shifts from one state to another: from alertness, to drowsiness, to sleep, and back again (Sander, 1975). Each of these states is unique psychologically and physiologically, and each has its purpose. But there is another marker that things are going well in this stage – one that is gleaned entirely through the emotional tone of parents' interactions with their baby. A successful resolution of *basic regulation* is evidenced by increasing smiling, decreasing distress, and a good deal of direct face-to-face contact, as well as the baby's ability to turn off, turn away, and relax between bouts of social interaction. By the age of 2½–3 months, babies become a lot more attentive and a lot more social, indicating the consolidation and retrieval of complex sensorimotor schemes. With this success, they no longer have to worry about making their bodies and brains work properly, and now they can have some fun being in the world. Also, due to their rapidly growing preoccupation with human faces, they become a lot more fun to be with. The famous "social smile" begins to appear regularly by this age, and that is a true reward for parents' hard work.

In sum, the *basic regulation* phase is a time when body and brain systems become connected to each other, synchronized with the rhythms of parents and other family members, and coordinated with the conditions of the world they live in, to fashion complex and fluid sensorimotor schemes. Because these schemes depend for their consolidation on routines that the baby can recognize and anticipate, infants need predictability, especially concerning the physical aspects of care. Emotional responses at this age (e.g., smiling at the sight of mother's approach) depend on the infant's capacity to hold the spatiotemporal features of important events in mind, through the application of a single sensorimotor scheme. Thus, even at this young age, their emotions derive from their cognitive activities, not just from the physical sensations of pleasant and unpleasant properties. However, babies at this young age have minimal capacities for regulating their emotions. Therefore, parents are advised to maintain positive, comforting, soothing interactions with their infants as much as possible. Once they are aware that their infant's emotional and cognitive acquisitions derive from the quality of their ministrations, they can be encouraged to maintain predictable habits, even at the price of considerable personal sacrifice. Parenting a young infant is difficult and challenging. Sleep and recreation go out the window. But the successful resolution of *basic regulation* helps to usher in the next phase, *interpersonal attention,* which brings with it a new set of rewards.

Phase 2: Interpersonal Attention

By 2½–3 months, until about 4 or 4½ months, the baby's full-bore attention to people and their activities marks a new stage of emotional development. We refer to this short period as *Interpersonal attention,* because it is a time when bodily habits, coordinated between the mother and the baby, have finally become consolidated, and the infant can now turn his attention to the most exciting things in the world outside his body: other people. At this age (which corresponds with the second half of the *sensorimotor consolidation* substage), babies' limited set of skills includes grasping, sucking, and gazing at objects and people for long periods. But more importantly, this age is marked by the initiation of "reciprocal exchange," as noted by Sander (1975), because it involves prolonged gazing at the mother and other family members who inevitably gaze back at the infant. The baby now gazes at the mother, smiles, coos, and delights in the ensuing changes in the mother's face and voice. The mother, in turn, becomes fascinated by her baby's facial expressions and smiles – especially the smiles that seem to be a response to her own expressions and actions. As described by Daniel Stern, this feeling of being noticed, being important, being a source of excitement and pleasure for the baby is highly rewarding to the mother, who gazes at the baby while vocalizing in exactly the way babies find most interesting (called *Motherese*). The baby notices mother's gaze and vocalizations, as well as the changing facial expressions that accompany them, and incorporates them into the scheme representing interpersonal exchanges. This interpersonal scheme becomes a dominant representation for most infants, who stare at mother's face for long periods while cooing and gooing (a phrase we borrowed directly from Robbie). From about 2½ to 4 months, episodes of mutual gazing stretch out longer and longer, and they become a fundamental source of excitement and joy for both partners. Scottish theorist Colwyn Trevarthen describes this as a state of "intersubjectivity" between the infant and caregiver. There is a sense, not only of each partner responding to the other, but also of both partners sharing a world in which "we are here together."

Many developmentalists see the 3- to 4-month period as the fruition of a "love affair" between the infant and the caregiver. Robbie was quite taken with this idea. In fact, mostly through his students, he absorbed some of the key insights of object relations theory, with its emphasis on the mother's highly emotional impact on the infant's internal world at this age. Robbie rarely underestimated the power of emotion in organizing developmental outcomes, and he was even content to place emotion in the driver's seat with respect to cognitive processes – at least sometimes. What surprised his colleagues was that Robbie's interest in emotion led him to respect many of the tenets of psychoanalytic theory. Robbie's flirtation with object relations theory, and especially the work of Melanie Klein, was partly inspired by those of his students who studied with Otto Weininger. Weininger, a brilliant but eccentric psychoanalytic scholar, inhabited the Department of Applied Psychology along with Case (but at the opposite end of the building!) for many years, and he provided a potent, often affectionate, counterpoint to Robbie's emphasis on cognitive processes. The impact of motivational forces on cognition, championed by Weininger, and of cognitive structure on motivation, argued by Robbie, set up a creative tension for students who studied with them both, including the authors of this chapter. In fact, this was a potent springboard to our theoretical development. However, both men agreed on the big picture of development to a surprising extent, and the idea of the young baby's love affair with the mother was included in their common vision.

We may call the mother–infant bond a love affair, but according to Case's theory it's a love affair with the qualities of a still life. It does not *progress* from moment to moment, and that's because babies aren't keeping track of what to expect, what happens next, at this stage of their development. The cognitive software simply isn't there yet – not until the commencement of the substage of *unifocal coordination*. That's why, regardless of how intensely infants gaze at their mothers, there is no disappointment when the interaction ends – as long as it is followed by something else the baby can attend to. Even when left alone in a baby seat, 2½- to 4-month-old infants will generally not fuss when their mother leaves the room.

This may seem counter-intuitive, and when Marc was doing hands-on research with young infants for his graduate work, he was more than a little surprised to see this lack of a reaction first hand. The camera was on, Mother was instructed to "talk" with her 3-month-old as she normally would, and then, after 3 minutes of interaction, she was to get up and leave the room without looking back. A chime sounded at 3 minutes, and the moms did what they were supposed to do. But when we examined the video record of the baby's face and body over the next few minutes, almost all showed the same dramatic response: they did nothing at all. Robbie and Marc sat together in a viewing room watching these tapes, and marveling over the utter absence of distress. According to Robbie, there was no distress because there was no coordination. Nothing to expect, and thus nothing to lose. To paraphrase another paraphrase: no frustration without representation.

The fact that infants of this age cannot cognize expectancies about future events does not mean that their cognitive system is devoid of emotional meaning. We must emphasize that, prior to 4 months, infants are very much aware of *changes* in familiar interactions as they occur. In a classic experiment designed to manipulate infants' emotions had mothers stop interacting with their infants in the middle of an interpersonal exchange. Infants aged 2–4 months became upset when they noticed that their mothers had turned off, and this distress led to a phase in which babies looked away from their mothers, apparently ignoring them. This experiment demonstrated what the object relations theorists had long assumed: that 3 to 4-month-old infants have a rich repertoire of emotional responses to their interactions with mother. To reconcile this picture with Case's approach, we suggest that, even at this young age, babies' emotions are a function of their cognitive interpretations. One sensorimotor scheme may be sufficient to maintain a sense of the interpersonal exchange with the mother, such that an abrupt end to that exchange violates the scheme, providing the occasion for frustration and distress.

Despite Tronick's observed distress, being stuck in the present shields the 2- to 4-month-old infant from the emotional trauma that might otherwise stem from the sudden disappearance of loved ones. And that is something the object relations theorists would not have predicted. Rather than being intensely sensitive to mother's comings and goings, the infant in the phase of *Interpersonal attention* is more protected and resilient than she will be in another month or two. This is a period of dawning interpersonal excitement, affection, and sharing, but without the sense of "what comes next" that is such a fundamental platform for most human interactions. Due to this resilience, this low-cost affection, changes in household routines, especially concerning parents' whereabouts, are less likely to be traumatic, from 2½ to 4½ months, than in the following phase, *Interpersonal expectancy.*

Phase 3: Interpersonal Expectancy

The budding reciprocity, positive emotionality, and sustained attention infants display at 3–4 months soon usher in a major stage transition in cognitive development and a parallel suite of social–emotional changes that are both challenging and rewarding for parents. While reciprocal gazing may begin as early as 2–3 months, it continues to grow toward a climax that takes place between 4 and 5 months, kicking off a phase we call *Interpersonal expectancy.* The climax of mother–infant reciprocity at about 4½ months is described as a key transition point by Margaret Mahler, an infant observer with a background in the psychoanalytic approach to development. Now begins a phase of "differentiation" of the infant from the mother, according to Mahler, marked by a mushrooming sense of autonomy: a sense of a self – an *I* – who can act on the world *out there.* Yet autonomy does not mean that the bond with the parent is over. Rather, Mahler emphasizes that the baby's sense of a unique, separate self forms the basis of a new kind of bond with the primary caregiver – a bond between two partners, rather than a fusion in which mother and baby act as parts of a single organism. (Note, however, that the notion of self–other fusion was persuasively overturned by Stern [1985] and others.)

Infants now begin to interact with their caregivers in a back-and-forth fashion (not quite turn-taking, as that implies planning and waiting for a response). They may look at their father's face, make a noise, a squawk, or grunt or squeak, and then notice that father smiles too and perhaps reaches down to tickle the baby or manipulate his limbs in a playful fashion. The baby may now squawk again, anticipating father's response, and so begins a chain of actions in which each partner does something the other partner is likely to appreciate, and each responds to the other in an ongoing exchange. Also at this age, infants begin to initiate play and wait for the parent to respond to them. So the onset of *differentiation* at 4½ months is a time of both budding autonomy and increased interpersonal engagement, leading to true play for the first time ever. The time babies spend gazing at mother's face now begins to decline, but their attraction to game-playing skyrockets. Almost any kind of game will do, as long as it involves some repetitive, expectable activity. By 5 months, infants love the feeling of excited anticipation they get while waiting for the parent to swoop down, pat or tickle them, or throw them up in the air (a speciality of fathers everywhere, despite the mother's anxiety).

This new phase of emotional development, marked by interpersonal play and growing autonomy, corresponds almost perfectly with the first half of the *unifocal coordination* substage in Case's theory of sensorimotor development. This transition is marked by the infant's new capacities to coordinate two sensorimotor schemes, such as a scheme to control gazing (or visual tracking) with one to control reaching, or one to control reaching with another to control grasping. (Note that each of these is a *sensorimotor* scheme, containing both sensory and motor elements. It is incorrect to think of a sensory scheme being coordinated with a motor scheme. Neither exists in isolation at any level of analysis.) This capacity for scheme coordination allows for a new kind of approach to the world: one in which the infant's actions are propelled by a wish for and anticipation of some outcome, permitting intentional or goal-directed behavior.

Robbie's favorite example of the acquisition of two-part expectations was the observation that 5-month-old infants begin to rotate their heads to look for an object that is slowly moved around behind them. For this task, the examiner would suspend an object from a string and slowly move it around the infant's head in an ongoing circle. Prior to 4 months, infants invariably lost track of the object when it went behind them, disappearing at one edge of their visual field, and they would shift their gaze to something novel at that moment. By 5 months, however, most infants would swing their gaze around to the opposite edge of their visual field, anticipating the object's imminent reappearance. For Robbie this made perfect sense: one scheme representing the object's disappearance at location A, another scheme representing its reappearance at location B. The capacity for coordination permits the integration of these two schemes into a visual act connecting the two locations.

But for Robbie, the hallmark of *unifocal coordination* was the dawning of intentional behavior. Infants could now coordinate an action with an outcome, and therefore act with the *intention* of producing a change in their relation with the environment. The anticipation of outcomes on the basis of actions was referred to by Piaget as magico-phenomenalistic causality in his description of the same period of development. According to this idea, the infant now seems to expect that the world will be changed – magically – as a result of her acts. Actions are not merely executed to maintain a current state of affairs, as was the case in the previous substage. Rather their purpose is to initiate a *new* state of affairs. Thus, for both Piaget and Case, actions are motivated by an expectation of their *effect* beginning at the age of 4–5 months.

How should we conceptualize the link between cognitive and the social–emotional changes at this point in development? Infants at 4–5 months act to produce an outcome, not only on *things* in their environment but also on *people*. Consequently, when they make a noise directed at a parent, they anticipate a response from that parent as an outcome. When they make a noise, and mother or father respond, they connect the noise to the response. They coordinate these events in their working memory. And the next time they make a similar noise, they *expect* a similar response. Without the new cognitive software, this expectancy would not exist. Now, by keeping track of both parts of a social exchange – their own vocalization and the other person's smile, coo, or tickle – babies can engage in true reciprocity, reciprocity that goes beyond mutual gazing in a prolonged still life. They can now participate willingly and consciously in a *chain* of actions, each of which is a response to a previous action by the other partner.

However, at the same time that these social skills are emerging, infants are learning how to act on the *physical* world in a way that is highly rewarding as well. Instead of flailing their arms about, and grabbing whatever their hands happen to touch, they can now direct their reach according to their gaze, and they can grasp an object just as their hand reaches it. With these skills, infants can reach for, grab, play with, and suck on the dozens or hundreds of things they see around them. . .intentionally. The world of toys and objects now becomes highly appealing and compelling, drawing attention away from the reciprocal exchanges they engage in with their parents. So, the "love affair with the parent" soon has to compete with a "love affair with the world," giving rise to a tension or conflict between the interpersonal realm and the realm of inanimate objects. For most babies, this tension is resolved at approximately 5–6 months, when the physical world generally wins out.

What are the implications of interpersonal expectancies for the parenting bond in general and for interpersonal stresses and frustrations in particular? The baby at this age expects parents to be available when she is ready to play. In fact, just the parent's presence may seem to be an invitation to begin some new game. And when the parent is heard but not seen, the baby may call out, *expecting* a reply, and getting frustrated when nothing comes back. There is some evidence that separation reactions become more intense, at least briefly, around the period of 4–5 months. In his graduate work with Robbie, Marc studied separation–reunion reactions around this age and discovered that separation distress changes its meaning at right about $4\frac{1}{2}$ months. Distress prior to this age did not seem to result from the cessation of a play episode or parental separation, as noted above. But distress after this age did. This difference in the meaning of distress led to some interesting predictions. As detailed in several papers, distress prior to 4 months predicted lower cognitive proficiency both concurrently (Lewis, 1993b) and 4 years later (Lewis, 1993a). But why? Robbie and Marc argued over the interpretation of these findings many times. Robbie's favorite explanation was a simple one – cognitively proficient infants were more likely to notice and be disturbed by the loss of the mother following the onset of *unifocal coordination*. Marc's less conventional interpretation was that more potent emotional exchanges between infant and mother, at the beginning of this stage, actually pushed cognitive development ahead for some infants. In other words, Robbie saw the correlation as an index of an underlying but static state of affairs. Marc saw it as a window onto a process that altered cognitive competencies. No studies have been conducted to test these competing explanations, but over the years, Marc has come over to Robbie's view for the most part. It now seems clear that cognitive proficiency and emotional sensitivity or engagement are two sides of the same coin, and that the emotional and cognitive sides of the same coin were being measured independently. As is often the case in psychological research, the simpler explanation is probably best.

This research was never replicated, and it is premature to draw conclusions from this one sample of children. However, at the very least, these studies complement what theory and observation already suggest about developmental timing: that 4–5 months is a period of rapid cognitive and emotional change, in which new cognitive coordinations permit the anticipation of interpersonal responses to the infant's bids and thereby result in a concomitant change in emotional responsiveness. Consequently, 4–6 months would not be the best time to embark on interpersonal challenges, especially those that concern the parent's whereabouts. When it comes to parent education, we would advise parents not to introduce major changes to interpersonal routines involving time spent together, feeding and sleeping routines, and the general rhythm of parents' presence and availability during the day or night. In other words, we would not advise parents to begin daycare, go back to work, or shift the infant to more isolated sleeping arrangements during the 4- to 6-month period.

Phase 4: Motor Initiative

The infants' emotional life settles down quite noticeably in the next month or two, and indeed this phase, which we are calling *Motor initiative* after Sander, is a period characterized by autonomy, independence, and resilience. From $5\frac{1}{2}$ to $7\frac{1}{2}$ months, the new skills coming on-line with *sensorimotor coordination* become practiced and efficient (see Fig. 1). And as they do, the physical world opens up to the infant in a way that we can barely imagine. The profusion of glittering surfaces, splotches of color, and regular and novel movements must have seemed like a highly intricate decoration scheme – fun to look at but not very practical – to the younger infant. Now, the capacity to coordinate schemes allows infants to reach out, touch, hold, and bring to their mouths everything they lay their eyes on. This is why the physical world wins out over the social world. Infants have already learned what to expect from faces, fascinating though they are. But they have only begun to learn about what's out there in the world. Sander (1975) calls this the period of "infant initiative." Infants now reach out into the physical world almost continuously, trying to grab what they see. They seem compelled and driven to explore every object within their reach, first with their hands and then with their mouths. They touch corners, surfaces, indentations, and protrusions, explore textures with their fingers and move their bodies in new and untested ways to get at things that are just out of reach. And then they suck or chew on whatever they can get to their mouths, exploring these objects with the tactile surfaces they enjoy most – their lips and tongues. The same period is described by Mahler as the phase of "practicing." By this she means simply the repeated, energetic actions that infants engage in to get to know the physical world. Very few infants can crawl by 6 months, but some can roll, creep, or move their bodies in the most remarkable ways to get closer to what they want to explore. The point is that everything they do is motivated by the excitement generated by their approach to objects in their environment.

There is little to say about social–emotional development in the $5\frac{1}{2}$–$7\frac{1}{2}$ month period, except that it is highly stable. The game-playing routines acquired by about 5 months continue to proliferate. These routines become more complex, more interesting, and more involved, but their fundamental nature does not change. Infants still see other people as playmates in simple back-and-forth rituals. They neither see them as agents who might be recruited to fulfill their needs, nor as other beings with their own habits and preferences. Perhaps most interesting in this period, infants' reactions to loss are rather muted. They may become frustrated if a toy falls on the floor and can't be retrieved. But their distress is usually short-lived or completely eclipsed by some distraction or other. And if a person suddenly disappears from view, they may gaze intently at the location where she was last seen. Or, they may gaze around the room, knowing that the person must be here somewhere. But at this age infants have no idea how to find what's missing. As a result, they don't try very hard, and soon their attention passes on to other, more accessible attractions.

This is a very important point when it comes to parenting. No matter how engaging and thoughtful one's child may appear, and no matter how good he is at noticing details he never noticed before, the 5½- to 7½-month-old infant does not search for people who have gone missing, at mothers who have just gone downstairs or fathers who have just gone out for groceries. And because they do not search, they are not frustrated by the failure that comes from searching for someone who can't be found. This stable and relatively imperturbable 5½- to 7½-month-old infant is thus a good candidate for beginning daycare, sleep-training, or other changes in fundamental routines that involve increased separations from parents. However, once babies near the age of 8 months, this window of opportunity disappears once again.

Phase 5: Social Referencing

As will be obvious by now, social–emotional development consists of a patchwork of phases, each with its own unique character, rather than a smooth progression of increasing or decreasing sensitivity, attunement, or anything else. In fact, this patchwork has the character of a pendulum swing: periods of emotional sensitivity and social vulnerability are interspersed with periods of greater independence, tolerance, and stability. And the nesting of the first four social–emotional phases in the first two cognitive substages follows a simple logic: each sensorimotor substage can be divided into a front half, housing a more sensitive period of social–emotional development (*Basic regulation* and *Interpersonal expectancy*), and a back half, in which social–emotional dynamics are more stable and resilient (*Interpersonal attention* and *Motor initiative*). Indeed, for the purposes of parent education, the phase of *Motor Initiative* was a honeymoon in social–emotional development. The baby at this age was resilient enough to be left alone to play for long periods, happy to go on car rides, and tolerant of sudden changes in routines. But now, at 8 months, the honeymoon is over. Now the baby is more sensitive to parents' whereabouts, their comings and goings, their presence, and especially their absence, than ever before.

Like many other phases of social–emotional development, but more conspicuously than most, this phase depends for its character on a dramatic transition in cognitive development: the advent of *bifocal coordination*. This transition allows the infant to represent, not only one sensorimotor coordination (say between a scheme for reaching and one for grasping), but a second coordination (say between a scheme for calling to the parent and one for the parent's expected response). The former coordination controls the infant's goal of accessing a desired toy. The latter coordination controls the infant's capacity to enlist the parent's attention. The coordination of these two coordinations permits the recruitment of the parent's attention for the benefit of the infant's acquisition of the toy. And this allows the parent to fulfill the child's bid by supporting his attempts to achieve his goal. As with Case's modeling in general, the two coordinations are hierarchically embedded to form a single cognitive operation – one which achieves the baby's goals *through* a communicative exchange with another person.

What is critical about this cognitive advance for the social–emotional realm is not only that other people serve as an effective means for achieving what the baby wants to achieve, but that this partnership produces a sense that both infant and parent are participating together in the same dance, sharing attention to the same object, or embarked on the same agenda. So, if the baby wants to play with an object she can't reach, she will look to the parent to retrieve it. She may tug on the mother's dress, she may point, and she may look back and forth between the object and the parent. But one way or another, she will act on the parent in order to get the parent to act on the object – that's the bifocal coordination that links the child's needs and wishes with the activities of other humans. That coordination is what allows the child to experience another person paying attention not only to her, but also *with* her, to her goals. This insight can be seen as the first blush of truly *social* cognition, and it serves as the first step in a series of acquisitions leading to a full-fledged theory of mind by the age of 3 or 4 years (Tomasello, 1995).

Let's add to this basic formula a number of specific skills and propensities that emerge around 8–9 months, also resulting from *bifocal coordinations* in the social realm. Babies learn to point, an operation that combines a hand gesture directed at an object with attention to the target of the other person's gaze. They also learn to look where someone else is pointing, combining their attention to the pointing hand with their attention to objects at some distance out there in the world. Pointing doesn't make sense unless someone is looking where you're pointing, or you're looking where someone else is pointing, and it is not until the capacity for *bifocal coordination* that the infant can represent both parts of this equation. Babies also learn to retrieve hidden objects. The child can now keep track of the location of a vanished object, say behind some barrier, while at the same time reaching for the barrier in order to remove it. The capacity to retrieve hidden objects makes it sensible to search for them, just as the capacity to look where someone is pointing makes it sensible to point. The dawning of object retrieval was a cornerstone of Piaget's portrayal of this stage of development (Sensorimotor Stage 4), although he assumed that the infant forgot about the existence of the object after it disappeared. For Case, the retrieval of hidden objects depended, not on maintaining the existence of the object in memory, but on constructing a representation of how to retrieve it by first removing the barrier which obscured it – a representation that relies on two distinct coordinations, one hierarchically nested in the other. As we see, the 8- to 11-month-old's obsession with retrieving hidden objects is fundamental to a major change in social development: the dawning of separation distress based on an obsession with retrieving hidden parents.

Another social habit that emerges at this age is gazing at other people, usually parents, for cues as to the *meaning* of a situation. This is called *social referencing,* the phrase we've used to label this phase of social–emotional development. The classic experiment to test social referencing involves a piece of apparatus called the visual cliff, in a paradigm developed by Campos and his colleagues (e.g., Campos &

Stenberg, 1981). This is a plexiglass (see-through) surface that covers an actual cliff – a drop of several feet – often composed of brightly colored checks for easy visibility. The infant is invited to crawl across the flat, plexiglass surface, which he very often does with little prompting. Although there is no real danger, it appears to the infant that the floor is about to drop away from under him as he approaches the cliff. Prior to 8–9 months, babies (at least those who can creep or crawl) usually move blithely across the visual cliff, whether trusting in some divine protection or just plain dumb. But now, at this age, they generally stop, search for their mother's face, and register her facial expression. The experiment is usually designed with instructions for mother to either smile encouragingly or to frown and look discouraging. Starting at 8–9 months, infants' actions depend very much on mother's expression. If she is smiling, they proceed across the visual cliff. If she is frowning, they stop, and treat the cliff as dangerous. The point of the experiment is to show that the older infant decides whether to cross or not based on the parent's nonverbal communication. Their interpretation is contingent on the parent's social cues. Campos (e.g., Campos et al., 2000) theorizes that it is the capacity to crawl, rather than any general advance in cognitive development, that provides the baby with the insight to gaze toward the mother in order to get information about the physical world. However, on this Case takes the extreme opposite view. For him, it is a general advance in cognitive abilities that fans out to these component acquisitions, not the other way around.

If we combine what we know about pointing and social referencing, both of which show up at about 8–9 months, we get a deeper perspective on what's unique about this phase of social–emotional development. Infants are entering a new kind of awareness of other people, which we call "social." What babies now experience with other people is the advent of *joint attention,* which means an understanding that both the infant and the adult are attending to the same thing. In the case of pointing, the infant understands that both are attending to the object being pointed at. In the case of social referencing, he understands that both are attending to whatever novel or uncertain aspect of the situation (e.g., the visual cliff) needs to be evaluated. According to Tomasello, it is this special capacity for joint attention that provides a springboard to other critical features of development under the rubric of *theory of mind.* If the infant can glean what the other person is attending to, she can also begin to infer what aims the other person has, what goals he is pursuing, what he wishes, what he wants. The understanding of others' goals is perhaps the bedrock feature of human social cognition. It is, more than anything else, what makes us *socially intelligent.* The understanding of others' intentions is the first step on the pathway to theory of mind, and it may be one of the fundamental capacities that autistic children lack. As we will see, this understanding of others' intentions is still at a preliminary stage at 8–12 months. According to Tomasello and others, not until the period of 18–24 months do infants acquire a more objective and accurate understanding of others' goals, as part and parcel of the onset of symbolic understanding across many domains.

But perhaps the aspect of social–emotional development most important for parent education is the onset of separation distress. Now that hidden objects can be found, so can hidden mothers. If it's a toy that's hidden, the two-part coordination required to retrieve it involves the removal of a barrier or container. But if it's a parent that's missing, the action required is to call out and demand her return. Prior to this age, calling out was not in the service of. . .anything. The two-part coordination required to retrieve a missing mother is thus expressed by the heartfelt demand, uttered, as often as not, in a high-pitched wail, to get back here! And sure enough, the few studies that have looked carefully at the timing of separation distress in infancy find a spike at about 9 months (e.g., Emde, Gaensbauer, & Harmon, 1976). Babies become more clingy, more demanding, and more emotionally aroused when there is any indication that the parent is about to leave, or when they look around and find that the parent is further away than expected. Any kind of separation, either anticipated or actual, will challenge the 9-month-old baby's new social sensibilities, and set the occasion for trying to reverse it. Thus, separation protests are functional behaviors that express negative emotions resulting from a novel cognitive appraisal – part and parcel of the infant's emerging capacity for bifocal coordinations in the social realm.

Unfortunately, 9 months is an age when parents frequently do return to work and initiate some kind of daycare arrangement. This timing often results in bouts of anxiety and distress, sometimes leading to the complete breakdown of emotional stability with one or both parents. It is also an age when many parents initiate sleep-training and attempt to leave their infant to fall asleep on his or her own. Sleep-training may be well advised for many parents. But 9 months is the wrong age to start. Now is the time when the infant's social–emotional concerns are centered on a sense of connection and shared perceptions. Now is when negative emotions arise from violations of those concerns. If developmental theory can influence parents' decisions about critical life events, this is one age at which there should be little ambiguity. And putting theory into practice in this phase would be an excellent way to make use of the insights derived from Robbie's understanding of development while honoring his commitment to educational practice based on psychological knowledge.

Phase 6: Motor Practice

Just when we begin to think that our babies are entirely ruled by their needs, their vulnerabilities, their desire for nurturance, and their concerns for safety and interpersonal closeness, the developmental game-plan sets us straight once again. The pendulum swings once more and we are reminded that babies (in fact, children in general) are just as taken with the joy of being free agents, exploring the world, as they are with their needs for security. The period of 12–16 months, which we dub *Motor practice,* is one such period. This phase has many of the same qualities as the phase of *Motor initiative*, which transpired between 5½ and 7½ months. Both phases followed a period of rapid and dramatic cognitive change paralleled by emotional vulnerabilities centered around other people. Both phases are characterized by relative independence, autonomy, and emotional resilience. And both phases borrow much of their thrust from the pure excitement and joy of exercising a newly emerging motor capacity. In the case of *Motor initiative,* the new capacity consisted of coordinations among gazing, reaching, and grasping, allowing the baby to manipulate and explore the vast array of objects in his immediate environment. Now, beginning at 12 months, the new game in town is upright locomotion.

Of course, babies vary in the age at which they begin to walk. Some start walking as early as 10 months, others not until 14 or 15 months or even later. But 12 months is typical. And walking is not the infant's first stab at locomotion. Crawling, which emerges for many babies around 8–9 months, also brought with it a new sense of mobility and freedom. But there is something unique about walking. You can cover a lot more ground, a lot more quickly, while at the same time enjoying a bird's-eye view of the world. Margaret Mahler described the advent of walking as the period of "late practicing" – not a very evocative title. But Mahler was right in viewing the "practicing" infant as gleeful, independent, and fully enamored of the non-social world. This staggering, loping, adventurous little creature cares little about the respite offered by loving arms, until she becomes tired or hungry – or scared. Until then, she is a free agent, gliding about on a landscape of novel possibilities.

The cognitive-developmental changes ushering in the stage of motor practicing are not as dramatic as those that triggered the previous phase. According to Case, infants in the substage of *elaborated (sensorimotor) coordinations* are especially interested in reversible operations, such as putting objects into a container and dumping them back out again, or taking the phone off the hook and putting it back on again. Through these reverse operations, they are able to streamline and systematize the *bifocal* coordinations which continue to be the fundamental building blocks of this period. They do so by consolidating connections among each of the component schemes. But two advances are particularly relevant for social–emotional development. The first one is the use of single-word utterances to express simple ideas. These simple words are mostly nouns: names of foods, "Mama," "Pappa," and other proper nouns, and simple prepositions and adjectives such as "up" and "down" or "cold" vs. "hot." The capacity to use even single words to express one's wishes, goals, or thoughts, helps to consolidate the sense of a shared world that began in the previous stage. Indeed, the capacity for joint attention, first seen at about 9 months, might be the prerequisite for any language use, because the use of words takes as its premise the idea that both people are listening to the same sound and deriving from it the same meaning. This is, after all, the basis of language. If joint attention gives language its first boost, then language also helps to extend and consolidate joint attention. In other words, the shared meaning of simple words establishes for the infant a sense that self and other really are paying attention to the same thing. Baby shouts "up!" and Dad picks her up. That confirms, with utter certainty, that Dad knows what you want, knows what you are thinking about, knows what you intend. The second advance is one we have already introduced: upright locomotion itself. While we don't usually consider walking a "cognitive" advance, a lot of concentration, practice, repetition, and refinement go into the baby's efforts to get herself off the floor and gliding on two feet. This may require the same kind of practice that goes into many of the novel abilities of the 12- to 16-month period.

The main point is that the new capabilities to arrive on the scene soon after 12 months create a novel, exciting, and gleeful world for the infant – the infant who can now be properly called a toddler. To be able to walk, even run from place to place, opens up great opportunities to explore the world. Now the child has taken his place as a bona fide member of the family, to whom the floor is no longer a prison, and for whom each room in the house presents a new invitation to play and explore. To be able to use single words to express ideas increases the child's sense that his wishes not only matter, are not only shared by others, are not only understood, but also have the power to harness the adult's attention and will. What the child says has tremendous impact on other humans, gets his needs met quickly and accurately, adding to his sense of being in command of a new set of capabilities and his sense of being socially important, central, not to be ignored. These acquisitions spell emotional confidence. The needy child of the 8- to 11-month period has vanished, only to be replaced by someone who is robust, independent, confident, even proud, and who tackles the world with a certain amount of glee, optimism, and authority. This happy and resilient child is solid enough to handle the challenges of daycare and other extended separations better than his 8- to 11-month-old predecessor, and may take to sleep-training more easily as well. So, the 12- to 16-month period provides another window when social challenges can be faced with a minimum of distress and succeeded with a minimum of effort.

Phase 7: Social Negotiation

By 17 or 18 months begins the most profound developmental change to occur in the lifespan so far: a major transition in cognitive development, and a transformation in social–emotional development to match it. This is the true watershed between infancy and early childhood – the hatching of the child from a preoccupation with physical reality to an appreciation of symbolic reality. The beginning of language and all that that entails, and the consolidation of a social relationship with parents based on an understanding of doing things together, achieving joint goals, cooperation versus defiance, and a sense of the self as a social being who is part of a family. This transition also represents a distinct swing of the pendulum back toward dependency needs and social vulnerability. Becoming a new kind of human being – a truly social being – brings with it enormous uncertainties about how to connect with parents in a way that neither threatens the child's independence nor his or her needs for safety and security.

According to Case, 18–20 months is the average age at which children move from the sensorimotor stage to the interrelational stage. The fundamental building blocks of their cognitive operations are no longer sensorimotor schemes, representing motor actions and sensory transformations. Rather, they are schemes that represent the relationships between *kinds* of things, schemes that represent relations between agents, actions, object classes, goals, and other types or categories encountered by the toddler. These relations are entirely semiotic or symbolic in nature, and hence subject to rapid generalization within classes of events. They stand not for the entities in the world but for the ways in which entities relate to one another, the ways in which they can be described or used or classified. This definition is admittedly difficult to grasp, but we will provide examples that make it more accessible. There are three kinds of relational links that Robbie would emphasize as typifying interrelational cognition: language, roles, and goals. Language relies on the coordination of verbal categories like the subject and predicate of a sentence. Roles stand for relations people have with one another. And goals describe relations between actors and their desires. Here we discuss each of these interrelational categories in terms of its implications for social–emotional development.

The first advance is language itself. Children shift from using words in isolation to embedding words in small sentences. The simplest of these sentences may be only two words in length, consisting of a subject (e.g., Mama) and a predicate (e.g., come), or a predicate (e.g., Go) and an object (e.g., home). But the outcome is profound. By saying "Mama come" or "Go home" children are referring not only to a single object or isolated feature of the world, but to a situation, an event, which is a more or less accurate read-out of what they are actually thinking, imagining, or wishing. The ability to string words together to communicate full, complete ideas and wishes, and the naming explosion that comes with it, provide the child of 17–21 months with the most powerful tool available for interacting with other people: true language.

What is so special about language? When discussing the phase of *Social referencing* (8–11 months) we spoke of the dawning of joint attention and of the baby's sense of people as having goals or intentions. But these intuitions were still vague and ill-defined. The advent of language clinches the deal. When the child says "Mama come" and Mama listens and comes over to where the child is located, there is absolute assurance that both parent and child are focused on the same words and, more than that, on the *idea* that the words express. Their attention is synchronized and their intentions are synchronized. They are thinking about the same thing and they are sharing the same goal. This is a major improvement over the dawning of a sense of joint attention at 9 or 10 months. Instead of just looking to where the child is pointing, the parent is showing that her thoughts and goals are accessible and incontrovertibly linked with the child's thoughts and goals. It's obvious that language provides an incredibly powerful way to achieve one's goals, and this is not lost on little people who don't always have enough skill or know-how to achieve their own goals. But besides getting her needs met quickly and effectively, the language-using child now begins to understand that she is a social being, a person, in a world of other persons, who share a matrix of thoughts, feelings, goals, and desires. The child finally sees herself as she really is: part of a group of beings who share a world of meanings and actions.

Now this realization in itself brings on both confidence and doubt. It's handy to convey your goals to the adults in your life, to harness their attention for a moment or two. But it doesn't always work. Parents aren't always listening. And what if they don't listen? What if their attention drifts away again? It is typical to observe toddlers of this age saying the same thing over and over, or making the same demand repeatedly: "Mama? Mama? Mama? Mama?" . . .until mother turns her head and finally asks, "Yes? What do you want?" Or "More, more, more!" with escalating anxiety, not knowing if the parent will actually fulfill the child's cherished goal of attaining more raisins for his snack. So, even the glories of being a language user, and the satisfaction of finding your place in the world of thoughts and actions shared with your parents, have their dark side. Words have to be heard, and messages have to be received, or else the child is helpless, isolated, and worse off than before: a language user who can't communicate!

The second advance of this period is the understanding of social roles, and in particular the coordination of two roles that are complementary with each other. The child who can understand complementary roles sees himself as either part of the program or not. If mom wants to dress you this morning (as she does most mornings), then your complementary role would entail pushing one hand and then another through your sleeves, and raising each foot to receive its sock and shoe. There is nothing sweeter than observing toddlers engaged in these complementary roles, and very often they are happy to play along. But not always. If roles can fit together then they can also not fit together. This provides a hinge-point between autonomy and cooperation. The 18-month-old toddler becomes aware of this tension, because it spells a challenge for his sense of self. Playing a social role means submerging the self in a larger plan, for the larger good, but at the expense of doing whatever comes to mind. The result is a potential stand-off. Complementary roles serve to organize the fabric of a relationship in a way that pleases both participants. When roles don't correspond, somebody gets left out, somebody gets mad, or sad, or insecure. Which means that social roles become parts to play in the family drama with distinct emotional consequences. Play your part, and everyone will be happy. Refuse and there's going to be trouble. Toddlers at this age can't formulate this logic quite so precisely, but they can sense the consequence of their refusal to comply.

The third cognitive advance has much in common with role relationships. It is the understanding toddlers gain at 18–20 months of competing goals. As we explained earlier, infants begin to see people as intentional agents at 8–9 months. And they manipulate those intentions with a pointed finger, or with a demand – a scream or shout – to get parents to do their bidding. However, this understanding of people's goals is implicit, intuitive, and lacking in clarity (Tomasello, 1995). At the end of the first year, the infant has a sense that other people's actions have a direction that somehow spells volition, or intention, or desire, but that's as far as they get. In order to really understand goals, as symbolic entities that can be influenced or manipulated, shared or blocked, one has to be able to hold in mind two goals, or two forms of a goal, or competing goals. That's what is made possible by cognitive development at this age. I can only understand your desire to pay for dinner if I see it in relation to your abhorrence of feeling that you're in my debt. A goal is, after all, a choice between alternatives – a choice one holds in mind as a guide for action. At about 18 months, according to Robbie, toddlers acquire the working memory capacity to consider two possible goals, perhaps competing goals, or to compare the success vs. failure of a goal. So their understanding of goals is now explicit and objective.

At this age, understanding goals is as much a part of social–emotional development as understanding role relationships. Toddlers in this phase of development recognize that their goals are often in competition with yours. You want them to go to bed. They don't want to go to bed. You want them to eat their potatoes. They don't want to eat their potatoes. You want them to come inside. They want to stay outside. Congruent goals spell approval and positive emotion, much like congruent roles. But competing goals spell conflict, which can be the harbinger of anger, rejection, and the withdrawal of parental affection. Given these ominous possibilities, why not comply? Why doesn't the child just shift his goals to line up with those of mom and dad? For two reasons. First, because he really does have his own goals, and he can't necessarily re-write them. A toddler's desires are incredibly strong and not usually subject to modification. And second, because there is still this issue of autonomy. Perhaps it's a holdover from the previous phase, when the "practicing" toddler so enjoyed being his own agent. Perhaps giving in to the parent's goals means that the child is inevitably relinquishing his or hers. And toddlers in this stage like to be loved, they like to please their parents, but they have no taste for ignoring their own wishes in order to do so. And that's why the one word we inevitably expect to emerge in the toddler's vocabulary at this age is "No!" And why 18 months is often considered the beginning of the "terrible twos."

Other changes in social cognition are part of this sweep of novel thought patterns at 17–21 months, including a dawning sense of territoriality. There is little doubt that the declaration "Mine!" will first be heard during this period, along with "No!" – signaling the child's understanding that possession is nine-tenths of the law. It isn't enough to have a cracker when you can hang on to the whole bag. That's another example of getting ahead of the competition in the toddler's sense of the world. All of these advances share the same flavor: they further elaborate the child's understanding of a social order in which he must participate, through the use of language and gestures, in order to assume his position in the family and maintain some chance of getting his way. But the emotional tone of these social advances should now be clear: this is an age of negotiation. The child at this age is like someone who has just joined a club that, once joined, can never be left. It is a club that provides its members with a road map showing how the social world really works, that bestows on its members the power to influence others in order to achieve one's wishes and needs, that promises its members a profound sense of both inclusion and control. It is a club that one would never willingly leave – because it offers its members a steady stream, not only of resources, but of true affection, understanding, acceptance, and love. Then shouldn't this be a time of social confidence? No! Because, while the toddler would never voluntarily leave the club, she never knows when one of the club managers will tell her she's on probation, she's breaking the rules, her status is being revoked until she gets her act together. So there is negotiation about how much you have to comply, to behave, to agree, to acquiesce, in order to maintain your good standing in the club.

Thus, the child at this age, though feisty and independent, is also insecure. And her insecurity, while easily triggered by physical separations, as was the case at

9 months, is really about psychological separations: the loss of affection, understanding, shared intentions, and support. Children this age will cling to their parent, refusing to allow her to move out of range. But that's not because they are afraid they won't be able to find her again – physically. It's because there is no better assurance of that parent's ongoing approval and care than the feeling of being cuddled up against her skin, or basking in her smile. We may never grow out of the need for that most fundamental reassurance, but it first makes the scene during this stage.

Given the powerful emotional vulnerabilities of this stage of development, and given the importance of the social communication, complementarity, and understanding into which the child is inducted at this age, we see this as one of the worst times for introducing new challenges. Now is not the time to begin daycare, to announce your impending divorce, to take a sabbatical in Libya, or to move the child into or out of the family bed. All of these perturbations will disrupt the toddler's need for proximity, shared routines, tokens of affection and support, and assurances of continued emotional connection. Now is a time to comfort and reassure, not to challenge or demand. We are not suggesting that parents have to comply with every wish their child expresses, at this or any other age, or to fashion a cushioned environment hived off from the bumps of day-to-day life. But sharing, intimacy, and both physical and psychological security should not be challenged at this transitional age any more than is necessary. The child will soon find his *interrelational* "sea legs" and learn how to negotiate his needs and wishes without so much emotional turmoil.

Phase 8: Social Stabilization

About halfway through the substage of *unifocal (interrelational) coordination*, around 22 months or so, club membership becomes the status quo, and the toddler starts to feel more assured that his compelling goals and needs will go on being met, at least most of the time. He starts to recognize that conflicting roles and goals will not be the end of him. From about 22–28 months, no major new cognitive acquisitions come along to stir things up. The toddler is able to settle down with his new set of skills and build up a repertoire – of expressions, habits, gestures, ways of getting attention, and ways to soothe himself when the parent's attention is elsewhere. This period of *Social stabilization* comes on like a holiday from the "terrible twos," providing a temporary respite to parents until the next substage transition hits with a vengeance.

One of the main pastimes of this period is the continued growth of language facility. Like other cognitive skills, the acquisition of two-part sentences soon becomes so ingrained that it doesn't take a lot of mental effort or working memory to initiate. Rather, cognitive resources can be put to other uses, like building up a vocabulary and putting nouns and verbs together in new combinations. But why is talking so attractive? Why bother? Because talking is fun, and the more words you have at your disposal, the more seamlessly you can communicate, without thought, without planning, and let others know just what's passing through your mind right now. Meanwhile, language allows toddlers to assemble a fundamental coping response, and one that is terrifically challenging for children of all ages: impulse control. Joseph wants his yoghurt now, not later, but his mom wants him to finish his carrots first. So she says: *Wait.* You can have yoghurt *soon!* "Wait. . .soon" provides a structure for containing his desire for another 5 minutes. And because this is a tall order, Joseph sees fit to repeat the verbal structure, and the gesture that goes with it, over and over, telling himself there's a pot of gold – or at least of yoghurt – at the end of this particular rainbow.

Thus, the 22- to 28-month-old toddler uses the mental software of *unifocal coordination,* which he has now been practicing for several months, to improve his facility to communicate with others and to alleviate his own negative emotions – in this case, anxiety – by taking advantage of freed up cognitive resources. The second of these skills is particularly important, because it demonstrates how each cognitive stage has a double impact on social–emotional development: downloading new cognitive software changes the way situations are interpreted in the first place, giving rise to new emotional constellations. But it also changes children's facility for coping with those emotional constellations. Joseph is using language and gesture to over-write what he actually feels with an alternative construction: instead of focusing on the immediate desire for yoghurt, he is focusing on a division drawn in time, delineating a "before" and an "after." The *before* is a time to wait; the *after* is a time to get the goods you've been longing for. The way these two-part episodes fit together, and the declaration of "Wait" that stands for their connection, epitomizes how toddlers use *unifocal (interrelational) coordination* to reconfigure reality, making their needs less oppressive and compelling.

Beyond this practice of symbolic constructions – both those shared with others and those directed at the self – there are no major new acquisitions during this period. This is a time of consolidation, increasing social facility, increasing social confidence, and a partial return to the freewheeling, easy sense of self that characterized the phase of *Motor practicing.* Toddlers' anxiety about separations diminishes during this time, and some of their stubbornness – not all, but some – gets folded back into the pleasure they get from cooperating with others. Also, at about this age, individual differences start to play a larger role in parents' decisions and successes with challenging life events such as daycare, the birth of a sibling, sleep-training, and so forth. Regardless, all other things being equal, the 6-month period of *Social stabilization* can offer parents another chance to initiate challenging emotional events without the trauma, tears, and exhaustion that are relatively familiar in toddlerhood overall.

Phase 9: Social Comparison

The next phase of social–emotional development, from roughly 28 months (about $2\frac{1}{2}$ years) to roughly 36 months (3 years), gets its name from two new constellations: the ability to interact with others based on a prediction of how one's behavior affects them, and the first gleanings of true jealousy. Let's discuss the first of these. According to Judy Dunn (e.g., Dunn, 1988), a prolific researcher into the social side of early childhood, children this age begin to coordinate their newfound knowledge of people's goals with their growing awareness of household rules. At the age of about 28 months, on average, Case's substage of *bifocal (interrelational) coordination* begins to upgrade children's mental capacities. Toddlers become capable of a double coordination of the symbolic units now held in mind. Taking one coordinated social concept, the notion of a rule that can be obeyed or violated, and linking it with a second one, the concept that happiness depends on achieving one's goals, allows the child significantly more insight and control. Parents' goals demand that you follow the rules. The child can now understand how accepting or breaking rules asserts his own power over parents' goals and hence their emotional states – no small advance in the diplomatic halls of family life. In fact, this understanding provides the child with a new level of social sophistication, social influence, and capacity for manipulation. The "terrible twos" now descend once again.

Toddlers will now test the limits, not only to see what they can get away with, not only to satisfy their basic need to assert independence, but to go a step further, to see how much social influence they really have. They will find a way to touch and eventually ruin or ingest whatever parents least want them to handle: the kitchen knives, the computer, the bottles of detergent beneath the sink. But why do they do it? What could possibly motivate this Machiavellian twist? It isn't because they are truly evil – although we sometimes wonder. It isn't because they really want to wreck your day, or be rushed to the hospital. It's because they need to know how much control they have over the thing that matters most: how other people are feeling. They need to understand what lies behind bad emotions as well as good ones. They are exploring the workings of the emotional lives of those they love and depend on.

But the toddler's newfound capacity to be so influential – and such a pest! – is offset by another coordination that can be deeply painful. During the phases of *Social negotiation* and *Social stabilization,* toddlers were capable of understanding that their hopes of getting their wishes met depended on their ability to capture and hold their parent's attention. They left no stone unturned in their efforts to get you to pay attention to them, by repeated calls, interruptions, or demands. At that age they were also capable of seeing how parents would often pay attention to other things and other people, following their own mysterious whims. Toddlers of this age could see that mom was helping dad, or dad was helping mom, and they may have had a vague sense that they were out of the picture for the duration of that episode. But with the onset of bifocal coordination, the toddler's bids for attention, and his ability to capture it by force, can now be *coordinated* with his understanding that mom is attending to someone else and helping *them* achieve *their* needs. This is the cognitive basis for jealousy. If I see that my need for your help or attention is in competition with that of someone else, say my little sister or brother, and if I see that you are helping them instead of helping me, then I can infer that their hold on you directly takes away from mine. Your wish or your decision to bestow your attention on the other person takes it away from me. And this has implications for the larger thrust of your preferences: who you really like, or love, the most. Why are you helping her and not me? Do you like her more? Is she cuter than me?

Jealousy is certainly one of the most painful of emotions, and Robbie was fascinated by its role in early emotional development. It was his student, Sonia Hayward, who clinched the timing of jealousy. Her experiment had mothers stop paying attention to their own child and bestow it on another child at a signal from her. Most of us laid bets that jealousy would emerge earlier – at about 1½–2. What Sonia discovered was that true jealousy, involving a negative response both to the other child and to the mother, was not evident until kids passed tasks involving *bifocal coordination*. For Robbie, this made perfect sense. This was the kind of double symbolic coordination that should rely on bifocal operations. As a supervisor, Robbie was always aware of the emotional dynamics at play in the lives of his students, and he followed them with concern and humor. As is often the case, our group experienced a certain amount of sibling rivalry. We vied for Robbie's attention and competed with each other to get it. All this was balanced by true affection and solidarity. Our connection with Robbie, and our sensitivity to his sometimes mercurial moods, was offset by our connection with one another. We considered ourselves both privileged to have Robbie as a supervisor and caught up in the need to please him, to excel in our work, and to make him proud. Which just went to show that jealousy, once let loose in one's interpersonal repertoire, required one's best efforts at regulation. And the ensuing soap opera gave Robbie both consternation and satisfaction. He knew he was loved.

To recapitulate, the stage of *Social comparison* brings with it two new emotional specialties. First is the child's ability to manipulate others' feelings by challenging their goals, in order to learn about her social power and its impact on the emotional world of the family. Second is the child's proclivity to jealousy, and its tendency to fester and grow into a conviction that she is left out and slighted because she is unimportant or even inferior. There are enormous differences in both these outcomes from child to child. Jealousy is particularly variable, differing as it does in frequency and intensity according to both personality and family constellation factors. Because of this variability, our advice to parents about the emotional challenges of this period is buffered by parents' assessment of their own child's vulnerabilities and capacities. But this is generally not an optimal age for changes that challenge the young child's sense of self. For two reasons. First, because the child's preoccupation with her social influence may exacerbate her reactions to major transitions. Second, and perhaps more important, because the child's capacity for jealousy can paint any personal challenge in the darkest of hues. This is particularly true concerning the advent of a new child in the family. For obvious reasons, this is a difficult age to welcome a new sibling.

Phase 10: Family Membership

As development continues to unfold in the third year of life, it becomes harder and harder to paint a normative picture of social–emotional issues and concerns. The "normal, average" child simply disappears over time, if it ever really existed. By this we mean that younger children's development follows a path of expectable stages at expectable ages that pretty accurately portrays most kids. They follow the sequence of cognitive and emotional changes with sometimes uncanny precision, as far as timing is concerned, and their abilities and habits fit nicely with the average picture for that age. But the older children get, the more they deviate from the norm in one way or another. The timing of changes begins to vary more and more, and so does the substance of these changes. Some children will follow one path of development, showing, say, a lot of defiance, jealousy, and negativity. Others will be more mellow, more content, and more concerned with cooperation than self-assertiveness. The fact that children become more and more distinct from one another makes sense. The reason, according to Robert B. McCall is that development has to be as "normal" as possible early on, so that children (and other animals) can accomplish what they need in order to survive. Too much deviation from the norm spells disaster. Most of the infants' behaviors are necessary to achieve the basic functions of physiological coordination, motor coordination, social engagement, protection, and nurturance. But once these basic functions are established, there's more room for variety, for individuality, for exploring the options. These variations take root in the world of the family. Parents adapt. And individual styles crystallize into stable human personalities. So, the older the child, the more we have to look at his individual profile instead of an age-based average in order to come up with an accurate description.

The phase of *Family membership,* from about 3 to 3½ years, occupies the second half of the substage of *bifocal coordination.* There are no major changes in children's cognitive capacities, but many minor changes, as certain abilities and habits get practiced and strengthened while others disappear. These variations are really the hallmark of this age. But here we focus on what many, if not most, kids do have in common at this age. First, they calm down. We call this the phase of *Family membership* because children now accept their status as fully functioning members of the family. They know the rules, they have the capability to follow them, and they are not driven to test the limits in the ways younger children were. Second, they're smarter about emotions – both their own and other people's. They know what kinds of events cause anger and distress, and they can adjust their behavior, and sometimes the behavior of others, to minimize these negative emotions. They can follow the rules in order to maintain their status as family members in good standing. And they are better at regulating their emotions. For example, impulse control was the biggest single challenge to the 2-year-old. But by the age of 3, children are able to wait until they blow out the candles before opening their presents. They are able to stop themselves from grabbing someone else's toy or bite back on their anger before they hit or kick. Third, children at this age have enormous verbal facility compared to children even 6 months younger. They use more words, in more complex sentences, but nearly all their speech is about social activities, events, and stories, using well-practiced "scripts" that are familiar and evocative. Those verbal talents come in handy when children have to share, or to wait their turn, or play with someone else, or just talk to their stuffed animal because they need someone to talk to and everyone else is busy. Fourth, the same verbal abilities usher in a major acceleration in sociodramatic play. Pretend games, where dinosaurs face off against each other, do battle, or wash the dishes together, now flourish. Children of this age don't need as much adult contact because they are often quite happy to play with their animals and dolls, where they can enact whatever scenarios interest them without having to get someone else involved. Each animal and doll has its own voice, its own position in the social hierarchy, and even its own personality. And the personalities they bestow on their animals and dolls, the love they feel for them, provide an additional means for coping with emotions such as loneliness and separation anxiety.

In sum, the phase of *Family membership* is often a happy time in the life of young children. Before the arrival of false-belief understanding, which we'll discuss in the next section, they are not terribly prone to shame. While there is considerable variation from child to child at this age, most 3-year-olds don't worry much about what others think of them, and they often assume their parents' approval without much in the way of proof. They are not, as a rule, insecure. They are chatty and social. They love to interact through drawn-out conversations with real and imagined others, and they rarely feel lonely or left out. For these reasons, the 3- to 3½-year-old child is relatively malleable and resilient when it comes to accepting new rules and other social–emotional challenges. It is therefore a good age to introduce emotional challenges such as the beginning of full daycare or the birth of a sibling.

Stage 11: Self-Consciousness

The last pendulum swing we cover in this chapter takes place for most children at 3½–4 years of age. As described in the last section, individual variability is now the rule. Children's styles, temperaments, and personalities promote a wide spectrum of differences in language and social development, in habits of self-control, and in interpersonal skills ranging from toilet training to cooperative play. Children are now feeling like members in good standing in their families. They have developed the critical skills of impulse control, and they can use these skills to ward off or modify their feelings of anger, frustration, greed, and jealousy. Things are going well for the average child at this age. And then along comes another cognitive advance, rocking the boat once more.

By this age, cross-domain or general changes in development are not as evident as they were in previous years. As far as we know, Robbie never fully tackled this truism of child development. He freely acknowledged that education has an increasing impact on child development as children grow. It perhaps follows that individual differences would increasingly be the rule in children's development, as their exposure to social agents of knowledge and change must vary with circumstances and opportunities the more time they spend in formal or informal learning environments. However, Robbie stuck to his guns when it came to the hypothesis of parallel developments across domains. Even the incorporation of central conceptual structures into his theory in the early 1990s maintained cross-domain changes as the rule rather than the exception. However, one of the most important developmental transitions does show remarkable universality, and that is the advent of false-belief understanding at about 3½–4 years. Whether false-belief understanding relies on a more general change in cognitive competencies, one associated with the onset of *elaborated (interrelational) coordinations,* is an open question that has not to our knowledge been resolved or even properly tested.

False-belief understanding is the crowning achievement in the development of theory of mind, the awareness that other people have their own goals, feelings, internal states, thoughts, and opinions. With false-belief understanding, the child can now predict that other people will believe whatever they perceive through their own senses, regardless of whether it's true or false. Many studies have demonstrated that 4-year-old children understand this basic principle of human perception, while 3-year-olds do not. By the age of 3½–4, children can predict that a puppet will look for a hidden cookie where the puppet thinks it is located – where he last saw it hidden – rather than in a new location where it was hidden a second time, outside this puppet's awareness. When children can separate their own beliefs from the beliefs of others, they have undertaken a remarkable shift in social understanding. They have now begun to glean that each mind is like a chamber filled with its own perceptions of the world, and no two minds need ever see the world in the same way.

Understanding that your parents have minds of their own can be quite a shock to the 3- to 4-year-old child. Up until now, you took it for granted that Mom saw things the way you did. In fact, you didn't have to explain to her how you saw things, because there was only one way to see things: the way they really are. Now that people's beliefs are seen to be private affairs, carried around in their own heads and not accessible to others, a number of issues have to be worked out. One parent tells the story of his daughter Chloe who rode on the back of his bicycle to nursery school every day from her third birthday on. She would typically point to interesting sights as they rode by, saying, "That flower is blue! That boy has a funny hat!" and so forth. Around the age of 3 years and 4 months, however, her language changed. She began to phrase these comments as questions rather than statements: "Did you see the blue flower? Do you think that hat is funny?" She was clearly conceding that his reality was not the same as hers. But other changes were less cheerful in tone. At exactly the same age, Chloe would be sitting at the table eating her cereal when her father came downstairs, and Chloe would shout "Don't look at me!" While turning her head away or hiding behind her cereal box. What could possibly have prompted such outbursts? If your parents have minds of their own, and if you don't know what's inside them, then you might well worry. They *might* be looking at you, and they might be thinking that you just spilled your cereal, or that you were supposed to wait, or, more generally, that you're a bad, selfish little girl. How would you know?

In this way, false-belief understanding can be a ticket to a new suite of insecurities. A private mind, with its own thoughts and beliefs, might harbor thoughts about you that aren't very nice. This conjecture has been reinforced for us by many anecdotes. Parents of 3½-year-old children would tell us that their daughter suddenly stopped letting them hear her sing. "Go away! Don't listen!" Or "Don't look at me!" Or "Go away until I tell you!" This is also often the age where children suddenly stop letting their parents help them at the potty, if they've been potty-trained for a while. These reactions suggested extreme self-consciousness. These kids apparently worried about being seen, or being heard, because there was something about themselves that might not live up to such scrutiny. Something unpleasant, or greedy, or bad. In fact, false-belief understanding seemed to bring about a spurt of intense shame reactions.

To test this assumption, Marc conducted a study several years ago with Carla Baetz, his graduate student at the time. To see whether false-belief understanding brought about shame reactions, Carla went to the houses of 3- to 4-year-old children and conducted a shame-induction task. Carla pulled on the legs of an elasticized doll and encouraged the child to do the same. What the child didn't know was that the doll had been previously tampered with: one of its arms had been cut so it was ready to come off, and a little too much tension was sure to break it. Indeed, the enthusiastic kids pulled on the doll and ended up with an arm in one hand and the rest of the doll in the other. And then Carla would gaze at them intently while reciting a series of prompts: "Oh no. What happened? What did you do?" This psychological torment only lasted 60 seconds and was followed by a period of "debriefing" in which Carla assured the child that the doll was already broken. But by then we had our videotape, and that 60-second period was revealing! Younger children who did not pass false-belief tasks showed very little shame or remorse. The same was true of the older kids who passed false-belief tasks with ease. They might simply claim that the doll was a lousy toy. But those kids who passed some but not all false-belief tasks – in other words, who were making the transition into this stage of social understanding – showed shame reactions on the video. They scrunched down in their chairs, averted their gaze, held their arms in front of their faces, or said how sorry they were.

The point of the experiment was that the child's understanding that other people have independent minds, with their own thoughts and opinions, allows more than just mature perspective-taking. It promotes a new anxiety that people may think badly about oneself – an anxiety that reflects self-consciousness, embarrassment, and even intense shame. We see this shift in social–emotional dynamics as a double-edged sword. Its dark side is already obvious. But its bright side is a potential springboard along the path of moral development. Unless the child can experience shame about violating other peoples' expectations, unless he can feel self-conscious enough to want to fix his behavior, he won't be motivated to conform to the norms and standards of his family and his society. The self-consciousness that makes its debut with false-belief understanding may be a necessary, in fact crucial, aspect of children's social–moral development. But for at least a few months, while this insight is still fresh, before the child has developed skills for coping with the anxieties it promotes, the child may be particularly vulnerable to feelings of insecurity, lapses in self-confidence, and concerns about being admired, liked, or loved.

This pendulum swing back toward sensitivity and insecurity is the occasion for a variety of social–emotional concerns. These include the emergence of irrational fears, such as a recurring fear of the dark, or the worry that some person (or animal) is angry at the child for some small wrongdoing. This is an age when bad dreams and night terrors can proliferate. It is also an age when kids become highly compulsive, needing to act out each step in a detailed ritual when putting on their clothes, going to the bathroom, or going to bed (Evans, Lewis, & Iobst, 2004). In short, anxieties seem to increase in kind and in frequency at the age of 3½–4 years, and many of them involve concerns about being seen as "bad" by others. For all these reasons, the phase of *Self-consciousness* at 3½–4 (and beyond) requires parents' reassurance, comforting, and ability to read their child's mind. Now is when they need to be sensitive to children's anxieties, not to exacerbate them. So, the period right around the onset of false-belief understanding should be viewed as a hiatus in social–emotional challenges. This is an age when challenges to the young child's sense of self should be avoided, if at all possible, at least until her regulatory capacities have a chance to catch up to her newly acquired social cognitions.

Conclusion

This completes our depiction of the phases of social–emotional development over the first 4 years of life. We have seen that these phases correspond, for the most part, with advances in cognitive development that provide new ways of interpreting the world, giving rise to new emotional responses and new capacities for controlling those responses. And we have seen how these phases describe a pendulum swing back and forth between periods of sensitivity and periods of resilience. Finally, we have touched on the implications of each of these phases for parents' decisions about when to initiate challenging life events. The richness of social–emotional development and its interface with the stages of cognitive development provide insights into many more issues than those we have covered in this chapter. Indeed, social–emotional development constitutes not one domain but a cluster of developmental domains, some of which follow more or less normative schedules while others are highly individual in their content and timing. However, our goal in this chapter has been to provide a simplified picture of normative social–emotional development of use to scholars, clinicians, and parents, and to show how Case's account of normative cognitive acquisitions suggests a scaffolding that makes sense of the obscure trajectory of children's emotional habits, concerns, capacities, and vulnerabilities throughout early childhood. The clarity and precision with which this translation can be made attests to the power and reach of Robbie's theory more generally. And we emphasize that the application of that theory to emotional development was a goal that captivated Robbie throughout his lifetime, providing inspiration and direction for his students and colleagues.

References

Beauregard, M., Lévesque, J., & Bourgouin, P. (2001). Neural correlates of conscious self-regulation of emotion. *The Journal of Neuroscience: The Official Journal of the Society for Neuroscience*, *21*, 6993–7000.

Campos, J. J., Anderson, D. I., Barbu-Roth, M. A., Hubbard, E. M., Hertenstein, M. J., & Witherington, D. (2000). Travel broadens the mind. *Infancy*, *1*, 149–219.

Campos, J. J., & Stenberg, C. R. (1981). Perception, appraisal and emotion: The onset of social referencing. In M. E. Lamb & L. R. Sherrod (Eds.), *Infant social cognition: Empirical and theoretical considerations* (pp. 273–314). Hillsdale, NJ: Erlbaum.

Carver, L. J., & Vaccaro, B. G. (2007). 12-month-old infants allocate increased neural resources to stimuli associated with negative adult emotion. *Developmental Psychology*, *43*, 54–69.

Case, R. (1988). The whole child: Toward an integrated view of young children's cognitive, social, and emotional development. In A. D. Pellegrini (Ed.), *Psychological bases for early education* (pp. 155–184). New York: Wiley.

Case, R. (1991). Stages in the development of the young child's first sense of self. *Developmental Review*, *11*, 210–230.

Case, R., Hayward, S., Lewis, M. D., & Hurst, P. (1988). Toward a neo-piagetian theory of cognitive and emotional development. *Developmental Review*, *8*, 1–51.

Cunningham, W. A., Johnson, M. K., Raye, C. L., Gatenby, J. C., Gore, J. C., & Banaji, M. R. (2004). Separable neural components in the processing of black and white faces. *Psychological Science*, *15*, 806–813.

Dunn, J. (1988). *The beginnings of social understanding*. Cambridge, MA: Harvard University Press.

Emde, R. N., Gaensbauer, T. J., & Harmon, R. J. (1976). Emotional expression in infancy; a biobehavioral study. *Psychological Issues*, *10*, 1–200.

Evans, D. W., Lewis, M. D., & Iobst, E. (2004). The role of the orbitofrontal cortex in normally developing compulsive-like behaviors and obsessive-compulsive disorder. *Brain and Cognition*, *55*, 220–234.

Frijda, N. H. (1993). The place of appraisal in emotion. *Cognition and Emotion*, *7*, 357–387.

Lamm, C., Zelazo, P. D., & Lewis, M. D. (2006). Neural correlates of cognitive control in childhood and adolescence: Disentangling the contributions of age and executive function. *Neuropsychologia*, *44*, 2139–2148.

Lewis, M. D. (1993a). Early socioemotional predictors of cognitive competency at 4 years. *Developmental Psychology*, *29*, 1036–1045.

Lewis, M. D. (1993b). Emotion-cognition interactions in early development. *Cognition and Emotion*, *7*, 145–170.

Lewis, M. D. (1995). Cognition-emotion feedback and the self-organization of developmental paths. *Human Development*, *38*, 71–102.

Lewis, M. D. (1996). Self-organising cognitive appraisals. *Cognition and Emotion*, *10*, 1–25.

Lewis, M. D. (2000). The promise of dynamic systems approaches for an integrated account of human development. *Child Development*, *71*, 36–43.

Lewis, M. D. (2005). Bridging emotion theory and neurobiology through dynamic systems modeling. *Behavioral and Brain Sciences*, *28*, 169–194.

Lewis, M. D., & Granic, I. (1999). Who put the self in self-organization? A clarification of terms and concepts for developmental psychopathology. *Development and Psychopathology*, *11*, 365–374.

Lewis, M. D., & Granic, I. (Eds.). (2000). *Emotion, development, and self-organization: Dynamic systems approaches to emotional development*. New York: Cambridge University Press.

Lewis, M. D., Lamm, C., Segalowitz, S. J., Stieben, J., & Zelazo, P. D. (2006). Neurophysiological correlates of emotion regulation in children and adolescents. *Journal of Cognitive Neuroscience*, *18*, 430–443.

Monk, C. S., McClure, E. B., Nelson, E. E., Zarahn, E., Bilder, R. M., Leibenluft, E., et al. (2003). Adolescent immaturity in attention-related brain engagement to emotional facial expressions. *NeuroImage*, *20*, 420–428.

Ochsner, K. N., & Gross, J. J. (2005). The cognitive control of emotion. *Trends in Cognitive Sciences*, *9*, 242–249.

Ochsner, K. N., Ray, R. D., Cooper, J. C., Robertson, E. R., Chopra, S., Gabrieli, J. D. E., et al. (2004). For better or for worse: Neural systems supporting the cognitive down- and up-regulation of negative emotion. *NeuroImage*, *23*, 483–499.

Pessoa, L. (2008). On the relationship between emotion and cognition. *Nature Reviews Neuroscience*, *9*, 148–158.
Posner, M. I., & Rothbart, M. K. (1998). Attention, self-regulation and consciousness. *Philosophical Transactions of the Royal Society B: Biological Sciences*, *353*, 1915–1927.
Posner, M. I., & Rothbart, M. K. (2000). Developing mechanisms of self-regulation. *Development and Psychopathology*, *12*, 427–441.
Sander, L. W. (1975). Infant and caretaking environment: Investigation and conceptualization of adaptive behavior in a system of increasing complexity. In E. J. Anthony (Ed.), *Explorations in child psychiatry* (pp. 129–166). New York: Plenum.
Sander, L. W. (1983). Polarity, paradox, and the organizing process in development. In J. D. Call, E. Galenson, & R. L. Tyson (Eds.), *Frontiers of infant psychiatry*. New York: Basic Books.
Scherer, K. R. (1999). On the sequential nature of appraisal processes: Indirect evidence from a recognition task. *Cognition and Emotion*, *13*, 763–793.
Scherer, K. R. (2000). Emotions as episodes of subsystem synchronization driven by nonlinear appraisal processes. In M. D. Lewis & I. Granic (Eds.), *Emotion, development, and self-organization: Dynamic systems approaches to emotional development* (pp. 70–99). New York: Cambridge University Press.
Sroufe, L. A. (1979). Socioemotional development. In J. Osofsky (Ed.), *Handbook of infant development* (pp. 462–518). New York: Wiley.
Sroufe, L. A. (1995). *Emotional development: The organization of emotional life in the early years*. New York: Cambridge University Press.
Stern, D. N. (1985). *The interpersonal world of the infant*. New York: Basic Books.
Thatcher, R. W. (1991). Maturation of the human frontal lobes: Physiological evidence for staging. *Developmental Neuropsychology*, *7*, 397–419.
Thatcher, R. W. (1998). A predator-prey model of human cerebral development. In K. M. Newell & P. C. M. Molenaar (Eds.), *Applications of nonlinear dynamics to developmental process modeling* (pp. 87–128). Mahwah, NJ: Erlbaum.
Tomasello, M. (1995). Joint attention as social cognition. In C. Moore & P. J. Dunham (Eds.), *Joint attention: Its origins and role in development* (pp. 103–130). Hillsdale, NJ: Erlbaum.

Adolescent Narrative Thought: Developmental and Neurological Evidence in Support of a Central Social Structure

Anne McKeough and Stephanie Griffiths

Traditionally, narrative has served as an important means of understanding and knowing the social world. In this chapter, we review a representative sample of research that has mapped the role narrative has played in the development of children's and adolescents' social cognition. Following Case and Okamoto (1996), we argue that narrative knowing serves as a central conceptual structure that transforms developmentally and shapes thinking across a range of socially situated domains. We review studies with children that support this claim (Case & Okamoto, 1996) and briefly present data that support the existence of a central social structure in adolescence. We discuss these empirical findings in light of recent work in developmental neuropsychology, highlighting the biological basis of developmental central conceptual structures. Finally, we briefly outline implications for education.

The Development of Narrative Knowing

Long before the widespread use of written text, oral narratives recounted important events, posed problems, and offered ways of solving them (Bettelheim, 1976; Campbell, 1988). These stories, like printed stories, not only told of what had happened, but also what should happen, allowing them to reach in two directions, into the past and into the future, and so making them a very powerful means of understanding and transmitting personal and cultural knowledge and beliefs. Narrative knowing of this sort had traditionally been a subject of study in anthropology (e.g., Propp, 1928/1968) and literary theory (e.g., Culler, 1975, Scholes & Kellogg, 1966). With the notable exception of the work of Bartlett (1932), however, it did not feature prominently in psychological research until the advent of the cognitive revolution, when models of thinking and methods of analyses allowed work with complex connected discourse (Gardner, 1985).

Throughout the 1970s and 1980s, studies showed that stories were a rich source of information about children's developing cognitive competencies, illustrating

---

A. McKeough (✉)
Division of Applied Psychology, University of Calgary, Calgary, AL, Canada
e-mail: mckeough@ucalgary.ca

M. Ferrari, L. Vuletic (eds.), *The Developmental Relations among Mind, Brain and Education*, DOI 10.1007/978-90-481-3666-7_9,

changes in their capacity to generate and integrate the various syntactic and semantic elements (Peterson & McCabe, 1983; Mandler, 1984; Stein, 1988; Sutton-Smith, 1986). Subsequently, during the late 1980s and early 1990s, researchers and theoreticians expanded on the cognitive function ascribed to stories, positing that, by laying out the actions and thoughts of protagonists, stories link action and consequence, thus providing models of human action that, in turn, help us interpret human intentions and order the events of our own lives into meaningful experiences (e.g., McAdams, 1993; Palombo, 1991; Polkinghorne, 1988; Sarbin, 1986). Bruner saw narrative as one of two main ways that experience is ordered and understood, the other being what he termed paradigmatic thought. Whereas the paradigmatic mode of thought organizes the world into categories and concepts and is suited to scientific domains, the narrative mode "deals in human and human-like intention and action and the vicissitudes and consequences that mark their course" (Bruner, 1986, p. 13).

This growing awareness of narrative's interpretive function was reflected in its central role in a diverse range of research programs throughout the past two decades, including social and cultural factors (Bruner, 1990; Dickinson & Tabors, 2001; Heath, 1986; Leichman, Wang, & Pillemer, 2003; Michaels, 1981, 1991; Miller, Potts, Fung, Hoogstra, & Mintz, 1990; Miller, Wiley, Fung, & Liang, 1997), moral development (Tappan & Packer, 1991), memory (Fivush, & Haden, 2003; Fivush & Hudson, 1992; Haden, 2003; Hudson, Gebelt, Haviland, & Bentivegna, 1992; McCabe, Capron, & Peterson, 1991; Nelson, 1981, 2003), self knowledge (Neisser & Fivush, 1994; Polkinghorne, 1988), gender roles (1990, Nicolopoulou, 1997), literacy (Olson, 1990; Yussen & Ozcan, 1996), language (Bamberg & Damrad-Frye, 1991; Nelson, 2000; Stein, 1988; Sutton-Smith, 1986), processing capacity (McKeough, 2000; McKeough & Genereux, 2003; Pratt, Boyes, Robins, & Manchester, 1989), clinical psychology (e.g., Habermas & Bluck, 2000; McAdams, 1993; Runyan, 1982; Schaefer, 1981, 2004; Spence, 1982), and teaching (Case & McKeough, 1990; Egan, 1989; Hicks, 1994, McCabe, 1996; McKeough, Davis, Forgeron, Marini, & Fung, 2005; McKeough & Sanderson, 1996). In spite of the broad scope of topics, these researchers share a common view that "the fundamental function of narrative in human life is . . . to signal a perspective on events and create a satisfying pattern of themes one has drawn from one's various social traditions" (Gee, 1991, p. 20). Additionally, all acknowledge that the manner in which perspective and themes are constructed and displayed is linked to development. What is lacking in this diverse research context, however, is an agreed-on view of the structural constituents of narrative knowing and the transformations that characterize its development. Such a unifying framework would allow the comparison and integration of empirical work across research programs thus potentially creating a scaffold that would provide a new vantage point on the development of narrative thought.

Narrative Development and Central Conceptual Structures

One theoretical framework that offers considerable promise in this regard has been developed by Case and his colleagues (Case, 1992; Case & Okamoto, 1996).

Working within a neo-Piagetian tradition, Case proposed that common conceptual underpinnings among task-specific cognitive structures yield up superstructures. As is the case with all conceptual structures, central conceptual structures (CCS) are comprised of semantic nodes and relations that must be learned, may be culturally specific in content (especially at the more advanced developmental levels), and are thought to be subject to developmental constraints. CCSs are thought to apply to a range of tasks, transcend conventionally defined domains, and influence performance across a broad, yet delimited, range of tasks. The CCS discussed by Case that utilizes narrative thought is the central social structure (Case & Okamoto, 1996). That is, narrative thought and Case's central social structures are related in the following way: Culturally specific narratives are social meaning-making devices that children and adolescents gradually come to understand and apply in a range of contexts. Youths' growing understanding can be characterized as a series of central social structures (Case & Okamoto, 1996).

Considerable work has been done in mapping out the development of this central social structure throughout middle childhood (Case & Griffin, 1990; Case, Griffin, McKeough, & Okamoto, 1992; Case, Marini, McKeough, Dennis, & Goldberg 1986; Case & McKeough, 1990; Case & Okamoto, 1996; McKeough, 1992a; McKeough, Yates, & Marini, 1994, Porath, 1992). As with more narrowly defined conceptual structures, central conceptual structures become more complex as a result of increased working memory capacity. Throughout each of the four major developmental stages specified by Case (1985), there is a recursive progression through three substages, made possible by two factors: a functional increase in working memory (as a result of automatization) and experience in the domain. In the first substage (unifocal coordination), a new type of structure is assembled by coordinating two qualitatively different structures that were consolidated or chunked in the previous stage. This operation demands two working memory units. However, due to this working memory constraint, the structure can only be applied in isolation. In the second substage (bifocal coordination), a functional increase in working capacity to three units makes it possible for two such structures to be applied in succession. These structures cannot be successfully integrated, however, because of working memory capacity limitations. In the third substage (elaborated coordination), two or more such units can be integrated and applied simultaneously because automatization yields a further functional increase in working memory, adding a fourth unit. At this third substage, with practice, the four-unit structure chunks into a single unit, producing a consolidated structure that serves as a building block for the next major stage of development.

To illustrate this progression, consider the domain of oral storytelling. When storytelling, the typical 4-year-old generates a coherent scripted episode that is largely action based and tells of the physical world. This operation is hypothesized to require one consolidated working memory unit. In this same age range, children consolidate a structure for representing mental states (Astington, 2001; Pelletier & Astington, 2004). It is not until approximately 6 years of age, however, that children utilize these two different structures in a coordinated fashion in their stories. This cognitive operation yields a qualitatively different type of narrative – one that is goal or problem driven rather than scripted (McCabe & Peterson, 1991). We refer to these narratives as *intentional*, because the intentions of the characters drive the plot line. Stories with this level of structural complexity are hypothesized to have a working memory demand of two units. By approximately 8 years of age, a failed attempt or sub-problem is typically included in the plot line, which comprises a second coordinated action/mental state unit and is hypothesized to require a third unit of working memory. By age 10, four units of working memory are used to produce story components that are integrated in a more elaborate resolution (Case & McKeough, 1990; McKeough, 1992a). This structure is consolidated and serves as the basic building block for the next qualitatively different developmental change. Thus, during middle childhood, narrative is thought to be comprised of a series of causal relations between the external world of physical states and actions, on the one hand, and the internal world of feelings and mental states, on the other. This relationship is evident in children's story compositions, where characters' actions are motivated by a range of mental states, including feelings, thoughts, and desires (McKeough, 1992a; McKeough et al., 2005; Porath, 1992), and signals the emergence of what Bruner (1986) has termed narrative's dual landscapes, namely, the landscape of action (i.e., what characters do in the physical world) and the landscape of consciousness (i.e., what characters know, think, feel, or believe about the landscape of action).

Evidence of a social structure, in which actions are contextualized in the intentions of the characters, has also been found beyond the narrow domain of story composition in, for example, children's explanations of mothers' motivations (Goldberg-Reitman, 1992) and empathic response to peers (Bruchkowsky, 1992). Empirical support for the hypothesis that the intentional narrative structure is central to these sample tasks, as well as others, has been derived from factor analytic studies (Case & Okamoto, 1996). Instruction studies have further verified this view, demonstrating spontaneous transfer to, but not beyond, tasks hypothesized to share narrative underpinnings (Case, 1993; Case & Okamoto, 1996; Case & McKeough, 1990; McKeough, 1991, 1992b, 1995).

Although considerably less research has been done with adolescents' narrative knowledge, existing work has shown a shift to a more abstract level in both story interpretation and composition. Applebee (1978) was one of the first to document a trend toward analyzing and generalizing in the interpretation of fiction. Interpreting personal life experience has also been examined. Habermas and Bluck (2000) argued that not until adolescence does the cognitive capacity exist to construct a coherent life story. Other researchers have noted a shift to a psychological focus, accentuating characters' motivations and traits that drive their actions (e.g., Bamberg & Damrad-Frye, 1991; Beach, Appleman, Hynds, & Wilhelm, 2006; Beach & Wendler, 1987; Feldman, Bruner, Kalmar, Renderer, 1994; Genereux & McKeough, 2007; McConaughy, Fitzhenry-Coor, & Howell, 1984; McKeough & Genereux, 2003; Sun, 1998). To illustrate, developmental transformations that build on cognitive structures assembled in middle childhood have been identified throughout adolescence (Genereux & McKeough, 2007; McKeough & Genereux, 2003). Very briefly, research has demonstrated that a qualitative shift in narrative thought is evidenced between 10 and 12 years of age. According to Case (1985, 1992), children have entered the fourth major stage of cognitive development around 12 years of age and should demonstrate an emerging capacity to create a new structure by combining two of the narrative units they mastered as 10-year-olds. Whereas most 10-year-olds focus on immediate, proximal intentions and mental states, by age 12 storytellers begin to interpret the intentions of characters in terms of enduring, trans-situational mental states and character traits (McKeough, 2000; Yussen & Ozcan, 1996). To illustrate, a character's resistance to joining a group activity might lead to him being referred to as "a loner" and be explained in terms of a personal history of rejection and ridicule. Reference to such traits and prior social experiences suggests that, by age 12, adolescents are able to simultaneously consider two or more experiences that occurred at different times or in different situations and then extract a higher-order unit of meaning making, such as a personality trait or an enduring psychological state, from the two lower-level units. Such an operation is hypothesized to require two working memory units.

By age 14, a functional increase in working memory, to three units, makes possible the inclusion of additional enduring psychological states and traits, often creating a struggle within the characters as competing character traits war with each other. For example a story character might be torn between wanting to be part of the "cool" group and wanting to be alcohol and drug free. By 18 years, a fourth working memory unit allows adolescents to create a dialectic involving the protagonist's internal and external struggles and deal with the conflict in a coordinated and coherent fashion (McKeough, 2000; Yussen & Ozcan, 1996). Because a distinguishing feature of the adolescent organizational form involves the interpretation of characters' intentions, we have termed it *interpretive narrative* (Genereux & McKeough, 2007; McKeough, 1996, 2000; McKeough & Genereux, 2003).

Adolescent Central Social Structure: Empirical Evidence

If the interpretive narrative structure is "central" to a range of tasks beyond narrative composition, however, as was the case for the intentional structure in middle childhood, we should see evidence of the above developmental progression in other conceptually related but distinct task domains. To test this hypothesis we used a cross-sectional design to document the development of narrative thinking on four tasks and to determine if a common narrative structure can be articulated across the tasks.

Three hundred and ninety-nine academically average, middle socioeconomic status (SES) volunteers were selected from grade 5, 7, and 10 classrooms. Academic achievement was ascertained from existing standardized test scores and SES was established using the Socioeconomic Index for Occupations in Canada (Blishen, Carroll, & Moore, 1987). Academically average, middle SES students were used because the goal was to map out typical (not atypical) development.

We used four conceptually related pencil and paper tasks to assess narrative development. Tasks were administered to classroom grouping in random order.

Story Composition

Participants asked to write a story about a character who is approximately their age and who has a problem he or she wants to solve. Participants were also instructed to try to provide one of their best efforts.

Family Story Interpretation

Participants were given an explanation and example of a family story and asked to write one of their own. They were then asked to complete, in written form, as series of questions that probed the meaning the story holds for them, alternative interpretations that others might have, and the intentions of the teller.

Moral Reasoning

Two moral dilemmas were presented to participants and they were asked to respond in writing to a series of probes that aimed to have them interpret what the character in the dilemma should do and why. One scenario described a dilemma involving conflicting ownership rights that was likely to draw on justice-based reasoning whereas the other involved conflicting interpersonal responsibilities and was likely to draw on care-based reasoning.

Social Decision Making

This task, designed by Marini and Case (1994), measured subjects awareness of a characters' psychological make-up as a factor motivating actions in everyday situations. Participants read short descriptions of two adolescent characters' behavior in various social situations and responded, in writing, to a series of questions concerning how the characters will act in novel social situations and why.

Separate scoring schemes were applied to each task in order to tap in to the thinking demonstrated.[1] Although the scoring schemes reflected the different task demands, they shared a common structural organization based on Case's (1985) stage and substage progression, which is governed by a functional growth in working memory. A content-adapted version of this hypothesized developmental progression was utilized for the present study (McKeough & Genereux, 2003). That is, fifth-grade performance (i.e., elaborated intentional narrative thought) focused on action motivated by mental state, simple traits, and social rules; seventh-grade performance (i.e., coordinated interpretive narrative thought) focused on inner psychological states or generalized enduring traits and social rules, and tenth-grade performance (i.e., elaborated bifocal interpretive narrative thought) involved a social/psychological dialectic and dual psychological referencing.

Mean scores are displayed by task and age in Table 1. To test the hypothesis that narrative thought develops in complexity, a 3 (Grade levels) × 4 (Task) MANOVA

[1] The developmental scoring schemes are available from the first author on request.

Table 1 Means across grade levels

Tasks	Grade 4	Grade 7	Grade 10
Problem story	3.53	4.83	5.89
Family story	4.24	5.01	6.40
Moral reasoning	3.94	4.81	5.79
Social decision making	4.35	4.92	5.82

Table 2 Percent of participants' performance that reached predicted levels across task and grade

Grade	Problem story (%)	Family story (%)	Moral reasoning (%)	Social decision making (%)
4	48.2	51.2	84.7	74.5
7	75.2	53.8	78.6	54.8
10	83.3	31.6	76.3	51.9

was conducted. It revealed a significant main effect for grade and a grade-by-task interaction. On an average, the predicted developmental progression was verified, although participants performed differently across several tasks at certain grade levels. More specifically, there was variability across age levels and tasks in terms of the percent of participants who performed at the targeted level. Based on Case's theory (1985), participants at each age level were expected to perform at specific levels, as follows: grade 4 = level 4, grade 7 = level 5, and grade 10 = level 6. As Table 2 illustrates, participants' performance on the moral reasoning task was closest to the levels predicted by Case's theory. Fourth-grade performance on the problem story task and tenth-grade performance on the family story task fell below the 50% level. An inspection of the means presented in Table 1 reveals that fourth-grade performance on the problem story task fell almost a half level below the predicted level of 4, whereas tenth grade on the family story task fell almost a half level above the predicted level of 6. Further research is required to account for the variability across tasks and grade levels. Additionally, factor analysis was used to test the hypothesis that a single factor, narrative knowledge, accounted for a substantial portion of the variance. The results indicated a single factor with factor loadings for principal components ranging from 0.903 to 0.733 (see Table 3 for specific factor loadings for each task).

Table 3 Factor analysis loadings across four tasks

Tasks	Loadings
Problem story	0.863
Family story	0.777
Moral seasoning: Task 1 (Jesse)	0.903
Moral reasoning: Task 2 (Justin)	0.893
Decision making: Task 1 (Dennis)	0.733
Decision making: Task 2 (Cathy)	0.691

Cognitive Developmental Change

The results of the present study generally confirmed Case's developmental sequence for each of the four tasks. Although we do not claim that hypothesized increases in working memory impact the content of narrative thought, the current analysis demonstrates that it plays a central role in its rate of development. Importantly, however, other elements, such as the complexity of task demands and experience and familiarity with task content also impact performance. Nevertheless, within these patterns there is clear evidence that participants' performance on the four experimental tasks reflected an increase in complexity with age. Moreover, the four tasks loaded on a single factor, narrative thought, and so can be said to share a central conceptual underpinning. Next, we explore the neurobiological processes that might underlie the observed developmental changes in narrative thought in an effort to account for the existence of a central social structure that utilizes narrative thought.

Neurobiological and Neuropsychological Developmental Change

Given the empirical evidence in support of the stage-like development of central conceptual structures during childhood and adolescence, it is important to appreciate how neurological development might underlie these changes. Though discontinuous and marked by individual differences, human brain development progresses through predetermined stages, eventually forming efficient networks of neurons that function together to support cognitive processes. Although infants are born with close to their lifetime population of neurons, these neurons have inherent plasticity in their connections with one another, via synapses, and in the extent of myelination, which determines their speed of communication (Rivkin, 2000). Thus, maturational processes that affect neural functioning continue long after birth.

The malleability of synapses is, moreover, one important progenitor of functional specialization, whereby certain areas of the brain become responsible for specific cognitive functions during development (Desmurget, Bonnetblanc, & Duffau, 2007; Sakai, 2005). Functional specialization (Elston, 2003; Hutsler, 2003) has long been attributed to consistent and repeated communication between proximate groups of neurons, which gradually increases the strength of neural interconnections (e.g., Hebb, 1949) at regional and hemispheric levels of neural organization (Kelley, Baldo, Pratt, & Will, 2005; Klingberg, 2006; Posner & Rothbart, 2004; Stephan, Fink, & Marshall, 2007). Stronger connections, in turn, facilitate increasingly automatic neural processes. Indeed, Case's theory construes the automatization of cognitive processes as a major determinant of age-related increases in working memory or processing capacity (Case, 1985). Neurodevelopmentally, the timeline of functional specialization varies, such that brain regions subsuming sensory functions tend to mature first, followed by motor regions, and then by regions supporting more complex behavioral or cognitive processes (Volpe, 1995), such as early narrative thought.

The process of functional specialization is also supported by ongoing myelination. Neuroimaging studies of the developing brain describe non-linear declines in the volume of gray matter (i.e., neural cell bodies) and increases in white matter volume (i.e., myelin) with age (Jernigan & Tallal, 1990; Paus et al., 2001; Pfefferbaum et al., 1994; Steen, Ogg, Reddick, & Kingsley, 1997). Functionally, myelin tracts are thought to represent communication pathways within (Klingberg, 2006) and between brain regions (Mosenthal, 1995). The widespread neural myelination that occurs during development is thought to support age-related increases in the efficiency of neural communication and hence, cognitive processes. Although this type of neural plasticity has long been recognized as characteristic of early development, such processes have increasingly come to be construed as operating into adolescence and, indeed, across the lifespan (Satz, 1993). We suggest that these age-related increases in myelination and functional specialization are an important determinant of developmental changes in cognitive processes such as intentional and interpretive narrative. The construction of increasingly complex central conceptual structures, which relies on functional increases in children's working memory made possible through the chunking of information, may well depend upon these maturational processes.

During adolescence, cortical development also continues, as frontal and parietal maturation occurs (Sowell, Thompson, & Toga, 2004; Toga, Thompson, & Sowell, 2006). The frontal lobes, in particular, are thought to be involved in the most complex of cognitive functions and, not surprisingly, they mature later in the developmental timeline than areas related to more primary cognitive functions. Researchers consider the frontal lobes to play an important role in determining one's capacity to hold and integrate multiple streams of information, resist interference, and pursue goal-driven behavior (Miller & Cohen, 2001). The term, executive abilities, is often applied to these frontally mediated cognitive processes. These include initiation and inhibition of behavior, holding and manipulating information (i.e., working memory), self-monitoring, planning and organization, and social awareness (Grady & Keightley, 2002). The major shifts during adolescence in the ability to understand and use complex central social structures in narrative-based tasks reported in the current study are consistent with the protracted developmental timeline of the aforementioned executive functions. Moreover, recent evidence had suggested that the development of multifaceted cognitive processes is intertwined with the development of specific component abilities such as attentional control and working memory (Colom et al., 2006; Frangou, Chitins & Williams, 2004; Spencer et al., 2006; van Leeuwen, van den Berg, Hoekstra, & Boomsma, 2007). Thus it is reasonable to propose that interpretive narrative (where mental states are interpreted, past and future events are discussed and reconciled, and moral lessons are taught) likely relies heavily on the anatomical interconnections between brain regions responsible for executive functions.

Although the direct relationship between structural maturation and cognitive development (Casey, Tottenham, Liston, & Durston, 2005; Mall et al., 2005; Sowell, Thompson, Leonard, et al., 2004; Sowell et al., 2002), even for such complex and multifaceted constructs as intelligence (Romine & Reynolds, 2005; Shaw et al., 2006; Sowell et al., 2001) and executive abilities (Bunge & Wright, 2007; Rubia et al., 2006) is well established, there remains some debate as to whether age-related increases in the efficiency of these cognitive processes are primarily a product of the elimination of extraneous connections between neurons, the formation of new pathways, or both (Brown et al., 2005; Quartz & Sejnowski, 1997). Regardless of the mechanism, however, the increasing reliance on frontally mediated abilities during cognitive activities (e.g. Bjork et al., 2004; Ciesielski, Lesnik, Savoy, Grant, & Ahlfors, 2006; Kucian et al., 2007; Scherf, Sweeney, & Luna, 2006) is a widely recognized phenomenon. As noted, more sophisticated performance on interpretive narrative tasks comes 'on-line' as physiological maturation allows for increased recruitment of executive functions.

Other factors may also play a role in determining the developmental timeline of narrative proficiency. For instance, individual differences in cortical plasticity, or the capacity of specific populations of neurons to assume multiple functions or to demonstrate more dynamic age-related changes, has been suggested to account for some of the variance in the developmental timeline of cognitive skills like intelligence (Shaw et al., 2006). Similar considerations may also apply when considering the emergence of complex abilities such as interpretive narrative. As Mar (2004) pointed out, frontal cortical areas likely subserve the complex narrative operations of perspective taking, as well as selection and mental tracking of the progression of story elements, both of which are important elements of interpretive narrative (Genereux and McKeough, 2007; McKeough & Genereux, 2003). Other aspects of narrative formation, such as the use of figurative language in the narrative compositions of talented writers (McKeough & Genereux, 2003), may depend on both experience and the development of the ability to understand context, self-monitoring, and self-correction, as well as the appreciation of humor (Nippold & Taylor, 1995; Thoma & Daum, 2006). These self-regulating and metacognitive processes are intimately tied to frontal lobe functioning and would also be expected to show a gradual developmental trajectory (Romine & Reynolds, 2005). Therefore, the findings reported previously concerning the development of adolescent narrative thought, which indicate that the major shifts in complexity of central social structures occur during adolescence is consistent with our understanding of neurodevelopmental underpinnings of the associated cognitive abilities.

Educational Implications

Knowledge of the neuropsychological underpinnings of narrative thought utilized within the Central Social Structure offers educators a sense of certainty that teaching will support continued brain development. Over the past 10 years, considerable attention has been given to stimulating brain development from infancy, when brain plasticity is optiminal, to old age, when use of cognitive functions is seen as slowing cognitive decline. In short, understanding the neuropsychological basis of narrative thought tells educators that instruction is profitable.

Cognitive analysis of developmental change in narrative thought, as described in the present chapter, also tells educators what can be taught. The shift from intentional narrative thought to interpretive narrative thought suggests that adolescents' instruction can increasingly focus on why people experience specific feelings, hold particular beliefs, and experience unique desires. Adolescents' capacity to take a metaposition to these mental states allows them to, for example, appreciate literature at a deeper level (Applebee, 1978; Genereux & McKeough, 2007), create psychologically focused fiction that meaningfully integrates characters' past and present (McKeough & Genereux, 2003), understand the actions of others (Feldman, Bruner, Kalmar, & Renderer, 1993), and create an integrated life story (McAdams, 1993). Thus, it is reasonable to propose that educators can use knowledge of adolescents' interpretive narrative ability in a range of school contexts including curricular (e.g., study of literature and drama, as well as counseling supports) and extra-curricular (peer support, student governance, sports team cooperation) activities.

Our neo-Piagetian analysis, based on Case's theory (Case, 1985, 1992; Case & Okamoto, 1996), has also demonstrated that tasks as diverse as composition of fiction, interpretation of family stories, moral reasoning, and social decision making share conceptual underpinnings. Thus, narrative thought constitutes the basis of an adolescent Central Social Structure, which transcends conventionally defined domains. Potentially, then, the course discipline barriers that exist in many educational systems can begin to be broken down with the result that conceptually related subject matter is integrated. To illustrate, the study of history and literature has traditionally be joined only in terms of time periods (e.g., The Grapes of Wrath is taken up simultaneously with the study of the great depression). They can, however, be integrated conceptually, in terms of unique, context-specific perspective of the actors (e.g., Why were the parents of Romeo and Juliet unable to see beyond their narrow point of view until it was too late? Why were the early North American missionaries unable to see the rich culture of Aboriginal peoples?). By switching focus to conceptual commonalities (i.e., the interpretation of people's intentions) teachers of English literature and history would tap into learners' developing minds, with the probable result that school work would become more interesting and meaningful to adolescents.

Case's theory has been closely linked with instruction since the 1980s. Programs of instruction have been tested empirically for early story crafting (Case & McKeough, 1990; McKeough, Davis, Forgeron, Marini, & Fung, 2005), trickster tales (Jarvey, McKeough, & Pyryt, 2008), and numeracy (Griffin & Case, 1995; Griffin, Case, & Siegler, 1994). These programs of instruction that have practical utility for average functioning students as well as to those who are at risk academically. Although these instruction programs focus on middle childhood, rather than adolescence, they point to the potential for using Case's neo-Piagetian theory in the design of developmentally based instruction that is supported by neuropsychological research.

References

Applebee, A. (1978). *The child's concept of story*. Chicago: University of Chicago Press.

Astington, J. W. (2001). The paradox of intention: Assessing children's metarepresentational understanding. In B. F. Malle, L. J. Moses, & D. A. Baldwin (Eds.), *Intentions and intentionality: Foundations of social cognition* (pp. 85–103). Cambridge, MA: MIT Press.

Bartlett, F. C. (1932). *Remembering*. Cambridge, England: Cambridge University Press.

Bamberg, M., & Damrad-Frye, P. (1991). On the ability to provide evaluative comments: Further exploration of children's narrative competencies. *Journal of Child Language, 18,* 689–710.
Beach, R., Appleman, D., Hynds, S., & Wilhelm, J. (2006). *Teaching Literature to Adolescents.* Mahwah, NJ: Erlbaum.
Beach, R., & Wendler, L. (1987). Developmental differences in response to a story. *Research in the Teaching of English, 21*(3), 286–297.
Bettelheim, B. (1976). *The uses of enchantment: The meaning and importance of fairy tales.* New York: Vintage.
Bjork, J. M., Knutson, B., Fong, G. W., Caggiano, D. M., Bennett, S. M., & Hommer, D. W. (2004). Incentive-elicited brain activation in adolescents: Similarities and differences from young adults. *Journal of Neuroscience, 24,* 1793–1802.
Blishen, B. R., Carroll, W. K., & Moore, K. (1987). The 1981 socioeconomic index for occupations in Canada. *Canadian Review of Sociology and Anthropology, 24,* 465–488.
Brown, T. T., Lugar, H. M., Coalson, R. S., Miezin, F. M., Petersen, S. E., Schlaggar, B. L. (2005). Developmental changes in human cerebral functional organization for word generation. *Cerebral Cortex, 15,* 275–290.
Bruchkowsky, M. (1992). The development of empathic understanding in early and middle childhood. In R. Case (Ed.), *The mind's staircase: Exploring the conceptual underpinnings of children's thought and knowledge* (pp. 153–170). Hillsdale, NJ: Erlbaum.
Bruner, J. (1990). *Acts of meaning.* Cambridge, MA: Harvard University Press.
Bruner, J. (1986). *Actual minds, possible worlds.* Cambridge, MA: Harvard University Press.
Bunge, S. A., & Wright, S. B. (2007). Neurodevelopmental changes in working memory and cognitive control. *Current Opinion in Neurobiology, 17,* 243–250.
Campbell, J. (1988). The power of myth. New York: Doubleday.
Case, R. (1985). *Intellectual development: Birth to adulthood.* New York: Academic Press.
Case, R. (1992). *The mind's staircase: Exploring the conceptual underpinnings of children's thought and knowledge.* Hillsdale, NJ: Erlbaum.
Case, R. (1993). Theories of learning and theories of development. *Educational Psychologist, 28*(3), 219–233.
Case, R., & Griffin, S. (1990). Child cognitive development: The role of central conceptual structures in the development of scientific and social thought. *Developmental Psychology: Cognitive, perceptuo-motor, and neuropsychological Perspectives* (pp. 193–230). North Holland: Elsevier Science Publishers.
Case, R., Griffin, S., McKeough, A., & Okamoto, Y. (1992). Parallels in the development of children's social numerical, and spatial thought. In R. Case (Ed.), *The Mind's Staircase: Stages in the development of human intelligence* (pp. 269–284). Hillsdale, NJ: Erlbaum.
Case, R., & McKeough, A. (1990). Schooling and the development of central conceptual knowledge structures: An example from the domain of children's narrative. *International Journal of Education, 13*(8), 835–855.
Case, R., Marini, Z., McKeough, A., Dennis, S., & Goldberg, J. (1986). Horizontal structure in middle childhood: The emergence of dimensional operations. In S. Strauss and I. Levine (Eds.), *State and structure in children's development* (pp. 1–39). New York: Ablex.
Case, R., & Okamoto, Y. (1996). The role of central conceptual structures in the development of children's thought. *Monograph of the Society for Research in Child Development.*
Casey, B. J., Tottenham, N., Liston, C., & Durston, S. (2005). Imaging the developing brain: what have we learned about cognitive development? *Trends in Cognitive Sciences, 9,* 104–110.
Ciesielski, K. T., Lesnik, P. G., Savoy, R. L., Grant, E. P., & Ahlfors, S. P. (2006). Developmental neural networks in children performing a Categorical n-back task. *Neuroimage, 33,* 980–990.
Colom, R., Jung, R. E., & Haier, R. J. (2006). Distributed brain sites for the g-factor of intelligence. *Neuroimage, 31,* 1359–1365.
Culler, J. (1975). Structuralists Poetics: Structuralism, linguistics, and the study of literature. Ithaca, NY: Cornell University Press.

Desmurget, M., Bonnetblanc, F., & Duffau, H. (2007). Contrasting acute and slow-growing lesions: a new door to brain plasticity. *Brain, 130,* 898–914.
Dickinson, D. K., & Tabors, P. O. (Eds.) (2001). *Beginning literacy with language*. Baltimore, MD: Brooks.
Egan, K. (1989). *Teaching as storytelling: An alternative approach to teaching and curriculum in the elementary school*. Chicago, IL: University of Chicago Press.
Elston, G. N. (2003). Cortex, cognition and the cell: New insights into the pyramidal neuron and prefrontal function. *Cerebral Cortex, 13*(11), 1124–1138.
Feldman, C., Bruner, J., Kalmar, D., & Renderer, B. (1993). Plot, plight, and dramatism: Interpretation at three ages. *Human Development, 36*(6), 327–342.
Feldman, C., Bruner, J., Kalmar, D., & Renderer, B. (1994). Plot, plight, and dramatism: Interpretation at three ages. In W. F. Overton & D. S. Palermo (Eds.), The nature and ontogenesis of meaning (pp. 225–277). Hillsdale, NJ: Erlbaum.
Fivush, R., & Haden, C. A. (2003). *Autobiographical memory and the construction of a narrative self: Developmental and cultural perspectives*. Mahwah, NJ: Erlbaum.
Fivush, R., & Hudson, J. (Eds.). (1992). *Knowing and remembering in young children*. New York: Cambridge University Press.
Frangou, S., Chitins, X., & Williams, S. C. R. (2004). Mapping IQ and gray matter density in healthy young people. *Neuroimage, 3,* 800–805.
Gardner, H. (1985). *The mind's new science: A history of the cognitive revolution*. New York: Basic Books.
Gee, J. P. (1991). Memory and myth: A perspective on narrative. In A. McCabe, & C. Peterson, (Eds.), *Developing narrative structure* (pp. 1–26). Hillsdale, NJ: Erlbaum.
Genereux, R., & McKeough, A. (2007). Transformation in narrative thought during adolescence: The structure and content of narrative interpretation. *British Journal of Educational Psychology, 77* (3), 1–25.
Goldberg-Reitman, J. (1992). Young girl's conception of their mother's role: A neo-structural analysis. In R. Case (Ed.), *The mind's staircase: Stages in the development of human intelligence* (pp. 135–152). Hillsdale, NJ: Erlbaum.
Grady, C. L., & Keightley, M. L. (2002). Studies of altered social cognition in neuropsychiatric disorders using functional imaging. *Canadian Journal of Psychiatry, 47,* 327–336.
Griffin, S., & Case, R. (1995). Rethinking the primary school math curriculum: an approach based on cognitive science. *Issues in Education, 3,* 1–65.
Griffin, S., Case, R., & Siegler, R. (1994). Rightstart: Providing the central conceptual prerequisites for first formal learning of arithmetic to students at risk for school failure. In K. McGilly (Ed.), *Classroom lessons: Integrating cognitive theory and classroom practice* (pp. 25–49). Cambridge, MA: MIT/Bradford Books,
Habermas, T., & Bluck, S. (2000). Getting a life: The emergence of the life story in adolescence. *Psychological Bulletin, 126* (5), 748–769.
Haden, C. (2003). Joint encoding and joint reminiscing: Implications for young children's understanding and remembering of personal experiences. In R. Fivish & C. A. Haden, (Eds.). *Autobiographical memory and the construction of a narrative self: Developmental and cultural perspectives* (pp. 49–69). Mahwah, NJ: Erlbaum.
Heath, S. B. (1986). Taking a cross-cultural look at narrative. *Topics in Language Disorders, 7,* 84–94.
Hebb, D. O. (1949). *The organization of behavior*. New York: Wiley.
Hicks, D. (1994). Individual and social meanings in the classroom: Narrative discourse as a boundary phenomenon. *Journal of Narrative and Life History, 4*(3), 215–240.
Hudson, J. A., Gebelt, J., Haviland, J., & Bentivegna, C. (1992). Emotion and narrative structure in young children's personal accounts. *Journal of Narrative and Life History, 2*(2), 129–150.
Hutsler, J. J. (2003). The specialized structure of human language cortex: Pyramidal cell size asymmetries within auditory and language-associated regions of the temporal lobes. *Brain and Language, 86,* 226–242.

Jarvey, M., McKeough, A., & Pyryt, M. (2008). Teaching trickster tales. *Research in the Teaching of English, 42*(1), 42–73.
Jernigan, T. L., & Tallal, P. (1990). Late childhood changes in brain morphology observable with MRI. *Developmental Medicine and Child Neurology, 32,* 379–385.
Kelley, A. E., Baldo, B. A., Pratt, W. E., & Will, M. J. (2005). Corticostriatal-hypothalamic circuitry and food motivation: Integration of energy, action and reward. *Physiology and Behavior, 86,* 773–795.
Klingberg, T. (2006). Development of a superior frontal-intraparietal network for visuo-spatial working memory. *Neuropsychologia, 44,* 2171–2177.
Kucian, K., von Aster, M., Loenneker, T., Dietrich, T., Mast, F. W., & Martin, E. (2007). Brain activation during mental rotation in school children and adults. *Journal of Neural Transmission, 114,* 675–686.
Leichman, M. D., Wang, Q, & Pillemer. D. B. (2003). Cultural variations in interdependence and autobiographical memory: Lessons from Korea, China, India, and the United States. In R. Fivish, & C. A. Haden, (Eds.). *Autobiographical memory and the construction of a narrative self: Developmental and cultural perspectives* (pp. 73–97). Mahwah, NJ: Erlbaum.
Mall, V., Linder, M., Herpers, M., Schelle, A., Mendez-Mendez, J., Korinthenberg, R., et al. (2005). Recruitment of the sensorimotor cortex – A developmental fMRI study. *Neuropediatrics, 36,* 373–379.
Mandler, J. (1984). *Stories, scripts, and scenes: Aspects of story schema.* Hillsdale, NJ: Erlbaum.
Mar, R. A. (2004). The neuropsychology of narrative: Story comprehension, story production and their interrelation. *Neuropsychologia, 42,* 1414–1434.
Marini, Z., & Case, R. (1994). Development of abstract reasoning about the physical and social world. *Child Development, 65*(1), 147–159.
McAdams, D. P. (1993). *The stories we live by: Personal myths and the making of the self.* New York: William and Morrow.
McCabe, A. (1996). *Chameleon readers: Teaching children to appreciate all kinds of good stories.* New York, NY: McGraw Hill.
McCabe, A., Capron, E., & Peterson, C. (1991). The voice of experience: The recall of early childhood and adolescent memories by young adults. In A. McCabe and C. Peterson (Eds.), *Developing narrative structure* (pp. 137–173). Hillsdale, NJ: Erlbaum.
McCabe, A., & Peterson, C. (Eds.). (1991). *Developing narrative structure.* Hillsdale, NJ: Erlbaum.
McConaughy, S. H., Fitzhenry-Coor, I., & Howell, D. C. (1984). Developmental differences in schemata for story comprehension. In K. E. Nelson (Ed.), *Children's language* (Vol. 4, pp. 385–421). Hillsdale, NJ: Lawrence Erlbaum Associates.
McKeough, A. (1996). Changes in narrative knowledge across the school years: Evidence from typical and atypical populations. In A. Smorti (Ed.). *The self as text: Construction of stories and construction of the self* (pp. 275–307). Florence, IT: Giunti.
McKeough, A. (2000). Building on the oral tradition: How story composition and comprehension develop. In J. Astington (Ed.). *Minds in the making* (pp. 98–114). Cambridge, England: Blackwell.
McKeough, A. (1995). Teaching narrative knowledge for transfer in the early school years. In A. McKeough, J. Lupart, & A. Marini (Eds.), *Teaching for transfer: Fostering generalization in learning* (pp. 153–176). Hillsdale, NJ: Erlbaum.
McKeough A. (1992a). The structural foundations of children's narrative and its development. In R. Case (Ed.), *The mind's staircase: Stages in the development of human intelligence* (pp. 171–188). Hillsdale, NJ: Erlbaum.
McKeough A. (1992b). Testing for the presence of a central social structure: Use of the transfer paradigm. In R. Case (Ed.), *The mind's staircase: Exploring the conceptual underpinnings of children's thought and knowledge* (pp. 207–225). Hillsdale, NJ: Erlbaum.
McKeough, A. (1991). Neo-Piagetian theory goes to school: Program development and program delivery. *Exceptionality Education Canada, 1*(4), 1–16.

McKeough, A., Davis, L., Forgeron, N., Marini, A., & Fung, T. (2005). Improving story complexity and cohesion: A developmental approach to teaching story composition. *Narrative Inquiry, 15*(2), 96–125.
McKeough, A., & Genereux, R. (2003). Transformation in narrative thought during adolescence: The structure and content of story compositions. *Journal of Educational Psychology, 95*(3), 537–552.
McKeough, A., & Sanderson, A. (1996). Teaching storytelling: A microgenetic analysis of developing narrative competency. *Journal of Narrative and Life History, 6*(2), 157–192.
McKeough, A., Yates, T., & Marini, A. (1994). Intentional reasoning: A developmental study of behaviorally aggressive and normal boys. *Development and Psychopathology, 6,* 285–304.
Michaels, S. (1981). Sharing time: Children's narrative style and differential access to literacy. *Language in Society, 10,* 423–442.
Michaels, S. (1991). The dismantling of narrative. In A. McCabe & C. Peterson (Eds.), *Developing narrative structure* (pp. 303–351). Hillsdale, NJ: Erlbaum.
Miller, E. K., & Cohen, J. D. (2001). An integrative theory of prefrontal cortex dysfunction. *Annual Review of Neuroscience, 24,* 167–202.
Miller, P. J., Potts, R., Fung, H., Hoogstra, L., & Mintz, J. (1990). Narrative practices and the social construction of the self in childhood. *American Ethnologist, 17* (2), 292–311.
Miller, P. J., Wiley, A. R., Fung, H., & Liang, C. (1997). Personal storytelling as a medium of socialization in Chinese and American families. *Child Development, 68* (3), 557–568.
Mosenthal, W. (1995). *A textbook of neuroanatomy*. London: Taylor & Francis.
Neisser, U., & Fivush, R. (Eds.). (1994). *The remembering self: Construction and accuracy in the self narrative*. Cambridge, England: Cambridge University Press.
Nelson, K. (2003). Narrative and self, myth and memory: Emergence of the cultural self. In R. Fivish, & C. A. Haden, (Eds.). *Autobiographical memory and the construction of a narrative self: Developmental and cultural perspectives* (pp. 1–28). Mahwah, NJ: Erlbaum.
Nelson, K. (2000) The developmental psychology of language and thought. In M. Bennett (Ed.), *Developmental psychology: Achievements and prospects* (pp. 185–204). East Sussex, UK: Psychology Press.
Nelson, K. (1981). Social cognition in a script framework. In J. H. Flavell & L. Ross (Eds.), *Social cognitive development: Frontiers and possible futures* (pp. 97–118). Cambridge, England: Cambridge University Press.
Nicolopoulou, A. (1997). Children and narratives: Toward an interpretive and sociocultural approach. In M. Bamberg (Ed.), *Narrative development: Six approaches* (pp. 179–216). Hillsdale, NJ: Erlbaum.
Nippold, M. A., & Taylor, C. L. (1995). Idiom understanding in youth – Further examination of familiarity and transparency. *Journal of Speech and Hearing Research, 38,* 426–433.
Olson, D. R. (1990). Thinking about narrative. In B. K. Britton & A. D. Pellegrini (Eds.), *Narrative thought and narrative language* (pp. 99–111). Hillsdale, NJ: Erlbaum.
Palombo, J. (1991). Neurocognitive differences, self cohesion, and incoherent self narratives. *Child and Adolescent Social Work,* 8(6), 449–472.
Paus, T., Collins, D. L., Evans, A. C., Leonard, G., Pike, B., Zijdenbos, A. (2001). Maturation of white matter in the human brain: A review of magnetic resonance studies. *Brain Research Bulletin, 54*, 255–266.
Pelletier, J., & Astington, J. W. (2004). Action, consciousness and theory of mind: Children's ability to coordinate story characters' actions and thoughts. *Early Education and Development, 15* (1), 5–22.
Peterson, C., & McCabe, A. (1983). *Developmental psycholinguistics: Three ways of looking at a child's narrative*. New York: Plenum.
Pfefferbaum, A., Mathalon, D. H., Sullivan, E. V., Rawles, J. M., Zipursky, R. B., & Lim, K. O. (1994). A quantitative magnetic resonance imaging study of changes in brain morphology from infancy to late adulthood. *Archives of Neurology, 51,* 874–887.
Polkinghorne, D. E. (1988). *Narrative knowing and the human sciences*. Albany, NY: State University of New York Press.

Porath, M. (1992). Stage and structure in the development of children with various types of "Giftedness." In R. Case (Ed.), *The mind's staircase: Stages in the development of human intelligence* (pp. 303–317). Hillsdale, NJ: Erlbaum.
Posner, M. I., & Rothbart, M. K. (2004). Hebb's neural networks support the integration of psychological science. *Canadian Psychology, 45,* 265–278.
Pratt, M. W., Boyes, C., Robins, S., & Manchester, J. (1989). Telling tales: Working memory and the narrative cohesion of story retellings. *Developmental Psychology, 25*(4), 628–635.
Propp, V. (1968). *The morphology of the folktale.* Austin: University of Texas Press (Translated by L. Scott, 2nd edition. Revised by L. A. Wagner. Austin: University of Texas Press.)
Quartz, S. R., & Sejnowski, T. J. (1997). The neural basis of cognitive development: A constructivist manifesto. *Behavioral and Brain Sciences, 20,* 537–556.
Rivkin, M. J. (2000). Developmental neuroimaging of children using magnetic resonance techniques. *Mental Retardation and Developmental Disabilities Research, 6,* 68–80.
Romine, C. B., & Reynolds, C. R. (2005). A model of the development of frontal lobe functioning: Findings from a meta-analysis. *Applied Neuropsychology, 12,* 190–201.
Rubia, K., Smith, A. B., Woolley, J., Nosarti, C., Heyman, I., Taylor, E., et al. (2006). Progressive increase of frontostriatal brain activation from childhood to adulthood during event-related tasks of cognitive control. *Human Brain Mapping, 27,* 973–993.
Runyan, W. M. (1982). *Life histories and psychobiographies.* New York: Oxford University Press.
Sakai, K. L. (2005). Language acquisition and brain development. *Science, 310,* 815–819.
Sarbin, (1986). *Narrative psychology: The storied nature of human conduct.* New York: Praeger.
Satz, P. (1993). Brain reserve capacity on symptom onset after brain injury: A formulation and review of evidence for threshold theory. *Neuropsychology, 7,* 273–295.
Schaefer, R. (2004). Narrating, Attending, and Empathizing. *Literature and Medicine, 23*(2), 241–251.
Schaefer, R. (1981). Narration in psychoanalytic dialogue. In W. J. T. Mitchell (Ed.), *On narrative* (pp. 25–49). Chicago: The University of Chicago Press.
Scherf, K. S., Sweeney, J. A., & Luna, B. (2006). Brain basis of developmental change in visuospatial working memory. *Journal of Cognitive Neuroscience, 18* 1045–1058.
Scholes, R., & Kellogg, R. (1966). *The nature of narrative.* London: Oxford University Press.
Shaw, P., Greenstein, D., Lerch, J., Clasen, L., Lenroot, R., Gogtay, N., et al. (2006). Intellectual ability and cortical development in children and adolescents. *Nature, 440,* 676–679.
Sowell, E. R., Thompson, P. M., & Toga, A. W. (2004). Mapping changes in the human cortex throughout the span of life. *The Neuroscientist, 10,* 372–392.
Sowell, E. R., Thompson, P. M., Leonard, C. M., Welcome, S. E., Kan, E., & Toga, A. W. (2004). Longitudinal mapping of cortical thickness and brain growth in normal children. *Journal of Neuroscience, 24,* 8223–8231.
Sowell, E. R., Thompson, P. M., Rex, D., Kornsand, D., Tessner, K. D., Jernigan, T. L. , et al. (2002). Mapping sulcal pattern asymmetry and local cortical surface gray matter distribution in vivo: Maturation in perisylvian cortices. *Cerebral Cortex, 12,* 17–26.
Sowell, E. R., Mattson, S. N., Thompson, P. M., Jernigan, T. L., Riley, E. P., & Toga, A. W. (2001). Mapping callosal morphology and cognitive correlates – Effects of heavy prenatal alcohol exposure. *Neurology, 57,* 235–244.
Spence, D. P. (1982). *Narrative truth and historical truth: Meaning and Interpretation in psychoanalysis.* New York: W. W. Norton.
Spencer, M. D., Moorhead, T. W. J., Lymer, G. K. S., Job, D. E., Muir, W. J., Hoare, P., et al. (2006). Structural correlates of intellectual impairment and autistic features in adolescents. *Neuroimage, 33,* 1136–1144.
Steen, R. G., Ogg, R. J., Reddick, W. B., & Kingsley, P. B. (1997). Age related changes in the pediatric brain: Quantitative MR evidence of maturational changes during adolescence. *American Journal of Neuroradiology, 18,* 819–828.
Stein, N. L. (1988). The development of children's storytelling skill. In M. B. Franklin & S. S. Barten (Eds.), *Child language: A reader* (282–299). New York: Oxford University Press.

Stephan, K. E., Fink, G. R., & Marshall, J. C. (2007). Mechanisms of hemispheric specialization: Insights from analyses of connectivity. *Neuropsychologia, 45* 209–228.

Sun, L. (1998). The loss of narrative innocence: The development of narrative consciousness from child to adolescent. *Narrative Inquiry, 8(1),* 203–212.

Sutton-Smith, B. (1986). Children's fiction making. In T. R. Sarbin (Ed.), *Narrative psychology: The storied nature of human conduct* (pp. 67–90). New York: Praeger.

Tappan, M., & Packer, M. (Eds.). (1991). Narrative and storytelling: Implications for understanding moral development. *New Directions for Child Development, 54.*

Thoma, P., & Daum, I. (2006). Neurocognitive mechanisms of figurative language processing – Evidence from clinical dysfunctions. *Neuroscience and Biobehavioral Reviews, 30,* 1182–1205.

Toga, A. W., Thompson, P. M., & Sowell, E. R. (2006). Mapping brain maturation. *Trends in Neurosciences, 29,* 148–159.

van Leeuwen, M., van den Berg, S. M., Hoekstra, R. A., & Boomsma, D. I. (2007). Endophenotypes for intelligence in children and adolescents. *Intelligence, 35,* 369–380.

Volpe, J. J. (1995). *Neurology of the newborn.* Philadelphia: WB Saunders.

Yussen, S. R., & Ozcan, N. M. (1996). The development of knowledge about narratives. Issues in Education, 2, 1–68.

Disentangling the Complexity of Social Giftedness: Mind, Brain, Development, and Education

Marion Porath

This chapter explores the relationships between giftedness in the social domain, neuropsychological research, and education. The pattern of development of gifted children is complex, requiring an equally complex educational match. Neuropsychological research has identified links between distinctive activity in certain regions of the brain and intellectual giftedness that suggest neurocognitive underpinnings to advanced intellectual development and its attendant complexity of thought. Work on the nature of the "social brain" has implications for understanding advanced social intelligence. This research is explored in relationship to work on social intelligence conducted within Case's neo-Piagetian perspective.

As an educational psychologist with an interest in different forms of giftedness, my perspective in this chapter is one of exploration of how the social mind and brain may interact in development and what implications this interaction may have for education. These implications are explored largely through general recommendations and guiding questions since work on development and education of socially gifted learners is in its infancy. The relationship between education and the developing brain is part of the current zeitgeist in education, including education of gifted learners (e.g., Sousa, 2003), and individual differences in brain functioning have been identified as crucial to our understanding of a variety of talents (O'Boyle, 2000). This chapter puts Robbie Case's significant work in mapping development, work supported by neurobiological studies, at the conceptual center (Case, 1992a, 1998) of this exploration of what characterizes and underpins social giftedness.

Intellectual Giftedness

To set the stage for an exploration of social giftedness, the chapter begins with background on intellectual giftedness from the psychometric and neo-Piagetian perspectives. The neurocognitive underpinnings relevant to both perspectives on

---

M. Porath (✉)
The University of British Columbia, Vancouver, BC, Canada
e-mail: marion.porath@ubc.ca

M. Ferrari, L. Vuletic (eds.), *The Developmental Relations among Mind, Brain and Education*, DOI 10.1007/978-90-481-3666-7_10,

intellectual giftedness are described to inform the subsequent discussion of social giftedness.

The Psychometric Perspective

The study of giftedness has traditionally taken a psychometric perspective, focusing on individuals with high IQs. Similarly, the focus of neuropsychological research on individuals defined as gifted has been on relationships between the brain and IQ or between the brain and academic abilities strongly related to IQ (e.g., Scholastic Aptitude Test [SAT] scores or extraordinary mathematical ability). In summary, we know that intellectually gifted individuals demonstrate unusual reliance on the right hemisphere (RH) during information processing (O'Boyle, 2000), including during the performance of linguistic tasks which usually involve the left hemisphere (LH) (Alexander, O'Boyle, & Benbow, 1996; O'Boyle, Benbow, & Alexander, 1995). They also demonstrate superior and rapid elementary cognitive processing, the neurological underpinnings of which are less elevated alpha rhythms than average, implying increased brain activation (Alexander et al.; Jaušovec, 2000). Enhanced frontal lobe activity (Alexander et al.; O'Boyle, Benbow, & Alexander) and enhanced hemispheric coordination during high-level thinking (Alexander et al.; Jaušovec; O'Boyle) are also characteristics of highly intelligent individuals, as is greater cerebral plasticity (Jambaqué, 2004; Shaw et al., 2006)

Shaw et al.'s (2006) recent findings elaborate on the maturational pattern of development of the prefrontal cortex in relation to IQ. Intellectually gifted children have a "particularly plastic cortex" (Shaw et al., p. 676), in the sense that it is relatively thinner than that of children of high and average intelligence at about age 7, followed by a significant increase in cortical thickness at about age 11, as opposed to either a steady decline or a short increase, which peaked at about 7–8 years of age in children of average intelligence. In early adolescence, superior intelligence is associated with a more rapid rate and greater amount of cortical thinning as compared to the steady pattern of decline among those of high and average intelligence, possibly due to streamlined neural pruning (Asher, 2006; Giles, 2006; Shaw et al.) that results in specialization of abilities in adolescence. The longer phase of prefrontal cortical growth suggests an "extended 'critical' period for high-level cognitive cortical circuits" (Shaw et al., p. 678). Adolescents of superior intelligence thus have a "longer developmental window" (Asher) for the development of circuitry for high-level thinking.

The Neo-Piagetian Perspective

Work with intellectually gifted children framed within neo-Piagetian theory has focused on their conceptual understanding as described by structures of thought that develop in complexity in a hierarchical fashion. In logical–mathematical, narrative, and spatial–artistic domains, gifted children demonstrate levels of conceptual understanding that are approximately 2 years ahead of children of average ability, advancement that is less dramatic than that evident in their abilities tapped by intelligence and achievement tests. Their conceptual understanding is relatively constrained by working memory capacity and processing speed, both of which are heavily influenced by maturation (Case, 1992c). Case (1985, 1992c, 1995) proposed that working memory capacity was controlled by epigenetic factors and suggested mylenization – the thickening of the insulating layer of cells that surrounds axons and facilitates efficient transmission of impulses – as an explanatory variable for the increased speed of processing and amount of information processed and stored in working memory that occurs with maturation. These epigenetic factors vary little with IQ (Porath, 1992). Level of development is, thus, an index of "the endogenous growth of maturationally driven mental-attention mechanisms" (Pascual-Leone, 2000, p. 843), supporting the hypothesis that it is not stage advancement that is characteristic of giftedness but, rather, what is done with the available level of thought (Fischer & Pipp, 1984; Porath, 2006). Speed and amount of learning and the resultant elaboration and complexity within a level – the rich variation in the "constructive web" of development (Fischer & Bidell, 2006, p. 319) – account for individual differences (Case, 1992b; Fischer & Canfield, 1986; Porath, 1992).

Interrelating the Psychometric and Neo-Piagetian Perspectives to Explain Intellectual Giftedness

The extended critical period for cognitive development and superior cortical plasticity in children with superior IQs (Shaw et al., 2006) may account for the findings in neo-Piagetian studies of giftedness where greater facility with the conceptual schemas available to them has been suggested as characteristic of gifted development. At the same time, abilities that are considerably more advanced than those explained by a central conceptual structure – previously characterized as orthogonal to abilities with a conceptual base (Porath, 1992; Marini & Case, 1994) – may interact with conceptual understanding in complex ways (Case, 1996; Porath, 2006). Gifted children's application of conceptual understanding is markedly more complex and flexible than that of children of average ability (Porath, 2006). They appear to consolidate central conceptual structures associated with a particular stage of development quickly, allowing them to work flexibly with these structures and use advanced domain-specific knowledge and skills to create intricate elaborations on core understanding.

Case and Okamoto (1996) proposed a hierarchical feedback loop in which associative and conceptual learning "feed" on each other that may explain the mechanism that allows gifted children to accomplish the complex interaction described above. In this feedback loop, learning is "mediated by general understanding (which in turn is 'fed' by insights acquired in high-exposure situations)" (Case & Okamoto, p. 21). Gifted children appear to create their own high-exposure situations, in that their associative learning is rapid and extensive. They can, therefore, "feed" conceptual understanding in ways that result in complex central conceptual structures. These structures may be constrained to an extent by maturation but the feedback loop appears to show the kind of plasticity suggested by Shaw et al. (2006). The loop is iterative, such that "general conceptual benefits obtained in high-exposure situations should be 'passed on' to low-exposure situations via the mediation of the general structure" (Case, 1996, p. 160), thus further explaining the rapid and extensive learning of gifted individuals. Enhanced neural interactivity (Jambaqué, 2004; O'Boyle et al., 1995) also may contribute to complex integration of specific knowledge and conceptual understanding. Similarly, enhanced synaptogenesis – the formation of synapses across which information flows between neurons – is suggested by O'Boyle (2000) as a possible indicator of a "gifted brain." This enhancement may be part of the suggested superior hemispheric interaction underlying gifted performance.

As suggested by Shaw et al. (2006), "gifted brains" are better defined by their unique pattern of development rather than "more is better" or "faster is better" analogies. Some neurological differences may underpin advanced intellectual competencies while others (e.g., hemispheric dominance and/or coordination and integration of diverse cognitive functions) may be related to the richness of conceptual understanding demonstrated by gifted children on neo-Piagetian tasks tapping central conceptual structures (cf. O'Boyle et al., 1995). An additional possibility, however, is that these differences, primarily studied in early and middle childhood, may contribute to a greater degree of advancement in conceptual understanding in adolescence, the cumulative result of rich organization and/or flexible utilization of the brain's resources – perhaps in combination with the cortical thinning that results in earlier than average specialization. This hypothesis remains to be tested in studies of level and type of central conceptual thinking across domains among gifted adolescents.

Social Giftedness

Social intelligence has been of interest for over a century, at least since Baldwin (1898) studied the development of the social self and articulated the role of understanding the mind of the other in the development of social understanding (Müller & Runions, 2003). Piaget, too, despite being portrayed as neglecting social intelligence, was critically aware of its importance (Piaget, 1977/1995 [Sociological Studies]; DeVries, 1997; Suizzo, 2000). He emphasized the collective *and* individual nature of logical thought; in order to construct logical structures, one must be a "socialized person" (Piaget, 1965/1995, p. 154). However, little attention has been paid to those with high levels of social intelligence (Porath, 2000). It is only relatively recently that the importance of recognizing and supporting socially gifted individuals who demonstrate exceptional ability to ascertain and respond to others' thoughts, feelings, and intentions (Gardner, 1983) has been recognized (e.g., Bruner, 1996; Caprara, Barbaranelli, Pastorelli, Bandura, & Zimbardo, 2000).

There may be a unique neuropsychological foundation for social giftedness, as suggested by Gardner (1983) whose arguments for multiple separate intelligences based on neuropsychological evidence included interpersonal, or social, intelligence.

Implications of Neuroscience for Understanding Social Intelligence

Neural substrate of the "social brain" include the PFC (prefrontal cortex), amygdala, premotor cortex, orbito-frontal cortex, insular regions of the cortex, and superior temporal gyrus (Bar-On, Tranel, Denburg, Bechara, 2003; Baron-Cohen et al., 1999; Gallese, 2005). Baron-Cohen et al.'s work confirmed the modularity of social intelligence in an fMRI study of normal subjects and patients with high-functioning autism or Asperger syndrome. Their results support the extraction of socially relevant (i.e., mental state/emotional) information from visual stimuli and attribution of mental states as aspects of social intelligence linked to specific neural bases. Bar-On et al.'s work on the neurological substrate of emotional and social intelligence adds somatic state (emotional signaling) activation and personal judgment in decision making (behaving intelligently) to our understanding of what it means to demonstrate social intelligence. Bar-On et al. argue that "the complex cognitive processes that subserve social competence ... do not draw upon neural processes specialized for social information. Rather, these processes depend on known brain mechanisms related to emotion and decision making" (p. 1798).

Gallese's (2005) work on the neural underpinnings of intersubjectivity – "how people come to know what others have in mind and how they adjust accordingly" (Bruner, 1996, p. 161) – supports the involvement of the premotor cortex, the insula, and the amygdala in "S-identity" (p. 181), or the capacity to have meaningful relationships with others. While speculative, this involvement may involve mirror neurons, premotor neurons believed to fire when we act and when we observe others act (mirroring their actions), in action representations, and a similar "resonance mechanism" (p. 194) for emotions. Gallese introduced a conceptual tool, the *shared manifold of intersubjectivity*, as a way of integrating different levels of description of intersubjectivity – the phenomenological, or sense of similarity to others in our social communities (also defined as the empathic level); the functional, or "as if" modes of interaction (p. 195) that allow us to create models of self and other; and the subpersonal, or neuronal activity level. The shared manifold of intersubjectivity "enables and bootstraps mutual intelligibility" (p. 197). Gallese's shared manifold hypothesis is similar in some ways to Case's hierarchical feedback loop and the constructs and neurological mechanisms suggested as underlying intersubjectivity may be helpful in understanding social intelligence, as will be discussed later.

Social Giftedness and Neo-Piagetian Theory

Studies on social cognition within Case's theoretical perspective have emphasized the unique nature of understanding our social worlds (see Case, 1992a).

These studies identify a progression from understanding one's social world in terms of actions in early childhood, through increasingly sophisticated understanding of others' intentions in middle childhood, to taking an interpretive stance on the social–psychological world in adolescence (McKeough, 1992; McKeough & Genereux, 2003; Porath, 2003).

Social cognition is distinct from other domains of thought. It does, however, develop in ways similar to other domains. That is, the same general structure is apparent in the ways different domains of thinking are organized and the same hierarchical sequence is evident in the way aspects of making meaning in each domain build on one another, grow, and change over time (Case & Okamoto, 1996). Maturation both constrains and potentiates development across domains via growth of working memory capacity and patterns of EEG coherence (Case, 1992a, 1992c; Case & Okamoto). In Gallese's (2005) terms, the neo-Piagetian studies just described have concentrated on the phenomenological and functional levels of intersubjectivity. While they do not address candidates for a neuronal level of activity, the body of work is supportive of a brain–mind connection (Gibson, 2005) and the same sort of bootstrapping suggested by Gallese. Social learning and experiences are mediated by a central social structure which, in turn, is "fed" by specific social learning, which may, at least in part, be supported by the basic neuronal processes suggested by Gallese.

The Gifted Social Brain: Interrelated Explanatory Perspectives

In its gifted form, intersubjectivity, or interpersonal intelligence, is the ability "to read the intentions and desires – even when these have been hidden – of many other individuals and, potentially, to act upon this knowledge. . ." (Gardner, 1983, p. 239). Similar to the work on intellectual giftedness, studies on children who are considered gifted in the social domain demonstrate central conceptual structural abilities that are relatively constrained by maturation [understandings that are approximately 2 years in advance of their age peers, or one substage of development, as defined by Case (1985, 1992a)]. At the same time, they demonstrate other social abilities that are considerably more advanced, such as social skills, the language to talk about their social and emotional worlds, and the ability to decode subtle emotional cues (Porath, 2000, 2003). These abilities appear to result in rich and complex social conceptual understanding, such as was described for intellectual giftedness.

Developmental Implications

Currently, our knowledge of the social brain allows only speculation as to what may underlie the development of exceptional social ability. The following are suggested directions for thought and research:

- Articulate a social feedback loop following Case's (1996) mathematical modeling of the dynamic interplay between conceptual and associative learning, perhaps through constructs analogous to Gallese's (2005) shared manifold hypothesis.
- Investigate resonance mechanisms that may be implicated in social intelligence (Gallese, 2005). Gallese suggests that a whole range of resonance mechanisms may be at work in the brain. Building on our knowledge of the intellectual brain, might these show different developmental trajectories in socially gifted individuals? Perhaps socially gifted individuals have more well-developed resonance mechanisms and/or more interplay among resonance mechanisms.
- Investigate the degree to which neurological growth patterns and interactions differ in socially gifted individuals.
- Consider the interaction between general intelligence and social intelligence. In so doing, Anderson's (2005) discussion of the role of the PFC in novel task performance and Sousa's (2003) suggestion that earlier frontal lobe maturation in intellectually gifted students may be associated with earlier maturation of the limbic area which "generates, interprets, and stores emotional messages" (p. 52) may be important to consider.

Educational Implications

Much of the work on neuropsychology emphasizes the important role of the environment in the development of mind and brain. Jambaqué (2004) cites the influence of early, intense practice on the developing brains of musicians, and Alexander et al. (1996) and Fischer and Bidell (2006) note the necessity of a model that incorporates both biological and environmental factors. We must emphasize the mind and brain in interaction with environmental influences (Geake & Cooper, 2003). Barab and Plucker (2002) note that we need to move away from conceptions of giftedness that are in the heads of smart people (i.e., conceptions that concentrate on those who already demonstrate giftedness) and pay considerably more attention to "smart contexts." In essence, educational environments rich in opportunities to engage in social and emotional reasoning – smart contexts – may allow social giftedness to emerge.

We do not yet have a credible map of how environmental factors contribute to neurological developmental trajectories [cf. Shaw et al.'s (2006) notion of a critical period in the development of high-level cognitive cortical circuits], nor do we know how developmental trajectories play out across the lifespan. Byrnes (2001, p. 174) raises a number of other important questions that we should consider as we continue to probe the mind, brain, and education interplay, such as the meaning of readiness to learn, how information is represented as a neural assembly, and the probabilistic nature of links between mind and brain. However, we should not let the lack of a credible map delay our efforts to support the development of highly developed social cognition. Smart contexts for social development (cf. Collaborative for Academic, Social, and Emotional Learning, 2004) may, in fact, shape the social brain (cf. Doidge, 2007). We do, however, need to inform these efforts with coherent theoretical frameworks and systematically evaluate them (Eccles & Templeton, 2002; Farrell, Meyer, Kung, & Sullivan, 2001).

What we do know, and have evidence for, is that Case's model, a model compatible with brain development (Gibson, 2005), offers a strong link between development of mind, brain, and education. With the "design for development" (McKeough, Okamoto, & Porath, 2002) that Case's (1992a) theory affords, children can be assessed and then helped to consolidate their current understandings. Because Case and his colleagues have articulated the developmental sequence of conceptual understandings in a variety of domains, we have a blueprint for scaffolding children to the next level of development. This scaffolding, or bridging, also can be viewed as a transition from novice to expert understanding (Bereiter & Scardamalia, 1986). Essentially, the conceptual bridging approach is based on the nature of expertise at different stages and substages of development because of its spotlight on the *central conceptual understandings* in a domain. Experts have the sort of organized knowledge structures articulated by Case (1992a).

Research with preschoolers considered socially gifted informed an intervention that successfully helped other children develop more sophisticated social understanding through development and consolidation of central social understanding and expansion of "psychological vocabulary" (Porath, 2003, 2009). Socially gifted youngsters have complex central social understanding, exceptional social skills, and strong abilities to initiate and respond to social interactions. We can continue to learn from their expertise and their responses to their social environments to refine educational approaches for them and for all children.

Instructional approaches based on expertise lead to better developmental outcomes (Bransford, Brown, & Cocking, 2000; Meichenbaum & Biemiller, 1998). If skills alone are the instructional objective, we create more proficient novices (Bereiter & Scardamalia, 1986) rather than experts who understand at a meaningful, conceptual level. These guidelines are equally applicable to learners of all ability levels. The hierarchical feedback loop articulated by Case and Okamoto (1996) provides a model for an integrated approach to instruction that marries skills and conceptual understanding in a meaningful way. Research on the conceptual bridging approach to instruction shows positive effects (Griffin & Case, 1996; Griffin, Case, & Siegler, 1994; McKeough & Sanderson, 1996; Porath, 2009 and the potential to bootstrap meaningful social thought in the ways suggested by both Case and Okamoto and Gallese (2005). This approach can be used with socially gifted children (and children gifted in other domains) who need educational opportunities equivalent in complexity to their thinking. For gifted learners, the conceptual bridging approach can be enriched to allow for and encourage flexibility and elaboration in the use of central social structural elements (e.g., coordination of actions and intentions, coordination of multiple interpretations of behaviors). For example, children could be encouraged to elaborate on descriptions and explanations of their social worlds by incorporating multiple characters and/or settings, integrating these explanations in coherent ways, and building their repertoires of language to describe mental states. They could then be challenged to apply these abilities in exploration of other social worlds (e.g., the world of work) and social–cultural traditions.

Conclusion

Geake and Cooper (2003) raise a key question in thinking about the application of neuroscience to education: "What are the educational practices most conducive to the promotion of optimum social, cognitive, affective, and moral development of children and young people in ways that prepare them for active participation in post-industrial societies?" (p. 11). Geake and Cooper urge that we proceed with caution in thinking about how neuroscience may inform education, warning against a strictly neurological approach to making educational decisions. Similarly, Fischer and Daley (2007) argue for a reciprocal relationship between development, neuroscience, and education in which each field informs and learns from each other. Teachers should be involved in influencing the direction of cognitive neuroscientific research (Geake & Cooper), a suggestion that would have been applauded by Robbie Case whose work so admirably built on the real world of children and classrooms.

This chapter suggests that research on social giftedness be multifaceted, taking into account the interactions between mind, brain, development, and education. Case's neo-Piagetian perspective on the developing social mind provides a solid foundation from which to explore connections with neurocognitive research such as the developmental trajectories of brain growth in socially gifted individuals, neuronal mechanisms that underpin highly developed intersubjectivity, and the potential roles of general intelligence and its neurocognitive underpinnings in social giftedness. Mind, brain, and development must be considered in relationship to educational and personal contexts that may shape the brain and social behavior. Research must also be multifaceted in the inclusion of multiple points of view on social development, including teachers, parents, researchers, and children themselves.

References

Alexander, J. E., O'Boyle, M. W., & Benbow, C. P. (1996). Developmentally advanced EEG alpha power in gifted male and female adolescents. *International Journal of Psychophysiology, 23*, 25–31.

Anderson, M. (2005). Cortex forum on the concept of general intelligence in neuropsychology. *Cortex, 41*, 99–100.

Asher, J. (2006). *Cortex matures faster in youth with highest IQ*. National institute of mental health press release. Retrieved April 25, 2006 from http://www.nimh.nih.gov/press/youtcortexiq.cfm

Baldwin, J. M. (1898). *The story of the mind. Electronic reproduction*. Washington, DC: American Psychological Association. Retrieved from http://search.ebscohost.com/direct.asp?db=pzh&jid=%22200622795%22&scope=site

Barab, S. A., & Plucker, J. A. (2002). Smart people or smart contexts? Cognition, ability, and talent development in an age of situated approaches to knowing and learning. *Educational Psychologist, 37*, 165–182.

Bar-On, R., Tranel, D., Denburg, N. L., & Bechara, A. (2003). Exploring the neurological substrate of emotional and social intelligence. *Brain, 126*, 1790–1800.

Baron-Cohen, S., Ring, H. A., Wheelwright, S., Bullmore, E. T., Brammer, M. J., Simmons, A., et al. (1999). Social intelligence in the normal and autistic brain: An fMRI study. *European Journal of Neuroscience, 11*, 1891–1898.

Bereiter, C., & Scardamalia, M. (1986). Educational relevance of the study of expertise. *Interchange, 17*(2), 10–19.

Bransford, J. D., Brown, A. L., & Cocking, R. R. (Eds.) (2000). *How people learn: Brain, mind, experience, and school*. Expanded edition. Washington, DC: National Academy Press.
Bruner, J. (1996). *The culture of education*. Cambridge, MA: Harvard University Press.
Byrnes, J. P. (2001). *Minds, brains, and learning: Understanding the psychological and educational relevance of neuroscientific research*. New York: Guilford.
Caprara, G. V., Barbaranelli, C., Pastorelli, C., Bandura, A., & Zimbardo, P. G. (2000). Prosocial foundations of children's academic achievement. *Psychological Science, 11*, 302–306.
Case, R. (1985). *Intellectual development birth to adulthood*. New York: Academic Press.
Case, R. (1992a). *The mind's staircase: Exploring the conceptual underpinnings of children's thought and knowledge*. Hillsdale, NJ: Lawrence Erlbaum.
Case, R. (1992b). Neo-Piagetian theories of intellectual development. In H. Beilin & P. Pufall (Eds.), *Piaget's theory: Prospects and possibilities* (pp. 61–104). Hillsdale, NJ: Erlbaum.
Case, R. (1992c). The role of the frontal lobes in the regulation of cognitive development. *Brain and Cognition, 20*, 51–73.
Case, R. (1995). Capacity-based explanations of working memory growth: A brief history and reevaluation. In F. E. Weinert & W. Schneider (Eds.), *Memory performance and competencies: Issues in growth and development* (pp. 23–44). Hillsdale, NJ: Erlbaum.
Case, R. (1996). Modeling the dynamic interplay between general and specific change in children's conceptual understanding. In R. Case & Y. Okamoto (Eds.), The role of central conceptual structures in the development of children's thought. *Monographs of the Society for Research in Child Development, 61*(1–2, Serial No. 246) (pp. 156–188). Chicago: The University of Chicago Press.
Case, R. (1998). The development of conceptual structures. In W. Damon (Series Ed.) & D. Kuhn & R. S. Siegler (Vol. Eds.), *Handbook of child psychology: Vol. 2. Cognition, perception, and language* (5th ed., pp. 745–800). New York: John Wiley.
Case, R., & Okamoto, Y. (1996). The role of central conceptual structures in the development of children's thought. *Monographs of the Society for Research in Child Development, 61*(1–2, Serial No. 246).
Collaborative for Academic, Social, and Emotional Learning (2004). *CASEL The first ten years 1994–2004. Building a foundation for the future*. University of Illinois at Chicago.
DeVries, R. (1997). Piaget's social theory. *Educational Researcher, 26* (2), 4–17.
Doidge, N. (2007). *The brain that changes itself*. New York: Penguin.
Eccles, J. S., & Templeton, J. (2002). Extracurricular and other after-school activities for youth. In W. G. Secada (Ed.), *Review of Research in Education, 26*, 113–180.Washington, DC: AERA.
Farrell, A. D., Meyer, A. L., Kung, E. M., & Sullivan, T. N. (2001). Development and evaluation of school-based violence prevention programs. *Journal of Clinical Child Psychology, 30*, 207–220.
Fischer, K. W., & Bidell, T. R. (2006). Dynamic development of action and thought. In W. Damon & R. Lerner (Series Ed.) & R. M. Lerner (Vol. Ed.), *Handbook of child psychology: Vol 1.Theoretical models of human development* (6th ed., pp. 313–399). Hoboken, NJ: Wiley.
Fischer, K. W., & Canfield, R. L. (1986). The ambiguity of stage and structure of behavior: Person and environment in the development of psychological structure. In I. Levin (Ed.), *Stage and structure: Reopening the debate* (pp. 246–267). Norwood, NJ: Ablex.
Fischer, K. W., & Daley, S. G. (2007). Connecting cognitive science and neuroscience to education: Potentials and pitfalls in inferring executive processes. In L. Meltzer (Ed.), *Executive function in education: From theory to practice* (pp. 55–72). New York: Guilford.
Fischer, K. W., & Pipp, S. L. (1984). Processes of cognitive development: Optimal level and skill acquisition. In R. J. Sternberg (Ed.), *Mechanisms of cognitive development* (pp. 45–80). New York: W. H. Freeman.
Gallese, V. (2005). From mirror neurons to the shared manifold hypothesis: A neurophysiological account of intersubjectivity. In S. T. Parker, J. Langer, & C. Milbrath (Eds.), *Biology and knowledge revisited: From neurogenesis to psychogenesis* (pp. 179–203). Mahwah, NJ: Lawrence Erlbaum.
Gardner, H. (1983). *Frames of mind. The theory of multiple intelligences*. New York: Basic Books.

Geake, J., & Cooper, P. (2003). Cognitive neuroscience: Implications for education? *Westminster Studies in Education, 26*, 7–20.

Gibson, K. R. (2005). Human brain evolution: Developmental perspectives. In S. T. Parker, J. Langer, & C. Milbrath (Eds.), *Biology and knowledge revisited: From neurogenesis to psychogenesis* (pp. 123–143). Mahwah, NJ: Lawrence Erlbaum.

Giles, J. (2006). Scans suggest IQ scores reflect brain structure. *Nature, 440*, 588–589.

Griffin, S., & Case, R. (1996). Evaluating the breadth and depth of training effects when central conceptual structures are taught. In R. Case & Y. Okamoto (Eds.), The role of central conceptual structures in the development of children's thought. *Monographs of the Society for Research in Child Development, 61*(1–2, Serial No. 246), pp. 83–102. Chicago: The University of Chicago Press.

Griffin, S., Case, R., & Siegler, R. (1994). Rightstart: Providing the central conceptual prerequisites for first formal learning of arithmetic to students at risk for failure. In K. McGilly (Ed.), *Classroom lessons: Integrating cognitive theory and classroom practice*. Cambridge, MA: MIT Press.

Jambaqué, I. (2004). Contribution of developmental neuropsychology to the study of gifted individuals. *Psychologie Française, 49*, 267–276.

Jaušovec, N. (2000). Differences in cognitive processes between gifted, intelligent, creative, and average individuals while solving complex problems: An EEG study. *Intelligence, 28*, 213–237.

Marini, Z., & Case, R. (1994). The development of abstract reasoning about the physical and social world. *Child Development, 65*, 147–159.

McKeough, A. (1992). A neo-structural analysis of children's narrative and its development. In R. Case (Ed.), *The mind's staircase: Exploring the conceptual underpinnings of children's thought and knowledge* (pp. 171–188). Hillsdale, NJ: Lawrence Erlbaum.

McKeough, A., & Genereux, R. (2003). Transformation in narrative thought during adolescence: The structure and content of story compositions. *Journal of Educational Psychology, 95*, 537–552.

McKeough, A., Okamoto, Y., & Porath, M. (2002, April). *A design for development: The legacy of Robbie Case*. New Orleans, LA: Paper presented at the American Educational Research Association.

McKeough, A., & Sanderson, A. (1996). Teaching storytelling: A microgenetic analysis of developing narrative competency. *Journal of Narrative and Life History, 6*, 157–192.

Meichenbaum, D., & Biemiller, A. (1998). *Nurturing independent learners. Helping students take charge of their learning*. Cambridge, MA: Brookline Books.

Müller, U., & Runions, K. (2003). The origins of understanding self and other: James Mark Baldwin's theory. *Developmental Review, 23*, 29–54.

O'Boyle, M. W. (2000). A new millennium in cognitive neuropsychology research: The era of individual differences? *Brain and Cognition, 42*, 135–138.

O'Boyle, M. W., Benbow, C. P., & Alexander, J. E. (1995). Sex differences, hemispheric laterality, and associated brain activity in the intellectually gifted. *Developmental Neuropsychology, 11*, 415–443.

Pascual-Leone, J. (2000). Is the French connection neo-Piagetian? Not nearly enough! *Child Development, 71*, 843–845.

Piaget, J. (1965/1995). Logical operations and social life. In L. Smith (Ed.), *Sociological studies* (pp. 134–157). New York: Routledge.

Piaget, J. (1995) *Sociological studies*. London, UK: Routledge (L. Smith, chief trans. ed.). (Original work published 1933/1977)

Porath, M. (1992). Stage and structure in the development of children with various types of "giftedness". In R. Case (Ed.), *The mind's staircase: Exploring the conceptual underpinnings of children's thought and knowledge* (pp. 303–317). Hillsdale, NJ: Lawrence Erlbaum.

Porath, M. (2000). Social giftedness in childhood: A developmental perspective. In R. C. Friedman & B. M. Shore (Eds.), *Talents unfolding: Cognitive and developmental frameworks*, pp. 195–215. Washington, DC: American Psychological Association.

Porath, M. (2003). Social understanding in the first years of school. *Early Childhood Research Quarterly*, *18*(4), 468–484.
Porath, M. (2006). The conceptual underpinnings of giftedness: Developmental and educational implications. *High Ability Studies*, *17*, 145–158.
Porath, M. (2009). Fostering social expertise in early childhood. *Early Child Development and Care*, *179*, 93–106.
Shaw, P., Greenstein, D., Lerch, J., Clasen, L., Lenroot, R., Gogtay, N., et al. (2006). Intellectual ability and cortical development in children and adolescents. *Nature*, *440*, 676–679.
Sousa, D. A. (2003). *How the gifted brain learns*. Thousand Oaks, CA: Corwin Press.
Suizzo, M-A. (2000). The social-emotional and cultural context of cognitive development: Neo-Piagetian perspectives. *Child Development*, *71*, 846–849.

Mind, Brain, and Education in Socioeconomic Context

Martha J. Farah

Introduction

Ten years ago, when I was just becoming interested in the relation between child development and socioeconomic status, I attended a small workshop sponsored by the McDonnell Foundation to discuss new directions in developmental cognitive neuroscience. At the time I knew virtually nothing about development *or* SES but, since the meeting was so small and informal, I decided to present some ideas on the topic of "cognitive developmental neuro-sociology" for the sake of getting feedback from the experts present. Although everyone gave me a good-natured hearing, one person took me aside afterward and offered a wealth of information, advice, and encouragement. He continued to educate me through subsequent correspondence and a visit to his lab in Toronto. That person was Robbie Case. By guiding me to relevant literatures on socioeconomic disparities and childhood development, of which I had been embarrassingly ignorant, and by encouraging me to try working in this area, for which I was little prepared, he was instrumental in helping turn the vague musings of that small meeting into the program of empirical research described here.

What would a field with the inauspicious name "cognitive developmental neuro-sociology" be about? To me, it represented a new approach to the age-old problems of social stratification and the persistence of poverty. Why, in advanced societies that seem to offer opportunity for all, do some people remain poor? Why do many families remain poor across generations? These questions have occupied sociologists for as long as their field has existed, and have been answered in many ways.

Marxist approaches to the persistence of poverty emphasized purely economic factors that create and maintain social stratification (Marx, 1867). Functionalist accounts highlight the many ways in which society as a whole is served by the enduring presence of a lower class (e.g., Weber, 1923). The concept of a Culture of Poverty emphasizes causes within individuals and their subculture, rather than

M.J. Farah (✉)
Center for Cognitive Neuroscience, University of Pennsylvania, Philadelphia, PA, USA
e-mail: mfarah@psych.upenn.edu

M. Ferrari, L. Vuletic (eds.), *The Developmental Relations among Mind, Brain and Education*, DOI 10.1007/978-90-481-3666-7_11, © Springer Science+Business Media B.V. 2010

external societal forces, in perpetuating poverty across generations (Lewis, 1965). Each account undoubtedly captures some truth about the complex and multifactorial processes that confine children born of poor parents to lifelong poverty.

Cognitive neuroscience may offer yet another perspective on the problem by illuminating the ways in which the experience of growing up poor reduces people's ability to escape poverty. Neuroscience research on the effects of early experience on animal brain development suggests how childhood poverty might constrain human brain development. Specifically, the reduced opportunities for stimulating experience and increased stress of poverty would be expected to exert a negative influence on neurocognitive development. Without good neurocognitive development, intellectual and educational attainments are limited, which in turn limits upward socioeconomic mobility.

Education, Socioeconomic Status, and Child Development

In principle, education is an equalizer that provides all individuals in our society with the opportunity to fulfill their intellectual potential and prepare for worthwhile employment. In practice, these benefits of education are often less available to individuals of low socioeconomic status for a variety of reasons (see Arnold & Doctoroff, 2003, for a review). Schools attended by low-SES students are generally less well funded than other schools. This results in lower quality education and worse educational outcomes for students at such schools (Phillips, Voran, Kisker, Howes, & Whitebook, 1994; Pianta, La Paro, Payne, Cox, & Bradley, 2002). Attitudes of teachers and parents also play a role, with lower and more negative expectations of lower SES students (Alexander, Entwistle, & Thompson, 1987; Battin-Pearson et al., 2000; McLoyd, 1990). Finally, even before they enter school, low-SES children lag behind their middle-class counterparts by most measures of cognitive development (e.g., Bayley Infant Behavior Scales and IQ scores) and school readiness (e.g., preliteracy skills such as letter recognition) (Brooks-Gunn & Duncan, 1997). They enter the school system in need of an enriched educational experience, but often their lack of preparation is simply compounded by an inadequate school system (Arnold & Doctoroff, 2003).

The research summarized in this chapter is aimed at understanding the ways in which childhood poverty, including experiences prior to school entry, affect cognitive development. The correlations between SES and performance on standardized tests such as IQ tell us that SES must be related to brain development, as cognitive ability is a function of the brain. Yet little is currently known about the relationship between SES and brain development. Open questions include the specific neurocognitive systems that correlate with SES, the impact of these neurocognitive disparities on school readiness and school achievement, and the mechanisms by which these disparities emerge. The research summarized here includes work by me, my colleagues, and others, aimed at answering these open questions.

The Neurocognitive Profile of Childhood Poverty

For a cognitive neuroscience approach to be helpful in understanding cognitive development in poverty, the relations between socioeconomic status and the brain must be relatively straightforward and generalizable. The first question to be addressed is therefore: Can we generalize about the neurocognitive correlates of socioeconomic status, that is, the specific neurocognitive systems that are, and are not, correlated with SES?

Although most research on SES and child development has involved relatively broad-spectrum measures of cognition such as IQ or school achievement, there is evidence that points more specifically to associations with language development and executive function. The literature on language development is the most extensive in this regard, documenting robust SES disparities in vocabulary and phonological awareness among other linguistic abilities (see Whitehurst, 1997, for a review). SES disparities in executive functions associated with prefrontal cortex have also been noted. In the one such study, Mezzacappa (2004) tested a large group of urban 6-year-olds of varying SES on a computerized task that allows different components of attention to be assessed (the Attention Network Task, Rueda et al., 2004). He found the strongest relation with SES in what he termed "executive attentional" processes. Lipina, Martelli, Vuelta, and Colombo (2005) studied the development of working memory and inhibitory control in infancy by administering Diamond's (1990) "A-not-B" protocol to healthy infants from poor and nonpoor families. They found a significant disparity between the two groups.

These studies tell us that language and executive function, two types of ability that reflect the operation of specific neural systems, develop differently in children depending on SES. However, these studies do not tell us whether the SES disparities in cognition are limited to these neurocognitive systems, whether other specific systems are also affected, or whether the SES disparity in neurocognitive development is global, affecting all systems. To answer this question, it is necessary to assess the development of a set of different neurocognitive systems together in the same children. This is what we have done in a series of three studies.

In an initial study, we compared the neurocognitive performance of 30 low- and 30 middle-SES African-American Philadelphia public school kindergarteners (Noble, Norman, & Farah, 2005). The children were tested on a battery of tasks adapted from the cognitive neuroscience literature, designed to assess the functioning of five key neurocognitive systems. These systems are described briefly here:

- The *Prefrontal/Executive* system enables flexible responding in situations where the appropriate response may not be the most routine or attractive one, or where it requires maintenance or updating of information concerning recent events. It is dependent on prefrontal cortex, a late-maturing brain region that is disproportionately developed in humans.

- The *Left perisylvian/Language* system is a complex, distributed system encompassing semantic, syntactic, and phonological aspects of language and dependent predominantly on the temporal and frontal areas of the left hemisphere that surround the Sylvian fissure.
- The *Medial temporal/Memory* system is responsible for one-trial learning, the ability to retain a representation of a stimulus after a single exposure to it (which contrasts with the ability to gradually strengthen a representation through conditioning-like mechanisms), and is dependent on the hippocampus and related structures of the medial temporal lobe.
- The *Parietal/Spatial cognition* system underlies our ability to mentally represent and manipulate the spatial relations among objects and is primarily dependent upon posterior parietal cortex.
- The *Occipitotemporal/Visual cognition* system is responsible for pattern recognition and visual mental imagery, translating image format visual representations into more abstract representations of object shape and identity, and reciprocally translating visual memory knowledge into image format representations (mental images).

Not surprisingly, in view of the literature on SES and standardized cognitive tests, the middle-SES children performed better than the low-SES children on the battery of tasks as a whole. Also consistent with the literature just reviewed, the Left perisylvian/Language system and the Prefrontal/Executive system showed substantial disparities between the low- and middle-SES kindergarteners. Indeed, the groups differed by over a standard deviation in their performance composite on language tests, and by over two thirds of a standard deviation in the executive function composite. The other neurocognitive systems tested did not differ significantly between low- and middle-SES children, and in fact differed significantly less than the first two.

In a subsequent study we attempted to replicate and extend these findings in an older group of children with a different set of tasks. We tested 60 middle-school students, half of low and half of middle SES, matched for age, gender, and ethnicity (Farah et al., 2006). These children completed a new set of tests designed to tap the same neurocognitive systems as the previous study. In addition, instead of considering "prefrontal/executive" to be a single system, we subdivided it into three subsystems each with its own tests:

- The *Lateral prefrontal/Working memory* system enables us to hold information "on line" to maintain it over an interval and manipulate it, and is primarily dependent on the lateral surface of the prefrontal lobes. (Note that this is distinct from the ability to commit information to long-term memory, which is dependent on the medial temporal cortex.)
- The *Anterior cingulate/Cognitive control* system is required when we must resist the most routine or easily available response in favor of a more task-appropriate response and is dependent on a network of regions within prefrontal cortex including the anterior cingulate gyrus.

- The *Ventromedial prefrontal/Reward processing* system is responsible for regulating our responses in the face of rewarding stimuli, allowing us to resist the immediate pull of a attractive stimulus in order to maximize more long-term gains.

A second important difference between this and the previous study concerned the tests of the Medial temporal/Memory system. In both of the tasks used to assess memory in the previous study, the test phase followed immediately after the initial exposure to the stimuli and memory per se may not have been the limiting factor in performance. The tasks that we used in the second study included a longer delay between initial exposure to the stimuli to be remembered and later tested.

As with the younger children, sizeable and significant SES disparities were observed for language and executive function. In addition, it was possible to discern which aspects of executive function were most sensitive to SES. The Lateral prefrontal/Working memory and Anterior cingulate/Cognitive control subsystems showed SES disparities. Finally, with a longer delay between exposure and test in the memory tasks, we also found a difference in the Medial temporal/Memory system. SES was not associated with significant differences in the Parietal/Spatial cognition system, the Occipitotemporal/Visual cognition system, or the Ventromedial prefrontal/Reward processing system.

Finally, we assessed neurocognitive profile in 150 first graders of varying ethnicities whose SES spanned a range from low through middle (Noble, McCandliss, & Farah, 2007). As before, we used a battery of age-appropriate tasks designed to tap the different neurocognitive systems. Also as before, the Left perisylvian/Language system showed a highly significant relationship to SES, as did the Medial temporal/Memory system and the executive functions Lateral prefrontal/Working memory and Anterior cingulate/Cognitive control. In addition, there was an SES gradient in Parietal/Spatial cognition.

In sum, although the outcome of each study was different, there were also commonalities among them despite different tasks, different children, and different ages of testing. The most robust neurocognitive correlates of SES appear to involve the Left perisylvian/Language system, the Medial temporal/Memory system (insofar as SES effects were found in both studies that tested memory with an adequate delay) and the Prefrontal/Executive system, in particular its Lateral prefrontal/Working memory and Anterior cingulate/Cognitive control components. Children growing up in low-SES environments perform less well on tests that tax the functioning of these specific systems.

Neurocognitive Development and Academic Achievement

SES disparities in executive function, memory, and language would be expected to impact school success in a variety of ways, compounding the challenges faced by low-SES students in school. Abundant research has documented the importance of executive function for self-regulation and the importance of self-regulation, in turn, for school readiness and academic achievement more generally (e.g., Blair & Razza, 2007; Case, 1992; McClelland et al., 2007; Mischel, Shoda, & Rodriguez, 1989; Posner & Rothbart, 2005). The importance of memory ability for learning is obvious. Even when conceptual rather than rote learning is the goal, the ability to retain the particulars of facts or illustrations supports students' more abstract understanding. Finally, language is not only a subject of study in school but the medium through which most knowledge and skills are taught.

One pathway through which language ability affects school success is through its influence on reading ability. Kim Noble addressed the roles of language ability and SES on schoolchildren's reading ability in her dissertation research. She pointed out that, of the many aspects of language predictive of early reading, the most powerful predictor is "phonological awareness" (Bradley & Bryant, 1983; Wagner & Torgesen, 1987). This refers to our ability to attend to the sound structure of the language, as when we judge whether or not two words rhyme. Given earlier findings that phonological awareness is correlated with SES (Noble et al., 2005; Noble et al., 2007; Wallach, Wallach, Dozier, & Kaplan, 1977), we were led to ask: Does the SES gradient in phonological awareness account for the SES gradient in reading ability? By assessing SES, phonological awareness, and reading ability in the sample of first graders from our earlier study, we found that SES was correlated with reading ability above and beyond its correlation with phonological awareness.

Furthermore, SES and phonological awareness were not independent in their influences on early reading ability. At lower levels of SES, reading ability was well predicted by phonological awareness, whereas the relationship was weaker at higher levels of SES. Put another way, at higher levels of phonological awareness, all children mastered reading, whereas children with lower levels of phonological awareness were better readers if they came from higher levels of SES. The benefits of a higher SES background appear to buffer children against the effects of low phonological awareness (Noble, Farah, & McCandliss, 2006). A subsequent imaging study clarified the nature of this buffering effect. It might have reflected better functioning of the visual word decoding regions of the brain or other compensatory strategies used with a given level of visual word decoding. Our fMRI evidence showed that the visual word decoding area itself (in the left fusiform gyrus) was more active for higher SES children at a given level of phonological awareness, suggesting that the enriched literacy environment of higher SES homes affects the neural bases of visual word decoding per se (Noble et al., 2006).

Mechanism: Disentangling Causes and Effects

Why do different aspects of brain function come to be associated with SES? Do the associations discussed so far reflect the effects of SES on brain development, or the opposite direction of causality? Perhaps families with higher innate language, executive, and memory abilities tend to acquire and maintain a higher SES. Given that the direction of causality is an empirical issue, what data bear on the issue?

The methods of behavioral genetics research can, in principle, tell us about the direction of causality in the association between SES and the development of specific neurocognitive functions. However, these methods have yet to be applied to that question. They have been applied to a related question, namely the heritability of IQ and SES. Cross-fostering studies of within- and between-SES adoption suggest that roughly half the IQ disparity in children is experiential (Capron & Duyme, 1989; Schiff & Lewontin, 1986). If anything, these studies are likely to err in the direction of underestimating the influence of environment because the effects of prenatal and early postnatal environment are included in the estimates of genetic influences in adoption studies. Additional evidence comes from studies of when, in a child's life, poverty was experienced. Within a given family that experiences a period of poverty, the effects are greater on siblings who were young during that period (Duncan, Brooks-Gunn, & Klebanov, 1994), an effect that cannot be explained by genetics. In sum, multiple sources of evidence indicate that SES does indeed have an effect on cognitive development, although its role in the specific types of neurocognitive system development investigated here is not yet known.

Many different aspects of childhood SES could affect neurocognitive development. Some do so by their direct effects on the body and some by less direct psychological mechanisms. Three somatic factors have been identified as significant risk factors for low cognitive achievement by the Center for Children and Poverty (1997): inadequate nutrition, lead exposure, and substance abuse (particularly prenatal exposure).

The role of nutrition in SES disparities in brain development has been difficult to resolve because nutritional status is so strongly correlated with a host of other family and environmental variables likely to impact neurocognitive development, including all of the potential mechanisms of causation to be reviewed here. Although nutritional supplementation programs could in principle be used as an "experimental manipulation" of nutritional status alone, in practice these programs are often coupled with other, non-nutritional forms of enrichment or affect children's lives in non-nutritional ways which perpetuate the confound (e.g., children given school breakfast are less often late or absent). In addition, poor nutrition may synergize with other forms of childhood deprivation in impairing brain development. Iron-deficiency anemia is known to afflict about one quarter of low-income children in the United States (CHPNP 1998) and is known to impair brain development when severe.

Lead is a neurotoxin to which children of lower SES are more likely exposed. Even at relatively low levels of lead in the blood, under10 μg/dL, there is a systematic relationship between lead level and IQ (Surkan et al., 2007). As with nutrition, the effect of lead synergizes with other environmental factors and is more pronounced in low-SES children (Bellinger, Leviton, Waternaux, Needleman, & Rabinowitz, 1987).

Prenatal substance exposure is a third factor that affects children of all SES levels but is disproportionately experienced by the poor. Maternal use of alcohol, tobacco, marijuana, and other drugs of abuse have been associated with adverse cognitive outcomes in children (Chasnoff et al., 1998). Although the highly publicized phenomenon of "crack babies" might lead one to view prenatal cocaine exposure as a major contributor to the SES disparities noted here, there is little evidence that it plays a role. In her 2001 review of the literature on this topic, Frank offered the following tentative conclusion, pending new evidence: "there is no convincing evidence that prenatal cocaine exposure is associated with developmental toxic effects that are different in severity, scope, or kind from the sequelae of multiple other risk factors. Many findings once thought to be specific effects of in utero cocaine exposure are correlated with other factors, including prenatal exposure to tobacco, marijuana, or alcohol and the quality of the child's environment" (p. 1613). Indeed, we recently compared the performance of cocaine exposed and nonexposed children on the task battery used by Farah et al. (2006) and found no differences (Hurt et al., submitted).

The set of potentially causative somatic factors just reviewed is far from complete. There are SES gradients in a wide variety of physical health measures, many of which could affect children's neurocognitive development through a variety of different mechanisms (Adler et al., 1994). In addition, the typical psychological experiences of childhood differ sharply between poor and nonpoor families, and these differences also contribute to the differing neurocognitive outcomes for the children of these families.

Psychological Influences on Neurocognitive Development in Poverty

As with potential physical causes, the set of potential psychological causes for the SES gap in cognitive achievement is large, and the causes are likely to exert their effects synergistically. One difference between low- and middle-SES families that seems predictable, even in the absence of any other information, is that low-SES children are likely to receive less cognitive stimulation than middle-SES children. Their economic status alone predicts that they will have fewer toys and books and less exposure to zoos, museums, and other cultural institutions because of the expense of such items and activities. This is indeed the case (Bradley, Corwyn, McAdoo, & Garcia Coll, 2001) and has been identified as a mediator between SES and measures of cognitive achievement (Bradley & Corwyn, 1999; Brooks-Gunn & Duncan, 1997; McLoyd, 1998).

Such a mediating role is consistent with the results of neuroscience research with animals. Starting many decades ago, researchers began to observe the powerful effects of environmental stimulation on brain development. Animals reared in barren laboratory cages showed less well-developed brains by a number of different anatomical and physiological measures, compared with those reared in more complex environments with opportunities to climb, burrow, and socialize (van Praag, Kempermann, & Gage, 2000, Rosenzweig, 2003).

Other types of cognitive stimulation are also less common in low-SES homes, for example parental speech designed to engage the child in conversation (Hoff, 2003). The average number of hours of one-on-one picture book reading experienced by children prior to kindergarten entry has been estimated at 25 for low-SES children and between 1000 and 1700 for middle-SES children (Adams, 1990). In addition to material limitations, differing parental expectations and concerns also contribute to differences in the amount of cognitive stimulation experienced by low- and middle-SES children (Lareau, 2003).

Another major difference in the lives of low- and middle-SES individuals concerns levels of stress, and this has been related to differences in child development (Evans & English, 2002). The lives of low-SES individuals tend to be more stressful for a variety of reasons, some of which are obvious: concern about providing for basic family needs, dangerous neighborhoods, and little control over one's work life. Again, research bears out this intuition: Turner and Avison (2003) confirmed that lower SES is associated with more stressful life events by a number of different measures. The same appears to be true for children as well as adults, and is apparent in salivary levels of the stress hormone cortisol (Lupien, King, Meaney, & McEwen, 2001).

Why is stress an important consideration for neurocognitive development? Psychological stress causes the secretion of stress hormones, which affect the brain in numerous ways (Gunnar & Quevedo, 2007; McEwen, 2000). The immature brain is particularly sensitive to these effects. In basic research studies of rat brain development, rat pups are subjected to the severe stress of prolonged separation from the mother and stress hormone levels predictably climb. However, the effect of a brief handling (minutes per day), which also separates the animal from its mother, appears beneficial. Both prolonged maternal separation and brief handling affect later-life stress regulation ability and memory ability as a result of their impact on hippocampal development. The salutary effect of brief separations appears to result from the intensified nurturing behavior that follows the separation. The more a mother rat licks her pup following a brief stressor, the better regulated the pup's later response to stressors and the better its learning ability (Liu, Diorio, Day, Francis, & Meaney, 2000). This suggests that the high stress of poverty will take a toll on children's brain development, especially the development of the Medial temporal/Memory system, but that differences in parenting may strongly modulate those effects.

Our current research is attempting to make use of the description of the SES disparities in specific neurocognitive systems to test hypotheses about causal pathways. Drawing on the earlier findings indicating robust SES differences in Perisylvian/Language and Medial temporal/Memory systems, we are now testing hypotheses concerning the determinants of individual differences in the development of these systems in children of low SES (Farah et al., in press).

The participants in this research were 110 low-SES middle-school students from a cohort of children enrolled at birth in a study of the effects of prenatal cocaine exposure. Approximately half of the children have been exposed to cocaine prenatally and half have not. Maternal use of cocaine as well as amphetamines, opiates, barbiturates, benzodiazepines, marijuana, alcohol, and tobacco are ascertained by interview and medical record review at time of birth and, for all but the last three, maternal and infant urine specimens.

As part of the ongoing study of these children, a research assistant visited the home of each child at ages 4 and 8 and administered the HOME (Home Observation and Measurement of Environment, Caldwell & Bradley, 1984). The HOME includes an interview with the mother about family life and observations of the interactions between mother and child. The HOME has a number of different subscales relevant to different aspects of the child's experience. We combined a number of different subscales indicative of the amount of cognitive stimulation provided to the child to make a composite measure of Environmental Stimulation, and a number of different subscales indicative of the amount of social/emotional nurturance provided to the child to make a composite measure of Parental Nurturance. The subscales used for each composite, along with representative items, were as follows:

- The *Environmental Stimulation composite* for 4-year-olds was composed of *Learning stimulation* ("child has toys which teach color," "at least 10 books are visible in the apartment"), *language stimulation* ("child has toys that help teach the names of animals," "mother uses correct grammar and pronunciation"), *academic stimulation* ("child is encouraged to learn colors," "child is encouraged to learn to read a few words"), *modeling* ("some delay of food gratification is expected," "parent introduces visitor to child"), and *variety of experience* ("child has real or toy musical instrument," "child's art work is displayed some place in house"). For 8-year-olds, the subscales used for the cognitive stimulation composite were: *Growth fostering materials and experiences* ("child has free access to at least ten appropriate books," "house has at least two pictures of other type of art work on the walls"), *provision for active stimulation* ("family has a television, and it is used judiciously, not left on continuously," "family member has taken child, or arranged for child to go to a scientific, historical, or art museum within the past year"), *family participation in developmentally stimulating experiences* ("Family visits or receives visits from relatives or friends at least once every other week," "family member has taken child, or arranged for child to go, on a trip of more than 50 miles from his home").
- The *Parental Nurturance composite* for 4-year-olds: was composed of: *Warmth and affection* ("parent holds child close 10–15 minutes per day," "parent converses with child at least twice during visit") and *acceptance* ("parent does not scold or derogate child more than once," "parent neither slaps nor spanks child during visit"). For 8-year-olds, the subscales used were *Emotional and verbal responsivity* ("Child has been praised at least twice during past week for doing something," "parent responds to child's questions during interview"), *encouragement of maturity* ("family requires child to carry out certain self-care routines," "parents set limits for child and generally enforce them"), *emotional climate* ("parent has not lost temper with child more than once during previous week," "parent uses some term of endearment or some diminutive for child's name when talking about child at least twice during visit") and *paternal involvement* ("Father

[or father substitute] regularly engages in outdoor recreation with child," "Child eats at least one meal per day, on most days, with mother and father [or mother and father figure]").

Two other variables with the potential to account for differences in neurocognitive development included in our analyses were maternal intelligence and prenatal substance exposure. The former was measured by the Weschler Adult Intelligence Scale–Revised (WAIS–R). Maternal IQ could influence child neurocognitive outcome by genetic mechanisms or by its effect on the environment and experiences provided by the mother for the child. Prenatal substance exposure was coded for analysis on an integer scale of 0–4, with one point for each of the following substances: tobacco, alcohol, marijuana, and cocaine. Use of other substances was an exclusionary criterion.

We used statistical regression to examine the relations between the neurocognitive outcome measures and the predictor variables Environmental Stimulation, Parental Nurturance, maternal IQ, and polysubstance use, as well as the child's gender and age at the time of neurocognitive testing. Our results indicate that the development of different neurocognitive systems is affected by different variables.

Children's performance on the tests of Left perisylvian/Language was predicted by average Environmental Stimulation. This was the sole factor identified as predicting language ability by forward stepwise regression, and one of two factors identified by backward stepwise regression, along with the child's age. In contrast, performance on tests of Medial temporal/Memory ability was predicted by average Parental Nurturance. This was the sole factor identified as predicting memory ability by forward stepwise regression and one of three factors identified by backward stepwise regression, along with the child's age and prenatal substance exposure. The relation between memory and Parental Experience is consistent with the animal research cited earlier (Liu et al., 2000).

Our analyses did not reveal any systematic relation of the predictor variables considered here to Lateral prefrontal/Working memory or Anterior cingulate/Cognitive control function.

The relation between life experience and brain development for human beings is undoubtedly more complex than for animals, but we can nevertheless be guided by the animal research literature in formulating hypotheses to test. So far, the use of this strategy has shown that different aspects of life experience, cognitive stimulation, and parental buffering of stress act on brain development by different pathways and affect the different neurocognitive systems to different degrees.

Conclusions

Educators are increasingly incorporating the ideas and findings of neuroscience into their work, a trend that Robbie Case both foresaw and helped to bring about. Our growing understanding of normal brain development and atypical brain development is forming the basis for new and more effective educational practice. With regard to normal brain development, cognitive neuroscientists have only recently shifted from the study of commonalities among brains to the study of individual differences in brain function. Educators, who must teach students of varying ability, motivation, and cognitive style, will presumably not wait as long to apply the cognitive neuroscience of individual differences in their work.

The findings summarized in this chapter concern a major cause of individual differences in school readiness and academic performance, namely SES. The different kinds of childhood experience that students of lower and higher SES bring into the classroom affects what they learn there. Reciprocally, the different kinds of schools attended by children of lower and higher SES also affect the potential for learning. The neural mechanisms involved in these processes are important subjects for future research in neuroscience and education. Of course, it does not take a proverbial rocket scientist or, for that matter, a neuroscientist to realize that children should have access to stimulating experiences, be protected from high levels of stress, and go to good schools. Nevertheless, a better understanding of the ways in which childhood experience and classroom instruction shape brain function will suggest new ways of preventing and remediating some of the disadvantages suffered by poor children.

References

Adams, M. J. (1990). *Learning to read: Thinking and learning about print.* Cambridge, MA: MIT Press.

Adler, N. E., Boyce, T., Chesney, M. A., Cohen, S., Folkman, S., Kahn, R. L., et al. (1994). Socioeconomic status and health: The challenge of the gradient. *American Psychologist, 49*, 15–24.

Alexander, K., Entwisle, D., & Thompson, M. (1987). School performance, status relations, and the structure of sentiment: Bringing the teacher back in. *American Sociological Review, 52*, 665–682.

Arnold, D. H., & Doctoroff, G. L. (2003). The early education of socioeconomically disadvantaged children. *The Annual Review of Psychology, 54*, 517–545.

Battin-Pearson, S., Newcomb, M. D., Abbott, R. D., Kill, K. G., Catalano, R. F., Hawkins, J. D. (2000). Predictors of early high-school drop-out: A test of five theories. *Journal of Education and Psychology, 92*, 568–582.

Bellinger, D., Leviton, A., Waternaux, C., Needleman, H., & Rabinowitz, C. (1987). Longitudinal analyses of prenatal and postnatal lead exposure and early cognitive development. *New England Journal of Medicine, 316*, 1037–1043.

Blair, C. & Razza, R. P. (2007). Relating effortful control, executive function, and false-belief understanding to emerging math and literacy ability in kindergarten. *Child Development, 78*, 647–663.

Bradley, L., & Bryant, P. E. (1983). Categorizing sounds and learning to read – a causal connection. *Nature, 301*, 419–421.

Bradley, R. H., & Corwyn, R. F. (1999). Parenting. In C. L. B. Tamis-Lemonda (Ed.), *Child Psychology: A Handbook of Contemporary Issues* (pp. 339–362). New York: Psychology Press.

Bradley, R. H., Corwyn, R. F., McAdoo, H. P. & Garcia Coll C. (2001) The home environments of children in the United States. Part 1: Variations by age, ethnicity, and poverty-status. *Child Development, 72*, 1844–1867.

Brooks-Gunn, J., & Duncan, G. J. (1997). The effects of poverty on children. *The Future of Children, 7*, 55–71.

Caldwell, B. M., & Bradley, R. H. (1984). *Home Observation for Measurement of the Environment (HOME)*. Little Rock, AR: University of Arkansas.
Capron, C., & Duyme, M. (1989). Assessment of effects of socio-economic status on IQ in a full cross-fostering study. *Nature*, *340*, 552–554.
Case, R. (1992). The role of the frontal lobes in the regulation of cognitive development. *Brain and Cognition*, *20*, 51–73.
Chasnoff, I. J., Anson, A., Hatcher, R., Stenson, H., Iaukea, K., & Randolph, L. (1998). Prenatal exposure to cocaine and other drugs. Outcome at four to six years. *Annals of the New York Academy of Sciences*, *846*, 314–328.
Diamond, A. (1990). The development and neural bases of memory functions as indexed by the A(not)B and delayed response tasks in human infants and infant monkeys. *The Development and Neural Bases of Higher Cognitive Functions*. A. Diamond. New York: New York Academy of Science, 267–317.
Duncan, G. J., Brooks-Gunn, J., & Klebanov, P. K. (1994). Economic deprivation and early-childhood development. *Child Development*, *65*, 296–318.
Evans, G. W., & English, K. (2002). The environment of poverty: Multiple stressor exposure, psychophysiological stress, and socioemotional adjustment. *Child Development, 73*, 1238–1248.
Farah, M. J., Shera, D. M., Savage, J. H., Betancourt, L., Giannetta, J. M., Brodsky, N. L., et al. (2006). Childhood poverty: Specific associations with neurocognitive development. *Brain Research*, *1110*, 166–174.
Farah, M. J., Betancourt, L., Shera, D. M., Savage, J. H., Giannetta, J. M., Nancy, L., et al. (in press). Environmental stimulation, parental nurturance and cognitive development in humans. *Developmental Science, 15*, 793–801 (from her website).
Gunnar, M. R. & Quevedo, K. (2007). The neurobiology of stress and development. In S. Fiske (Ed.) *Annual Review of Psychology, 58*, 145–174.
Hoff, E. (2003). The specificity of environmental influence: Socioeconomic status affects early vocabulary development via maternal speech. *Child Development*, *74*, 1368–1378.
Hurt, H., Betancourt, L., Malmud, E. K., Shera, D. M., Giannetta, J. M., Brodsky, N. L., et al. (submitted). Effects of prenatal cocaine exposure at middle school age: A neurocognitive systems analysis.
Lareau, A. (2003). *Unequal childhoods: Class, race and family life*. Berkeley, CA: University of California Press.
Lewis, O. (1965). *La Vida*. New York: Random House.
Lipina, S. J., Martelli, M. I., Vuelta, B. L., & Colombo, J. A. (2005). Performance on the A-not-B task of Argentinean infants from unsatisfied basic needs homes. *Interamerican Journal of Psychology*, *39*, 49–60.
Liu, D., Diorio, J., Day, J. C., Francis, D. D., & Meaney, M. J. (2000). Maternal care, hippocampal synaptogenesis and cognitive development in rats. *Nature Neuroscience*, *3*(8), 799–806.
Lupien, S. J., King, S., Meaney, M.J., & McEwen, B.S. (2001). Can poverty get under your skin? Basal cortisol levels and cognitive function in children from low and high socioeconomic status. *Development and Psychopathology*, *13*, 653–676.
Marx, K. (1976 (first published in 1867)). *Capital* (Vol. I). New York: Penguin.
McClelland, M. M., Cameron, C. E., Connor, C. M., Farris, C. L., Jewkes, A. M., & Morrison, F. J. (2007). Links between behavioral regulation and preschoolers' literacy, vocabulary, and math skills. *Developmental Psychology*, *43*, 947–959.
McLoyd, V. C. (1990). The impact of economic hardship on black families and children: Psychological distress, parenting and socioemotional development. *Child Development*, *61*, 311–346.
McLoyd, V. C. (1998). Socioeconomic disadvantage and child development. *American Psychologist*, *53*, 185–204.
McEwen, B. S. (2000). The neurobiology of stress: From serendipity to clinical relevance. *Brain Research*, *886*, 172–189.

Mezzacappa, E. (2004). Alerting, orienting, and executive attention: developmental properties and sociodemographic correlates in an epidemiological sample of young, urban children. *Child Development, 75*, 1373–1386.

Mischel, W., Shoda, Y., & Rodriguez, M. L. (1989). Delay of gratification in children. *Science, 244*, 933–938.

Noble, K. G., Farah, M. J., & McCandliss, B. M. (2006). Socioeconomic background modulates cognition–achievement relationships in reading. *Cognitive Development, 21* (3): 349–368.

Noble, K. G., McCandliss, B. D., & Farah, M. J. (2007). Socioeconomic gradients predict individual differences in neurocognitive abilities. *Developmental Science, 10*(4): 464–480.

Noble, K. G., Norman, M. F., & Farah, M. J. (2005). Neurocognitive correlates of socioeconomic status in kindergarten children. *Developmental Science, 8*, 74–87.

Phillips D. A., Voran M., Kisker E., Howes C., & Whitebook M. (1994). Child care for children in poverty: opportunity or inequity? *Child Development, 65*, 472–492.

Pianta R. C., La Paro K. M., Payne C., Cox M. J., & Bradley R. (2002). The relation of kindergarten classroom environment to teacher, family, school, characteristics, and child outcomes. *The Elementary School Journal, 102*, 225–239.

Posner, M. I., & Rothbart, M. K (2005). Influencing brain networks: Implications for education. *Trends in Cognitive Sciences, 9*, 99–103 .

Rosenzweig, M. R., (2003). Effects of differential experience on the brain and behavior. *Developmental Neuropsychology*, 24, 523–540.

Rueda, M. R., Fan, J., McCandliss, B. D., Halparin, J. D., Gruber, D. B., Lercari, L. P., et al. (2004). Development of attentional networks in childhood. *Neuropsychologia, 42*, 1029–1040.

Schiff, M., & Lewontin, R. (1986). *Education and Class: The Irrelevance of IQ Genetic Studies*. Oxford, UK: Clarendon Press.

Surkan, P. J., Zhang, A., Trachtenberg, F., Daniel, D. B., McKinlay, S., & Bellinger, D. C. (2007). Neuropsychological function in children with blood lead levels <10 microg/dL. *Neurotoxicology, 28*, 1170–1177.

Turner, R. J., & Avison, W. R. (2003). Status variations in stress exposure: implications for the interpretation of research on race, socioeconomic status, and gender. *Journal of Health and Social Behavior, 44*, 488–505.

van Praag, H., Kempermann, G., & Gage, F. H. (2000) Neural consequences of environmental enrichment. *Nature Reviews Neuroscience, 1*, 191–198.

Wagner, R. K., & Torgesen, J. K. (1987). The nature of phonological processing and its causal role in the acquisition of reading skills. *Psychological Bulletin, 101*, 192–212.

Wallach, L., Wallach, M. A., Dozier, M. G., & Kaplan, N. E. (1977). Poor children learning to read do not have trouble with auditory discrimination but do have trouble with phoneme recognition. *Journal of Educational and Psychology, 69*, 36–39.

Weber, M. (1961 first published in 1923). *General economic history*. New York: Collier.

Whitehurst, G. J. (1997). Language processes in context: Language learning in children reared in poverty. In L. B. Adamson & M. A. Romski (Eds.), *Research on communication and language disorders: Contribution to theories of language development* (pp. 233–266). Baltimore, MD: Brookes.

Multiple Pathways to Bullying: Tailoring Educational Practices to Variations in Students' Temperament and Brain Function

Zopito A. Marini, Andrew V. Dane, and Richard E. Kennedy

In preparing this chapter, which like this entire book is dedicated to the memory of Robbie Case, we were guided by some of his best qualities as a powerful thinker and developer of grand theories. In a small way, we tried to emulate Robbie's adventurous spirit as he continuously searched to uncover developmental patterns, make predictions and test them, so that the end results could be put to the service of improving the lives of children. In addressing the issue of bullying, an area of concern to many school-age children, we tried to be cognitively adventurous by expanding our horizons and venturing across less-traveled research landscapes, to search for patterns and integrate different areas of research, perhaps the way Robbie would have done it.

Bullying and Its Educational and Psychosocial Consequences

Bullying is a major concern for educators in light of its substantial prevalence in schools, its considerable impact on the psychosocial adjustment of perpetrators and victims, and its adverse effect on the school environment. Bullying is a type of aggression characterized by repeated and systematic coercive use of power among peers (Marini, Dane, Bosacki, & YLC-CURA, 2006; Olweus, 2001; Smith, Pepler, & Rigby, 2004). Research has shown that involvement in bullying as a perpetrator, victim, or both is pervasive, with estimates ranging from as low as 10% to as high as 30% of the student population (Marini, McWhinnie, & Lacharite, 2004; Nansel et al., 2001). While the prevalence statistics are dependent on the way bullying is measured and the particular time frame used (i.e., 1 month vs. 1 year vs. lifetime), there is considerable agreement that about 10–15% of the student population are likely to report being bullied, with 5–10% reporting having bullied others (Nansel et al., 2001). In addition, there is an emerging group, ranging from

Z.A. Marini (✉)
Department of Child and Youth Studies, Brock University, St. Catharines, ON, Canada
e-mail: zmarini@brocku.ca

M. Ferrari, L. Vuletic (eds.), *The Developmental Relations among Mind, Brain and Education*, DOI 10.1007/978-90-481-3666-7_12,

10 to 15%, who are dually involved as both bully and victim (Craig, 1998; Marini, Dane, et al., 2006; Schwartz, Proctor, & Chein, 2001).

In childhood and adolescence, engagement in bullying is associated with a range of psychosocial problems including peer rejection, psychiatric difficulties such as Conduct and Anxiety disorder, and poor academic performance (Coie, Dodge, & Kupersmidt, 1990; Haynie et al., 2001; Loeber, Green, Lahey, & Kalb, 2000; Nansel et al., 2001; Olweus, 2001). Furthermore, several aspects of maladjustment in adulthood have been linked to childhood and adolescent aggression or bullying, including criminal convictions, unemployment, smoking and substance use, partner abuse, depression and anxiety, lower level of education, high-school drop out, and lower status occupation (Farrington, 1993; Moffitt, Caspi, Harrington, & Milne, 2002; Pepler, Jiang, Craig, & Connolly, 2008; Rigby, 2001). Students who are victimized often report an array of internalizing difficulties related to anxiety, depression, and self-esteem, as well as a heightened risk of suicide (Craig, 1998; Grills & Ollendick, 2002; Rigby, 2001).

In addition to the large array of psychosocial problems associated with bullying and victimization, incidents of aggression and bullying in the school may disrupt classroom activities and affect the overall school climate. Bullying may also disrupt classroom instruction; divert teachers', educational assistants', youth workers', and school psychologists' time from other students; and contribute to a classroom atmosphere that is not conducive to learning (Nucci, 2006). Educators must also tackle the issue of bullying because it is paramount that the school be a safe, secure environment for all students.

Although there are many programs that educators could obtain to address the issue of bullying in schools, research has shown that these interventions have had mixed results (Smith et al., 2004; Smith, Stewart, & Cousins, 2004). One possible reason for this limited success is these programs assume that children who bully are a homogenous group, whereas recent theoretical and empirical work suggests that children may follow different etiological pathways en route to bullying their peers. For example, some authors have proposed that children with two distinct clusters of temperament characteristics – callous-unempathic and emotionally dysregulated subtypes – follow two different pathways toward involvement in aggression and bullying (Frick & Morris, 2004; Nigg, 2006). Current etiological models emphasize that temperament features, such as impulsivity and fearlessness, may predispose children to greater engagement in aggression by influencing on-line actions, as well as making an indirect contribution by affecting transactions with socialization agents such as peers, parents, and teachers (e.g., Dodge & Pettit, 2003). Therefore, models of aggression and bullying, and interventions based on them, would be would be improved by greater attention to the role of temperament.

To enhance an appreciation of bullying as a heterogenous concept, the first aim of this chapter is to describe the characteristics of children with callous-unempathic and emotionally dysregulated temperaments and to discuss neural models that may account for individual differences along these temperamental dimensions. Second, we examine evidence of direct and indirect links between relevant temperament features and aggression in children and adolescents to determine whether empirical research supports the validity of theoretical work suggesting two distinct pathways to aggression and bullying for children with callous-unempathic and emotionally dysregulated temperaments. Finally, the practical implications of this research for educators are discussed.

Callous-Unempathic and Emotionally Dysregulated Temperaments

Temperament has been defined recently as constitutionally based individual differences in emotional, motor, and attentional reactivity and self-regulation that are relatively consistent across time and situations (Rothbart & Bates, 2006; for similar definitions see Kagan, 1998; Nigg, 2006; Putnam, Ellis, & Rothbart, 2002). Although a precise definition of temperament has been difficult to agree upon, there is a growing consensus that temperament characteristics are (1) biologically/constitutionally based; (2) early appearing, first surfacing in early infancy; (3) behavioral tendencies that constitute the core of personality and influence directions for development; (4) somewhat stable across time and situations; (5) an open system affected by developmental processes and social context; and (6) most readily observed in social interactions (Goldsmith et al., 1987; Nigg, 2006; Rothbart & Bates, 2006).

Although researchers have used a wide variety of terms to label temperament characteristics, a general consensus has been emerging recently about three or four basic dimensions of temperament that continually arise in factor analytic studies (Nigg, 2006; Putnam et al., 2002; Rothbart, Ahadi, & Evans, 2000). The first is related to surgency, extraversion, and positive affect, and individuals high in this dimension are particularly likely to approach and explore objects or situations that are perceived as novel or potentially rewarding. The second major characteristic involves negative affectivity, including fear, irritability, anger, and withdrawal. Although both fearful distress and irritable distress are considered to be components of negative emotionality, researchers are beginning to make a distinction between the two in infancy, toddlerhood, childhood, and adolescence (Nigg, 2006; Putnam et al., 2002). Effortful control is a third characteristic that features in most measures of temperament, which includes the regulation of attention; the inhibition of dominant responses to allow the activation of subdominant responses; as well as the activation of behaviors that are not immediately rewarding but provide longer-term positive consequences (Putnam et al., 2002). A fourth dimension, affiliativeness, includes warmth, agreeableness, friendliness, and sociability, but this dimension does not appear in the literature as consistently as the other three (Putnam et al., 2002).

Recently, researchers have been suggesting that exclusive emphasis on individual temperament variables may mask patterns among these variables (Nigg, 2006), and that specific clusters may be more predictive of adjustment outcomes than individual temperament features on their own. The first constellation, referred to as the callous-unempathic subtype, is characterized mainly by (a) low negative emotionality, especially low levels of fear, anxiety, sadness, and withdrawal and (b) low affiliation. The development of empathy and guilt is compromised in these individuals, possibly because fearlessness reduces their capacity to feel and recognize others' distress, and because irritability and hostility, opposites of affiliativeness, may interfere with feelings of compassion and remorse (Nigg, 2006; Rothbart & Posner, 2006), and hence people with callous-unempathic temperaments may be prone to psychopathic behavior. It was suggested that this pattern of temperament variables is predictive of proactive (planned, instrumental, and goal-directed) aggression, because their insensitivity to punishment and lack of regard for others' rights and feelings amplifies the likelihood that aggression may be used proactively to obtain instrumental rewards (e.g., tangible rewards, enhanced social status) without considering others' welfare (Frick & Morris, 2004; Nigg, 2006). The second combination is referred to as the emotionally dysregulated subtype and is characterized primarily by (a) high negative emotionality, including high fearfulness, anxiety, anger, frustration, and irritability; (b) high approach or surgency; and (c) low effortful control. This temperament pattern may be more predictive of reactive aggression (e.g., emotional, provoked, defensive) than proactive, and may ultimately result in major conduct problems. Emotionally dysregulated children may be prone to experiencing anger and frustration of high intensity and duration when their goals are blocked, or becoming fearful when they are facing stressful or threatening circumstances, which in combination with poor effortful control may predispose them to reactive aggression (Frick & Morris, 2004).

Neural Models of Temperament

Neural models of temperament, derived from physiological studies on animals, research on individuals with a brain injury, or brain imaging techniques, have outlined the function of three interrelated systems: (1) a positive affect or reward system variously called the Behavior Activation System (Gray & McNaughton, 2000) or the Behavior Facilitation System (Depue & Iacono, 1989) or Expectancy-Foraging System (Panksepp, 1998); (2) a negative affect system whose components include the Fight/Flight/Freeze and the Behaviour Inhibition systems (Gray & McNaughton, 2000), and the Rage system (Panksepp, 1998); and (3) a cognitive self-regulation system that has been described in terms of the Executive Attention Network or Anterior Attentional System (Derryberry & Rothbart, 2001; Posner and Rothbart, 2007).

The Behavior Activation System includes brain circuits that are dependent on the neurotransmitter dopamine, including the ventral tegmental area, nucleus accumbens, amygdala, hypothalamus, and prefrontal cortex (Gray, 1991; Gray & McNaughton, 2000). It responds to all appetitive stimuli signaling reward, and triggers voluntary approach behavior through motor systems in the cortex. Individual differences in the reactivity of this system have been linked to temperament dimensions relating to positive affect, including surgency and sensation seeking (Derryberry & Rothbart, 1997; Rothbart & Posner, 2006).

In contrast, the Fight/Flight/Freeze system is activated by aversive cues of punishment, which results in the emotion of fear and motivates defensive avoidance, freezing, or defensive aggression, depending on one's defensive distance from the perceived danger (McNaughton & Corr, 2004; Smillie, 2008). The primary neural components of the Fight/Flight/Freeze system include the periaqueductal gray, amygdala, hypothalamus, anterior cingulated cortex, and prefrontal cortex (McNaughton, 2006; Smillie, 2008), whose pathways are modulated by serotonin and noradrenaline. Variations in temperamental fearfulness are thought to be related in part to the reactivity of this system (Derryberry & Rothbart, 2001).

Although Gray and McNaughton (2000) discuss fearful and aggressive behaviors as being mediated by the Fight/Flight/Freeze system, Panksepp (1998) introduces a "rage system," that is separate from the fear system. It is proposed to underlie emotional experiences of frustration and anger, and to direct defensive aggression in the face of threat. He further proposed a connection between the rage system and the reward or positive affect system. Specifically, he suggested that the prefrontal cortex activates the circuitry of the rage system when expected rewards have not been detected, and the pursuit of reward is thwarted.

According to Gray and McNaughton (2000), the Behavior Inhibition System is another key circuit related to negative emotionality, which gives rise to feelings of anxiety. Specifically, this system is activated in the face of conflicting cues signaling both punishment and reward. It serves to inhibit approach and avoidance behavior, forestalling immediate action to allow a period of risk assessment during which one can determine whether it is safe to pursue a desired reward in a potentially dangerous environment. The Behavior Inhibition System is comprised of structures such as the periaqueductal gray, amygdala, hypothalamus, septo-hippocampal system, the posterior cingulate, and the dorsolateral prefrontal cortex, and its circuits depend upon the neurotransmitters serotonin and noradrenaline (McNaughton, 2006; McNaughton & Corr, 2004; Smillie, 2008).

The temperament characteristic of effortful control is thought to be related to neural activity in the anterior attention system (Derryberry & Rothbart, 2001; Posner, Rothbart, Sheese & Tang, 2007). The anterior cingulate cortex is the central feature of the attentional system, which receives input from systems processing affective-motivational (frontal cortex, amygdala, hippocampus), spatial (parietal cortex), object (temporal cortex), semantic (temporal and frontal cortex), and behavioral information (basal ganglia, supplementary motor area). Executive functions are performed by the attentional system, including the inhibition of dominant responses to perform a subdominant response, directing attention to semantic information, sustaining working memory, and error detection, which allow for more flexible decision making and planning.

Affiliativeness has been studied relatively less than other dimensions of temperament, and accordingly there is less literature discussing the neural circuits that may underlie it. However, Panksepp (1986) posited that opiate projections from the amygdala and cingulate cortex to the hypothalamus may promote social comfort, pair bonding, friendliness, trust, and helpful behavior, possibly by suppressing hostile and aggressive tendencies controlled by the central gray area of the brain stem. Individual differences in affiliation may be related to variations in endogenous opiates and the neuropeptide oxytocin (Panksepp, 1993).

Linking neural models to psychosocial theories of temperament, it seems that in children with callous-unempathic characteristics the Fight/Flight/Freeze system and the system underlying affiliativeness are relatively less responsive, whereas the reward or positive affect system (e.g., Behavior Activation System) and the anterior attention system function within normal limits. In contrast, an emotionally dysregulated temperament would appear to reflect hyperactivity in the three systems governing negative emotionality, including the Fight/Flight/Freeze system, the rage system, and the Behavior Inhibition System, as well as the Behavior Activation System. In addition, the emotional dysregulation likely reflects under-activity in the anterior attention system, leading to poor self-regulation.

Direct Links Between Temperament and Aggression

The purpose of this section is to examine whether research supports the conceptualization of temperament by Nigg (2006) and Frick and Morris (2004), by examining whether callous-unempathic and emotionally dysregulated temperaments are differentially linked to proactive and reactive aggression or bullying, respectively. Recent research has revealed that bullying is best characterized by heterogeneity in the forms used to carry out the attacks (e.g., direct vs. indirect; Marini, Dane, et al., 2006), the function (e.g., proactive vs. reactive) served for the attacker and the role (e.g., bullies, victims, bully-victims) of the participants (Little, Brauner, Jones, Nock, & Hawley, 2003; Marini, Koruna, & Dane, 2006). Thus, for instance, researchers have distinguished bullying with a proactive function from that which is a reaction to provocation. Reactive bullying involves a more immediate reaction to a perceived provocation, usually driven by frustration, instantaneous emotional release, defense against a perceived threat, and general lack of inhibition (Dodge & Coie, 1987; Poulin & Boivin, 2000). This type of abrupt reaction has also been labeled as self-defensive aggression and tends to be generally impulsive, accompanied by visible hostile expressions and a great deal of strong negative emotions (see Poulin & Boivin, 2000; Pulkkinen, 1996). In contrast, proactive bullying entails more deliberate and methodical planning of attacks, using aversive acts to obtain instrumental or social goals, such as stealing lunch money or bidding for popularity or social status (Camodeca, Goossens, Meerum-Terwogt, & Schuengel, 2002; Poulin & Boivin, 2000). In general, proactive bullying tends to entail unprovoked, goal-directed, predatory, and deliberate acts (Crick & Dodge, 1996; Pellegrini, Bartini, & Brooks, 1999). At this point, there is minimal research on temperament and bullying per se, although there is a considerable amount dealing with the closely related topic of temperament and aggression. Given that bullying is a specific form of aggression, this literature can illuminate the role that temperament plays in developmental pathways leading to bullying.

In general, less optimal temperament characteristics have been shown to correlate with later maladjustment in children and adolescents (Giancola & Parker, 2001; Ortiz & Gandara, 2006). With regard to aggression, the majority of research examining its connection to temperament refers to aggression or externalizing behavior (aggression, delinquency) in general without regard to subtypes. These data do not reveal whether there are differential outcomes associated with the two temperament subtypes, but they do nevertheless indicate that temperament dimensions related to the callous-unempathic and emotion dysregulation subtypes, such as surgency, fearlessness, emotional dysregulation, and effortful control, are associated with aggression and externalizing behavior in general (Barnow, Lucht, & Freyberger, 2005; Raine, Reynolds, Venables, Medrick, & Farrington, 1998; Rubin, Burgess, Dwyer, & Hastings, 2003; Schmidt, Fox, Rubin, Hu, & Hamer, 2002).

As shown in Table 1, there were seven studies that explicitly investigated direct links between temperament and proactive or reactive aggression. Seven of these papers consider aspects of temperament consistent with the emotion dysregulation subtype, (Barry et al., 2007; Bjornebekk, 2007; Pellegrini & Bartini, 2000; Raine et al., 2006; Shields & Cicchetti, 1998; Vitaro, Barker, Boivin, Brendgen, & Tremblay, 2006; Vitaro, Brendgen, & Tremblay, 2002). Consistent with the conceptualization of Nigg (2006) and Frick and Morris (2004), research demonstrated that reactive aggression was associated with a high level of fearfulness (reactivity, negative emotionality, emotional lability/negativity), high approach/surgency (BAS drive; approach–withdrawal; stimulation seeking), and low effortful control (low attention, high hyperactivity, high impulsivity). Notably, the measures of reactivity, negative emotionality, and emotional lability/negativity associated with reactive aggression are undifferentiated measures of emotionality, which would include both fearfulness and proneness to anger, irritability, or frustration, the latter of which may have a basis in high surgency and the concomitant sensitivity to reward.

There were four investigations that permitted an examination of whether the fearlessness aspect of the callous-unempathic temperament was associated with proactive aggression, as predicted by Nigg (2006) and Frick and Morris (2004). Consistent with this expectation, in two studies, behavior inhibition system sensitivity (e.g., sensitivity to punishment or negative consequences; Bjornebekk, 2007) and responsiveness to distressing stimuli (Kimonis, Frick, Fazekas, & Loney, 2006) were found to be inversely linked to proactive aggression in children and adolescents. In contrast, Vitaro and colleagues (2002; 2006) did not find proactively aggressive toddlers or children to be lower than average in negative emotionality or emotional reactivity, though they did find the expected distinction between proactive and reactive aggression in that only reactively aggressive participants were more fearful than other children. Low empathy is thought to be another component of the callous-unempathic temperament, and two studies included evidence of this characteristic, operationalized as psychopathy and callous-unempathic traits, being positively associated with proactive aggression (Barry et al., 2007; Raine et al., 2006). We did not find any research that explicitly examined whether individuals with a low degree of affiliativeness are more prone to proactive aggression, so this aspect of the proposed link between a callous-unempathic temperament and aggression could not be subjected to empirical scrutiny.

Table 1 Direct links between temperament subtypes and bullying subtypes

Author(s)	Methodology				
	N (Gender)	Age measures	Temperament measures	Aggression/bullying	Results
Direct Links Between Temperament and Aggression/Bullying Subtypes					
Barry et al. (2007).	160 (58 girls)	10 yrs 9 mon	Parent and impulsivity; teacher-rated impulsivity; narcissism; and callous-unempathic traits	Parent and teacher-rated proactive and reactive aggression	Impulsivity and narcissism positively associated with reactive aggression; narcissism positively linked with proactive aggression
Bjornebekk (2007)	48 (12 girls)	15.43 yrs	Self-report Behavior Inhibition System (BIS) and Behavior Activation System (BAS)	Self-reported proactive and reactive aggression	BAS positively associated with reactive aggression; BIS inversely associated with proactive aggression
Kimonis et al. (2006)	50 (23 girls)	9.3 yrs	Responsiveness to distressing or threatening stimuli (Dot-Probe Task)	Parent and child-rated proactive and reactive aggression	Proactive aggression negatively related to responsiveness to distressing stimuli
Vitaro et al. (2002)	3017 (1594 girls)	Long. 6–12 yrs	Mother-rated activity level, attention/distractibility withdrawal, rhythmicity, reactivity	Proactive and reactive aggression, teacher-rated	Reactively aggressive participants lower attention, higher approach-withdrawal, reactivity, activity than non-aggressive peers; proactively aggressive participants showed higher approach-withdrawal
Vitaro et al. (2006)	1516 (51% girls)	Long. 17 mon to 6 yrs	Parent-rated negative emotionality (at 17 mon)	Mother and teacher-rated reactive-proactive aggression (at 6 yrs)	Negative emotionality positively associated with reactive aggression

Table 1 (continued)

	Methodology				
Author(s)	*N* (Gender)	Age measures	Temperament measures	Aggression/bullying	Results
Raine et al. (2006)	503 boys	7 & 16 yrs	Self-report sensation seeking, impulsivity, hostility-aggression Childhood Psychopathy Scale	Reactive-proactive aggression questionnaire self-report	Stimulation-seeking significantly correlated with both proactive and reactive aggression; impulsivity correlated with reactive aggression
Shields and Cicchetti (1998)	228 (82 girls)	6–12 yrs	Parent and child-rated lability/negativity	Parent and teacher-rated reactive aggression	Emotional lability/negativity positively related to reactive aggression
Direct Links Between Temperament and Bully-Victim Status Subtypes					
Pellegrini and Bartini (2000)	138 (61 girls)	12.8 yrs (grade 5)	Teacher-rated emotional intensity	Senior Bully/Victim Questionnaire self-report	Emotionality positively associated with reactive and proactive aggression, and with aggressive victimization
Hess and Atkins (1998)	470 (231 girls)	7–9 yrs	Teacher-rated (TTQ-S) attention, approach, frustration tolerance, irritability, mood	Peer nominations of aggression and victimization	Compared to controls, aggressive victims are lower on attention, mood and frustration tolerance, and higher on irritability
Marini, Dane, et al. (2006)	7290 (3756 girls)	13–18 yrs	Adolescent-rated (DOTS-R) activity level, mood	Direct and indirect bullying and victimization checklist	Indirect and direct bully victims higher than uninvolved in activity level, and indirect bully-victims had less positive mood than uninvolved

Another way to confirm the validity of the concept of an emotionally dysregulated temperament is to examine the connection between these temperament characteristics and bully-victims, because their aggression tends to be reactive in nature (Salmivalli & Nieminen, 2002; Unnever, 2005). Although most studies have focused predominantly on bullies and victims, in a recent study it was found that about 33% of the students who reported high levels of experience with either bullying or victimization were dually involved in both (Marini, Dane, et al., 2006). Schwartz and his colleagues (see Schwartz et al., 2001) have suggested that the common risk factor predisposing bully-victims to both bullying and victimization is difficulty with the regulation of emotions. Since they are prone to emotional reactivity, they are likely to over-react to provocation such as peer teasing with an explosive outburst. Their predisposition to frustration and anger may render them more susceptible to being aggressive, whereas their emotional volatility may alienate peers and set them up as targets of bullying (Marini, Koruna, et al., 2006; Salmivalli, Kaukiainen, Voeten, & Sinesammal, 2004).

Three studies presented in Table 1 have examined the temperament of bully-victims. In all three studies, bully-victims were higher than uninvolved participants in various aspects of emotional reactivity, including emotionality, irritability, low frustration tolerance, and low positive mood (Hess & Atkins, 1998; Marini, Dane, et al., 2006; Pellegrini & Bartini, 2000). In addition, activity level was higher in bully-victims than in uninvolved participants, and attention regulation, suggesting a lower level of effortful control, a hallmark of individuals with an emotionally dysregulated temperament (Hess & Atkins, 1998; Marini, Dane, et al., 2006).

As a whole, this research supports the conceptualization that temperament characteristics reflecting emotional dysregulation may predispose children to reactive aggression. Specifically, temperament dimensions such as negative emotionality, emotional reactivity, emotional lability/negativity, low effortful control, and high surgency have been linked to reactive aggression and also to the probability of children being bully-victims, who primarily use aggression of a reactive nature. Although the amount of evidence was more limited, some research was consistent with the expectation that proactive aggression would be linked to low fear and low empathy; however, the possible link between instrumental aggression and low affiliation has not been empirically evaluated.

Interactive and Indirect Pathways from Temperament to Bullying

The challenge for teachers is to determine optimal strategies for managing and regulating the behavior of children with emotionally dysregulated or callous-unempathic temperaments. Recently, several studies have shown that children of different temperaments respond differentially to various behavioral control strategies used by parents, and are influenced dissimilarly by the parent–child relationship

(Collins, Maccoby, Steinberg, Hetherington, & Bornstein, 2000; Cumming, Davies, & Campbell, 2000). This research may have implications for teachers, who as socialization agents within the classroom, may need to be mindful of how emotionally dysregulated and callous-unempathic children may respond differently to behavior management strategies aimed at reducing bullying, and may respond in a unique fashion to the teacher–student relationships that develop over the course of a school year. An additional consideration that merits attention from teachers is how they themselves may react differently to emotionally dysregulated and callous-unempathic children in their daily interactions with them. Some insight into this issue may be gleaned from research on indirect links between temperament and aggression, mediated by the intermediate impact of temperament on the parents' parenting. A final benefit to examining literature on the relations among parenting, temperament, and aggression is some studies demonstrate that temperament can be shaped by parenting and is therefore amenable to change rather than being a fixed characteristic. Such investigations may provoke thoughts on how teachers may interact with emotionally dysregulated and callous-unempathic youngsters to curb their non-optimal tendencies and to promote more adaptive qualities. With these objectives in mind, we now turn to a brief review of literature on the interactive and indirect relations among parenting, temperament, and aggression.

Research on parent-temperament interactions is summarized in Table 2. One of the major patterns evident in this research is that children with emotionally dysregulated temperaments appear to react more adversely than other children to harsh forms of parental control and to negative parent–child relationships. With respect to parental control, harsh and inconsistent discipline was associated with aggression or conduct problems for children high in impulsivity (i.e., low effortful control) or fearfulness (Colder, Lochman, & Wells, 1997; Lengua, Wolchik, Sandler, & West 2000; Leve, Kim, & Pears, 2005), although the interaction between harsh discipline and impulsivity in the study by Leve and colleagues was significant only for girls. Problems with the parent–child relationship also seem to have a larger impact on emotionally dysregulated youngsters. In particular, children and adolescents who are uninhibited, low in effortful control, prone to anger, high in negative emotionality, or have a difficult temperament (defined as low inhibitory control, high frustration, high activity level, and low soothability) are more apt to experience behavioral problems if the parent–child relationship is characterized by avoidant attachment, maternal hostility, low maternal support, less positive parenting (low sensitivity, less positive and more negative affect, intrusiveness, detachment), and a lack of maternal sensitivity (Belsky, Hsieh, & Crnic, 1998; Burgess, Marshall, Rubin, & Fox, 2003; Carlo, Roesch, & Melby, 1998; Morris et al., 2002; van Aken, Junger, Verhoeven, van Aken, & Dekovic, 2007).

Two studies examined parenting by temperament interactions with respect to dimensions of the callous-unempathic temperament. Leve and colleagues (2005) found that harsh discipline increased girls' externalizing behavior when fear or shyness was low. In regard to the parent–child relationship, parental support was

Table 2 Interactive and indirect relations between temperament and aggression/bullying

Author(s)	Sample: *N* Gender	Sample: Age(s)	Temperament measure	Parenting measure	Aggression/bullying measure	Results
Parent-Temperament Interactions						
Burgess et al. (2003)	140	Longitudinal follow-up 14 mon to 4 yrs	Uninhibited temperament, -observed 24 mon, 4 yrs -heart rate; respiratory sinus Arrhythmia -maternal ratings 4 yrs	Mother-child attachment in strange situation – 14 mths	Mother-rated externalizing behaviors age 4	Avoidant attachment associated with externalizing behavior problems when uninhibited temperament high
Leve et al. (2005)	337; 163 girls	Longitudinal follow-up 5–17 yrs	Parent-rated fear/shyness, impulsivity at age 5	Mother and interviewer-rated maternal harsh discipline, age 5	Parent-rated externalizing behavior at ages 5, 7, 10, 14, 17	Harsh discipline predicted increases in girls' externalizing behavior only when impulsivity high or fear/shyness low.

Table 2 (continued)

Author(s)	Sample *N* Gender	Age(s)	Temperament measure	Parenting measure	Aggression/bullying measure	Results
Rubin et al. (2003).	104; 54 girls	Longitudinal follow-up to 4 yrs	Composite of observed effortful control and mother-rated emotion dysegulation at age 2.	Observed negative mothering (hostile affect, intrusive, negative control) at age 2.	Teacher-rated externalizing behavior at age 4	Behavioral/emotional under-control was associated with externalizing behavior for children with high and moderate levels of maternal negativity
Morris et al. (2002).	40	Mean 7.7 yrs	Mother-rated irritable distress, effortful control	Child puppet interview for maternal psychological control and hostility	Teacher-rated externalizing behavior	Maternal hostility associated with externalizing behavior for participants low in effortful control.
Carlo et al. (1998).	80	Mean 14.2 yrs	Parent-reported sociability and anger temperaments	Parent-rated support	Self-reported aggression and antisocial behaviors	Parent support inversely associated with aggression and antisocial behavior when sociability was low.

Table 2 (continued)

Author(s)	Sample N Gender	Sample Age(s)	Temperament measure	Parenting measure	Aggression/bullying measure	Results
						Maternal support inversely associated with aggression when anger was high and sociability low.
Rubin et al. (1998).	104; 52 girls	2 yrs	Observed and mother-rated dysregulated temperament	Observed maternal warmth and dominance	Mother-rated externalizing behavior observed aggression	Observed aggression and mother-rated externalizing behavior associated with dysregulated temperament only when boys' mothers were high in negative dominance.

Table 2 (continued)

	Sample		Temperament	Parenting	Aggression/bullying	
Author(s)	*N* Gender	Age(s)	measure	measure	measure	Results
Bates et al. (1998)	(Study 1) 139 44% girls	Study 1: Longitudinal follow-up from 13 mon to 10 yrs	Study 1: Mother-rated resistance to control; ages 13 mon and 24 mon	Study 1: Observed maternal restrictive control (prohibitions, warnings, scolding) at ages 6–24 mon	Study 1: Mother and teacher ratings of externalizing behavior, mean of measures.at ages 7, 8, 10.	Study 1: Resistance to control positively associated with teacher and mother-rated externalizing behavior only when mothers low in restrictive control
	(Study 2) 156 51% girls	Study 2: Longitudinal Follow-up 5–11 yrs	Study 2: Retrospective mother-rated resistance to control age 5 yrs	Study 2: Observed maternal restrictive control age 5	Study 2: Mother and teacher ratings of externalizing behavior, mean of measures. at ages 7, 8, 9, 10, 11.	Study 2: Resistance to control positively associated with teacher and mother-rated externalizing behavior only when mothers low in restrictive control.

Table 2 (continued)

Author(s)	Sample *N* Gender	Sample Age(s)	Temperament measure	Parenting measure	Aggression/bullying measure	Results
Belsky et al. (1998)	125 Boys	Longitudinal follow-up 12–37 mon	Parent-rated and observed infant negative emotionality at 12 mon	Observed positive parenting (sensitivity, positive affect, cognitive stimulation and detachment) and negative parenting (intrusiveness, negative affect) at 15–33 mon	Parent-rated externalizing behavior at 37 mon	Composite of maternal positive and negative parenting predictive of externalizing behavior only for infants high in negative emotionality.
Colder et al. (1997)	64 Boys	Fourth and fifth grade	Parent-rated activity level and fear; self-reported fear	Parent-rated involvement and monitoring, and harsh discipline.	Teacher-rated aggression	Poor monitoring positively associated with aggression only for high activity level boys; harsh discipline associated with aggression only for high and moderately fearful boys

Table 2 (continued)

Author(s)	Sample: N Gender	Sample: Age(s)	Temperament measure	Parenting measure	Aggression/bullying measure	Results
Paterson & Sanson (1999)	74; 40 girls	5–6 yrs	Parent-rated inflexibility (negative emotionality and adaptability); persistence (attention); and approach	Parent-rated physical punishment	Parent and teacher-rated externalizing behavior.	High inflexibility positively associated with externalizing behavior only for children exposed to high punishment.
Lengua et al. (2000).	231; 50.2% girls; divorced parents	9–12 yrs; mean 10.3	Child and mother-rated positive emotionality and impulsivity	Mother and child-rated rejection; inconsistent discipline	Child-rated conduct problems	Rejection more strongly associated with conduct problems for children low in positive emotionality Inconsistent discipline more strongly related to conduct problems for children high in impulsivity

Table 2 (continued)

Author(s)	Sample N Gender	Age(s)	Temperament measure	Parenting measure	Aggression/bullying measure	Results
Aken et al. (2007)	117 boys	Longitudinal follow-up 17–23 mon	Mother-rated inhibitory control, frustration, activity level and soothability	Observed maternal sensitivity and negative control	Mother-rated externalizing behavior	Lack of maternal sensitivity and high negative control positively associated with externalizing behaviors for children with a difficult temperament

Table 2 (continued)

Author(s)	Sample: N Gender	Age(s)	Temperament measure	Parenting measure	Aggression/bullying measure	Results
Parent-Temperament Indirect Effects						
Lengua and Kovacs (2005)	92; 54% Male	8–11 mean 9.9	Mother and child-rated fearfulness, irritability, positive emotionality and self-regulation.	Mother and child-rated acceptance, involvement and inconsistent discipline	Mother and child-rated externalizing problems.	Child irritability associated with greater inconsistent discipline, controlling for prior parenting. Child fearfulness and positive emotionality associated with greater maternal acceptance, controlling for prior parenting. Maternal inconsistent discipline predicted Higher fearfulness and irritability, controlling for

Table 2 (continued)

	Sample		Temperament	Parenting	Aggression/bullying	
Author(s)	*N* Gender	Age(s)	measure	measure	measure	Results
						prior temperament. Fearfulness, irritability, acceptance and inconsistent discipline uniquely associated with externalizing problems.
Eisenberg et al. (1999)	64; 33 girls	Longitudinal follow-up 58–132 mon	Parent-reported negative emotionality and self-regulation	Parent-reported distress, punitive responses and minimization responses to child negative emotions	Mother and father-rated problem behavior; teacher-rated social functioning (aggression/disruptive behavior minus socially appropriate behavior.	1)Age 6–8 self-regulation inversely related to age 8–10 parental punitive reactions age 8–10 punitive reactions positively associated with age 10–12 punitive reactions; age 10–12 punitive reactions positively related to age 10–12 problem behavior.

Table 2 (continued)

Author(s)	Sample N Gender	Sample Age(s)	Temperament measure	Parenting measure	Aggression/bullying measure	Results
						2) Age 6–8 parental distress inversely related to age 8–10 regulation age 8–10 regulation positively associated with age 10–12 regulation, which in turn was inversely associated with problem behavior.
Watson et al. (2004)	391 174 girls	Longitudinal follow-up; 7–13 yrs to 8–14 yrs	Mother-rated behavioral inhibition	Mother-rated negative family functioning	Mother and child-rated aggression	Negative family functioning associated with greater behavioral inhibition, which in turn was related to a higher level of aggression at 1-year follow-up.

Table 2 (continued)

Author(s)	Sample: *N* Gender	Sample: Age(s)	Temperament measure	Parenting measure	Aggression/bullying measure	Results
Finkenauer et al. (2005)	1359; 650 girls	12.3 yrs	Self-reported self-control	Self-reported acceptance/involvement, strict control, and psychological control	Self-reported undifferentiated aggression	Self-control partially mediated significant inverse relation between acceptance-involvement and aggression, and positive association between psychological control and aggression.

Table 2 (continued)

	Sample		Temperament	Parenting	Aggression/bullying	
Author(s)	*N* Gender	Age(s)	measure	measure	measure	Results
Zhou et al. (2004)	425; 236 girls	7 yrs, 8 mon	Parent and teacher-rated effortful control and anger/frustration	Parent-rated authoritative and authoritarian parenting	Parent and teacher-rated social functioning (which includes low aggression)	Positive relation between authoritative parenting and social functioning fully mediated by effortful control; inverse link between authoritarian parenting and social functioning partially mediated by effortful control.

Table 2 (continued)

Author(s)	Sample: *N* Gender	Sample: Age(s)	Temperament measure	Parenting measure	Aggression/bullying measure	Results
						Positive association between authoritative parenting and social functioning weakly mediated by anger/frustration; negative relation between authoritarian parenting and social functioning weakly mediated by anger/frustration
Shields and Cicchetti (1998)	228; 82 girls	6–12 yrs	Parent and child-rated lability/negativity	Parent-interview of maltreatment	Parent and teacher-rated reactive aggression	Positive association between maltreatment and reactive aggression

negatively linked with aggression and antisocial behavior only for children low in sociability, which relates to the lack of affiliativeness purported to characterize children with callous-unempathic temperaments (Carlo et al., 1998).

Other studies included data on temperament by parenting interactions, wherein the likelihood of a risky temperament characteristic predisposing a child to behavioral problems was altered by the kind of parenting experienced by the child. For example, three studies showed that youngsters with aspects of an emotionally dysregulated temperament, including low effortful control, high emotion dysregulation (i.e., approach, anger proneness), and negative emotionality, were more likely to evidence aggression or externalizing behavior when they experienced negative features of parental control or of the parent–child relationship, such as maternal dominance and negativity, and high parental physical punishment (Paterson & Sanson, 1999; Rubin, Hastings, Chen, Stewart, & McNichol, 1998; Rubin et al., 2003).

One explanation for these findings, provided by Rubin and colleagues (Rubin et al., 1998), is that children high in emotion dysregulation may have less effective internal mechanisms for exerting self-control, which places them at high risk for aggressive interactions with peers when parents limit opportunities for practicing self-regulation through intrusive forms of parenting (e.g., dominance). Paterson and Sanson (1999) suggest that emotionally dysregulated children are more likely to engage in coercive cycles when they encounter punitive parenting, by reacting adversely, escalating coercive exchanges until parents withdraw demands and negatively reinforce aggressive or externalizing behavior. Additional research by Bates and colleagues (Bates, Pettit, Dodge, & Ridge, 1998) also demonstrated a temperament by parenting interaction, except the link between resistance to control, which involves facets of emotional dysregulation and callous-unempathic characteristics, and externalizing behavior was moderated or offset by parental restrictive control. Consistent with the explanation advanced by Paterson and Sanson (1999), Bates and colleagues (1998) suggested that parents may avoid becoming involved in coercive cycles, wherein inappropriate behavior is inadvertently reinforced, with children high in aspects of emotion dysregulation (as well as some aspects of callous-unempathic temperaments, including low fear), by consistently restricting inappropriate behavior (and not giving in) in the face of defiance and oppositionality.

In addition to temperament by parenting interactions, three studies in Table 2 provide evidence of indirect effects, whereby temperament is indirectly linked to aggression through its intermediate impact on parenting. In accordance with the concept of evocative gene–environment correlations, whereby children with maladaptive temperaments are more likely than other youngsters to evoke negative parenting (e.g., Collins et al., 2000; Rutter, 1997), several studies indicated that children with emotionally dysregulated temperament features, such as high irritability and low self-regulation, appeared more likely to evoke negative forms of parental control including inconsistent discipline and punitive reactions, which in turn were uniquely associated with child behavior problems (Eisenberg et al., 1999; Lengua & Kovacs, 2005; Watson, Fischer, Andreas, & Smith, 2004).

However, several studies demonstrated that the reverse was also possible, in other words, that parenting could exacerbate or mitigate temperament qualities such as emotion dysregulation, which in turn may increase or decrease the risk of aggressive behavior. As shown in Table 2, negative aspects of parental control and the parent–child relationship, such as inconsistent discipline, parental distress to child behavior, negative family functioning, authoritarian parenting, psychological control, and parental maltreatment, were found to increase maladaptive temperament features such as fearfulness, irritability, emotional lability/negativity, poor self-regulation, uninhibited behavior, and low self-control (Eisenberg et al., 1999; Finkenauer, Engels, & Baumeister, 2005; Lengua & Kovacs, 2005; Shields & Cicchetti, 1998; Watson et al., 2004; Zhou, Eisenberg, Wang, & Reiser, 2004). These temperament characteristics were in turn uniquely associated with behavioral problems. On the other side of the coin, positive dimensions of parenting such as high acceptance-involvement and authoritative parenting were positively associated with self-control and effortful control, which in turn were linked with a reduced likelihood of negative social functioning (aggression and poor peer relations) and aggression (Finkenauer et al., 2005; Zhou et al., 2004). Notably, these studies provide evidence that parenting may shape facets of an emotionally dysregulated temperament, such as effortful control, proneness to irritability/frustration or fearfulness, but they do not speak as to whether the same is true for callous-unempathic characteristics. Since it is not clear whether it is possible to modify the problematic temperamental tendencies of callous-unempathic children through socialization, socialization agents instead may need to adopt strategies that compensate for or work around these temperamental limitations, as we discuss in greater detail below.

These findings are consistent with the contention of researchers that temperament is an open system subject to change (e.g., Rothbart & Bates, 2006), rather than being fixed or predetermined. Despite there being much theoretical agreement that temperament is malleable, the prospect of parenting exacerbating or reinforcing temperament characteristics is seldom studied (Lengua & Kovacs, 2005), and hence these results are quite notable.

Tailoring Educational Practices to Students' Temperament and Brain Function

Although existing research does not explicitly address the issue of temperament and aggression/bullying in a school context, the studies reviewed herein nonetheless have important implications for teachers dealing with bullying and disruptive behavior in their schools. The school is the setting in which the vast majority of bullying takes place, and moreover, processes relating to temperament and parenting may inform teachers since they too are important socializing agents. For example, teachers, like parents, may need to employ discipline strategies to manage student's behavior, and at the same time develop relationships with students as a means to engage, motivate, and maintain on-task and appropriate behavior.

Students with Emotionally Dysregulated Temperaments

The profile of individuals with emotionally dysregulated temperaments indicated by the research reviewed in this chapter suggests that certain strategies may be more effective for teachers working with these children. In summary, youngsters high in emotional dysregulation are prone to negative emotionality including irritability, frustration, anger, and fear due to the heightened sensitivity of the reward system that processes reward, positive affect, and frustration over blocked goals, and the system that governs fear responses to threatening or dangerous stimuli, in combination with poor effortful or cognitive control of those emotions due to limitations in prefrontal cortex functioning. Results from the empirical studies reviewed above indicated that emotionally dysregulated youngsters are susceptible to reactive aggression, and that they are at greater risk for behavioral problems than other children when they encounter harsh or ineffective forms of behavioral control (harsh or inconsistent discipline, physical punishment) or have relationships with parents characterized by insensitivity, hostility, dominance, negativity, attachment insecurity, or a lack of support. Additional evidence shows that emotionally dysregulated youngsters are likely to evoke negative parenting from parents. Moreover, negative parenting (e.g., inconsistent discipline, parental distress to child behavior, negative family functioning, authoritarian parenting, psychological control, and parental maltreatment) has been shown to exacerbate emotional dysregulation, whereas positive parenting with authoritative characteristics appears to improve self-control.

Taking these empirical findings and the temperamental profile of emotionally dysregulated children together, it appears that teachers may be able to make use of several strategies to better enable emotionally dysregulated children to exert cognitive control over their negative emotions and to reduce the negative emotionality itself through positive socialization. With regard to boosting effortful control over the behavioral expression of emotions, it is instructive to note that parenting characterized as authoritative or high in acceptance-involvement was associated with increased self-control. Some of the key elements of authoritative or highly involved parenting include good communication and the use of inductive discipline, which entails the use of reasoning and explanation to explain how others are affected by the child's inappropriate behavior (e.g., Gray & Steinberg, 1999). Teachers may take such an approach to dealing with behavioral infractions in the classroom or school yard, and in so doing, may give emotionally dysregulated children opportunities to reflect on how their emotional and behavioral outbursts affect other people. In other words, teachers may promote greater consideration of the negative consequences of emotionally volatile and reactively aggressive behavior, increasing the child's capacity to stop and think before acting out. Another quality of authoritative parenting is that children are granted an appropriate level of autonomy to make their own decisions and to solve their own problems, which in turn provides them with opportunities to learn how to regulate their own behavior rather than relying on the external regulation of adults (Gray & Steinberg, 1999). Teachers may facilitate such a process with emotionally dysregulated children as well, for example, by mediating conflict resolution between two students rather than dictating a solution, thereby helping to build self-regulation skills. Given their difficulties controlling emotions, it may be useful to enhance the self-regulation skills of emotionally dysregulated students by teaching self-instruction (e.g., counting to 10 before acting) or relaxation (e.g., deep breathing) techniques as a means to dampen emotional arousal, inhibit immediate, impulsive action, and to create space and time for more careful reflection.

Finally, it may be important for teachers to model appropriate self-control over their own emotions, given research showing a link between parental expression of distress to child behavior and decreased self-regulation abilities in children over time (Eisenberg et al., 1999). Further to this point, educators drawn into emotional or excessively punitive reactions by emotionally dysregulated students may precipitate an escalating exchange of aversive behavior. When teachers engage in a cycle of coercive behavior with these students, they may inadvertently reinforce inappropriate conduct, especially since they will likely have to back down to defuse the volatile confrontation. Indeed, the wisdom of exercising self-control in such situations is emphasized by research indicating children with emotionally dysregulated temperament features are more likely to exhibit behavioral problems when parents use heavy-handed tactics fraught with negative emotions to control their behavior, exemplified by maternal dominance and negativity or parental physical punishment (Paterson & Sanson, 1999; Rubin et al., 1998; 2003). Additional research by Bates et al. (1998) suggests that restricting inappropriate behavior through firm but unemotional admonitions may reduce problematic behavior effectively and prevent the escalation of coercive exchanges, which can unintentionally demonstrate that aggressive or bullying behavior can pay dividends.

To minimize emotionally dysregulated children's tendency toward negative emotionality, it may be helpful for teachers to avoid use of harsh, high-intensity behavior management strategies involving yelling, threatening, shaming, or guilt induction, in light of parenting research indicating that such control strategies tend to worsen the behavioral and emotional problems of emotionally dysregulated children. Instead, teachers may wish to employ more moderate behavior management strategies, such as privilege removal or inductive discipline, which provide consequences for inappropriate behavior that emphasize wrong doing, without overwhelming children who are prone to emotional reactivity. Because emotionally dysregulated children are temperamentally fearful, milder forms of behavior management should be sufficient to elicit an optimal level of anxiety in the face of these disciplinary encounters, which in turn should prompt attention to the moral message delivered by the teacher, and provide ample motivation for behavioral change (Kochanska, 1995). Consequently, higher intensity, more threatening forms of discipline would be unnecessary and likely counter productive. Putting such a practice into effect may be challenging, however, since research shows that irritable and unregulated children tend to evoke more punitive and inconsistent forms of discipline from parents (Eisenberg et al., 1999; Lengua & Kovacs, 2005), perhaps because their behavior can be unpredictable, disconcerting, and frustrating.

Emotional volatility may also be reduced through the cultivation of positive teacher–student relationships. As discussed earlier, emotionally dysregulated children seem to react more adversely to negative parent–child relationships than other children, being at heightened risk for behavioral problems in the face of hostility, insensitivity, detachment, controlling behavior, a lack of support, and insecure attachments. Speaking to negative emotionality more directly, increases in children's fearfulness have been shown to mediate or explain the positive association between negative family functioning and increased behavioral problems (Watson et al., 2004). Extrapolating from these results, it may be possible for teachers to lessen a child's emotional reactivity in the classroom, or at least not to aggravate the problem, by behaving in a kind, caring, warm, supportive, sensitive, and trustworthy manner with an emotionally dysregulated child. One strength of children with emotionally dysregulated characteristics is that they are not posited to have deficits in affiliativeness, and their being in the normal range with regard to warmth, friendliness, and sociability should aid teachers in their efforts to establish a positive relationship.

Students with Callous-Unempathic Characteristics

Teachers may need to address the bullying of callous-unempathic children using different levers. Recall that callous-unempathic characteristics included fearlessness, low interest in affiliation, and a lack of empathy or guilt. From the standpoint of neural models, the fearlessness, and to a certain extent the lack of empathy and guilt, stems from the Fight/Flight/Freeze system being relatively insensitive to cues of punishment, threat, or danger, such that in potentially threatening circumstances callous-unempathic children would have muted fear responses. Children with callous-unempathic characteristics appear more likely to be proactively aggressive, using aggression as a means to obtain instrumental and social rewards without regard for the victim's welfare. Although research addressing the parenting of youngsters with this temperamental profile is scant, one study indicated that a lack of parental support was more strongly linked with aggression when children were low in sociability, a key callous-unempathic characteristic (Carlo et al., 1998).

Considering all of these findings together, there would appear to be two major strategies that teachers could use to address the bullying of callous-unempathic students. First, it may be helpful for teachers to recognize that these youngsters may have difficulty feeling emotions that would normally motivate a person to inhibit an inappropriate action. For example, in light of having a relatively insensitive fear system, such students may be able to use physical intimidation to take money from another student, or to humiliate a weaker student on the playground, without feeling empathetic about the victim's distress, guilty about the behavior being wrong, or fearing possible punishments that might result, such as a school suspension or having privileges removed at home by parents. It is not clear from a theoretical or empirical standpoint what could be done to change the emotional experiences of callous-unempathic children, and thus it might be best for teachers to help them at a cognitive level, providing scaffolding to assist with the development of perspective taking or problem-solving skills, so that the child learns to exert cognitive control over harmful actions driven by the desire for tangible or instrumental rewards. In other words, the teacher may help a child to develop beliefs whereby he "knows" that a bullying behavior is wrong and harmful, even if he does not "feel" that this is so as other children do intuitively. To provide an example, teachers may try an approach akin to inductive discipline, using reasoning and explanation following a bullying incident to point out the negative consequences for the bully and the victim. This strategy may be coupled with a problem-solving exercise through which alternative solutions to a social problem might be identified, illuminating tactics that may accomplish a desired goal in a less harmful way. Current educational initiatives, such as "Character Education," may help in this regard as long as greater emphasis is given to enhancing cognitive control mechanisms (e.g., perspective taking) rather than taking an approach that relies solely on building moral emotional responses such as empathy and guilt. In working on the development of cognitive control in callous-unempathic children, teachers would be taking advantage of the fact that their effortful control capabilities are more or less normal, as they are not as impulsive as students with emotionally dysregulated temperaments. Speaking from the standpoint of neural models, the anterior attention system of callous-unempathic youngsters appears to be fully functional and can perhaps be recruited to exert cognitive control over aggressive behavior resulting from the weak inhibitory role played by the Fight/Flight/Fear system, centered in the subcortical, limbic, and brainstem regions of the brain.

From the point of view of behavior management in the classroom and on the playground, harsh, high-intensity strategies such as yelling, threatening (i.e., harsh discipline), shaming, and guilt induction (i.e., psychological control) are unlikely to be effective, since callous-unempathic children are relatively fearless and less sensitive to punishment. However, on a more positive note, the dopaminergic pathways underlying the neural systems that process reward and positive affect (e.g., Behavior Activation System) appear to function normally in these youngsters and this may provide teachers with a mechanism for motivating appropriate behavior. Specifically, students with callous-unempathic characteristics may not inhibit inappropriate behavior out of fear of punishment, but they may activate appropriate actions to please the teacher, if they find the relationship with that teacher to be rewarding and positive. Thus, developing a mutually positive relationship with such students may provide a foundation for mutually respectful behavior. This possibility is consistent with the aforementioned finding that children with callous-unempathic characteristics are less likely to be aggressive or to engage in antisocial behavior when they have a supportive relationship with their parents (Carlo et al., 1998).

Conclusion

School bullying remains a serious problem for educators, but recent research, reviewed in the foregoing chapter, has suggested that its etiology and prevention may be better understood through careful consideration of the different pathways toward aggression and bullying that may be taken by children with emotionally dysregulated and callous-unempathic temperaments. Looking at the bigger picture, we hope that this chapter illustrates how individual differences in brain function and structure may affect students' psychosocial and behavioral adjustment in the school setting, and how educators may capitalize on this knowledge to tailor educational programs and their personal interactions with these children to best meet the particular needs of each student. It is our hope that the foregoing chapter embodies Robbie Case's multidisciplinary approach to the study of children, in that we tried to integrate elements of diverse areas of theory and research, including neuropsychology, developmental psychology, psychopathology, and education. Perhaps the synthesis of these broad areas of research, and the subsequent application of these ideas to educational practice, will in some small way facilitate the socialization and education of children, particularly those whose temperaments present challenges to parents and educators.

Acknowledgment The preparation of this manuscript was supported, in part, by a grant from the Social Sciences and Humanities Research Council of Canada to The Youth Lifestyle Choices Community-University Research Alliance (YLC-CURA). We gratefully acknowledge the support we received from Teena Willoughby and Heather Chalmers, co-directors of the YLC-CURA.

References

Barnow, S., Lucht, M., & Freyberger, H. J. (2005). Correlates of aggressive and delinquent conduct problems in adolescence. *Aggressive Behavior, 31*(1), 24–39.

Barry, T. D., Thompson, A. R., Barry, C. T., Lochman, J. E., Adler, K., & Hill, K. R. (2007). The importance of narcissism in predicting proactive and reactive aggression in moderately to highly aggressive children. *Aggressive Behavior, 33*, 185–197.

Bates, J. E., Pettit, G. S., Dodge, K. A., & Ridge, B. (1998). Interaction of temperamental resistance to control and restrictive parenting in the development of externalizing behavior. *Developmental Psychology, 34*, 982–995.

Belsky, J., Hsieh, K., & Crnic, K. (1998). Mothering, fathering, and infant negativity as antecedents of boys' externalizing problems and inhibition at age 3 years: Differential susceptibility to rearing experience. *Development and Psychopathology, 10*, 301–319.

Bjornebekk, G. (2007). Dispositions related to sensitivity in the neurological basis for activation of approach-avoidance motivation, antisocial attributes and individual differences in aggressive behavior. *Social Behavior and Personality: An International Journal, 35*, 1251–1263.

Burgess, K. B., Marshall, P. J., Rubin, K. H., & Fox, N. A. (2003). Infant attachment and temperament as predictors of subsequent externalizing problems and cardiac physiology. *Journal of Child Psychology and Psychiatry, 44*, 819–831.

Camodeca, M., Goossens, F. A., Terwogt, M., & Schuengel, C. (2002). Bullying and victimization among school-age children: Stability and links to proactive and reactive aggression. *Social Development, 11*, 332–345.

Carlo, G., Roesch, S. C., & Melby, J. (1998). The multiplicative relations of parenting and temperament to prosocial and antisocial behaviors in adolescence. *Journal of Early Adolescence, 18*, 266–290.

Coie, J. D., Dodge, K. A., & Kupersmidt, J. B. (1990). Peer group behavior and social status. In S. R. Asher & J. D. Coie (Eds.), *Peer rejection in childhood: Cambridge studies in social and emotional development* (pp. 17–59). New York: Cambridge University Press.

Colder, C. R., Lochman, J. E., & Wells, K. C. (1997). The moderating effects of children's fear and activity level on relations between parenting practices and childhood symptomatology. *Journal of Abnormal Child Psychology, 25*, 251–263.

Collins, W. A., Maccoby, E. E., Steinberg, L., Hetherington, E. M., & Bornstein, M. H. (2000). Contemporary research on parenting: The case for nature and nurture. *American Psychologist, 55*, 218–232.

Craig, W. (1998). The relationship among bullying, victimization, depression, anxiety and aggression in elementary school children. *Personality and Individual Differences, 24*, 123–130.

Crick, N. R., & Dodge, K. A. (1996). Social information-processing mechanisms in reactive and proactive aggression. *Child Development, 67*, 993–1002.

Cummings, M. E., Davies, P. T., & Campbell, S. B. (2000). *Developmental psychopathology and family process: Theory, research, and clinical applications*. New York: Guilford.

Derryberry, D., & Rothbart, M. K. (1997). Reactive and effortful processes in the organization of temperament. *Development and Psychopathology, 9*, 633–652.

Derryberry, D., & Rothbart, M. K. (2001). Early temperament and emotional development. In A. F. Kalverboer & A. Gramsbergen (Eds.), *Brain and behavior in early development* (pp. 967–990). Dordrecht, The Netherlands: Kluwer Academic Publications.

Dodge, K. A., & Coie, J. D. (1987). Social-information-processing factors in reactive and proactive aggression in children's peer groups. *Journal of Personality and Social Psychology, 53*, 1146–1158.

Dodge, K. A., & Pettit, G. S. (2003). A biopsychosocial model of the development of chronic conduct problems in adolescence. *Developmental Psychology, 39*, 349–371.

Depue, R. A., & Iacono, W. G. (1989). Neurobehavioral aspects of affective disorders. *Annual Review of Psychology, 40*, 457–492.

Eisenberg, N., Fabes, R. A., Shepard, S. A., Guthrie, I. K., Murphy, B. C., & Reiser, M. (1999). Parental reactions to children's negative emotions: Longitudinal relations to quality of children's social functioning. *Child Development, 70*, 513–534.

Farrington, D. P. (1993). Understanding and preventing bullying. In M. Tonry (Ed.), *Crime and justice* (Vol. 17, pp. 381–458). Chicago, IL: University of Chicago.

Finkenauer, C., Engels, R., & Baumeister, R. (2005). Parenting behavior and adolescent behavioral and emotional problems: The role of self-control. *International Journal of Behavioral Development, 29*, 58–69.

Frick, P. J., & Morris, A. S. (2004). Temperament and developmental pathways to conduct problems. *Journal of Clinical Child and Adolescent Psychology, 33*, 54–68.

Giancola, P. R., & Parker, A. M. (2001). A six-year prospective study of pathways toward drug use in adolescent boys with and without a family history of a substance use disorder. *Journal of Studies on Alcohol, 62*, 166–178.

Goldsmith, H. H., Buss, A. H., Plomin, R., Rothbart, M. K., Thomas, A., Chess, S., et al. (1987). Roundtable: What is temperament? Four approaches. *Child Development, 58*, 505–529.

Gray, J. A. (1991). The neuropsychology of temperament. In J. Strelau & A. Angleitner (Eds.), *Explorations in temperament: International perspectives on theory and measurement*. New York: Plenum Press.

Gray, J. A., & McNaughton, N. (2000). *The neuropsychology of anxiety*. Oxford, UK: Oxford University Press.

Gray, M. R., & Steinberg, L. (1999). Unpacking authoritative parenting: Reassessing a multidimensional construct. *Journal of Marriage and the Family, 61*, 574–587.

Grills, A. E., & Ollendick, T. H. (2002). Peer victimization, global self-worth, and anxiety in middle school children. *Journal of Clinical Child and Adolescent Psychology, 31*, 59–68.

Haynie, D. L., Nansel, T., Eitel, P., Crump, A. D., Saylor, K., Yu, K., et al. (2001). Bullies, victims, and bully/victims: Distinct groups of at-risk youth. *Journal of Early Adolescence, 21*, 29–49.

Hess, L. E., & Atkins, M. S. (1998). Victims and aggressors at school: Teacher, self, and peer perceptions of psychosocial functioning. *Applied Developmental Science, 2*, 75–89.

Kagan, J. (1998). Biology and the child. In W. Damon (Ed.), *Handbook of child psychology:* (5th ed., Vol. 3, pp. 177–235). New York: Wiley.
Kimonis, E. R., Frick, P. J., Fazekas, H., & Loney, B. R. (2006). Psychopathy, aggression, and the processing of emotional stimuli in non-referred girls and boys. *Behavioral Sciences & the Law, 24*, 21–37.
Kochanska, G. (1995). Children's temperament, mothers' discipline, and security of attachment: Multiple pathways to emerging internalization. *Child Development, 66*, 597–615.
Lengua, L. J., & Kovacs, E. A. (2005). Bidirectional associations between temperament and parenting and the prediction of adjustment problems in middle childhood. *Journal of Applied Developmental Psychology, 26*, 21–38.
Lengua, L. J., Wolchik, S. A., Sandler, I. N., & West, S. G. (2000). The additive and interactive effects of temperament and parenting in predicting adjustment problems of children of divorce. *Journal of Clinical Child Psychology, 29*, 232–244.
Leve, L. D., Kim, H. K., & Pears, K. C (2005). Childhood temperament and family environment as predictors of internalizing and externalizing trajectories from ages 5–17. *Journal of Abnormal Child Psychology, 33*, 505–520.
Little, T. D., Brauner, J., Jones, S. M., Nock, M. K., & Hawley, P. H. (2003). Rethinking aggression: A typological examination of the functions of aggression. *Merrill-Palmer Quarterly. Special Issue: Aggression and Adaptive Functioning: The Bright Side to Bad Behavior, 49*(3), 343–369.
Loeber, R., Green, S. M., Lahey, B. B., & Kalb, L. (2000). Physical fighting in childhood as a risk factor for later mental health problems. *Journal of the American Academy of Child and Adolescent Psychiatry, 39*, 421–428.
Marini, Z. A., Dane, A., Bosacki, S., & CURA-YLC. (2006). Direct and indirect bully-victims: Differential psychosocial risk factors associated with adolescents involved in bullying and victimization. *Aggressive Behavior, 32*, 551–569.
Marini, Z. A., Koruna, B., & Dane, A. (2006). Individualized interventions for ESL students involved in bullying and victimization. *Contact,* (Spring Issue), 1–15.
Marini, Z. A., McWhinnie, M., & Lacharite, M. (2004). Preventing school bullying: Identification and intervention involving bystanders. *Teaching and Learning, 1*, 17–21.
McNaughton, N. (2006). The role of the subiculum within the behavioral inhibition system. *Behavioral Brain Research, 174*, 232–250.
McNaughton, N., & Corr, P. J. (2004). A two-dimensional neuropsychology of defense: Fear/anxiety and defensive distance. *Neuroscience and Biobehavioral Reviews, 28*, 285–305.
Moffitt, T. E., Caspi, A., Harrington, H., & Milne, B. J. (2002). Males on the life-course-persistent and adolescence-limited antisocial pathways: Follow-up at age 26 years. *Development and Psychopathology, 14*, 179–207.
Morris, A. S., Silk, J. S., Steinberg, L., Sessa, F. M., Avenevoli, S., & Essex, M. J. (2002). Temperamental vulnerability and negative parenting as interacting predictors of child adjustment. *Journal of Marriage and Family, 64*, 461–471.
Nansel, T. R., Overpeck, M., Pilla, R. S., Ruan, W. J., Simons-Morton, B., & Scheidt, P. (2001). Bullying behaviors among US youth: Prevalence and association with psychosocial adjustment. *JAMA: Journal of the American Medical Association, 285*, 2094–2100.
Nigg, J. T. (2006). Temperament and developmental psychopathology. *Journal of Child Psychology and Psychiatry, 47*, 395–422.
Nucci, L. (2006). Education for moral development. In M. Killen & J. Smetana (Eds.), *Handbook of moral development* (pp. 657–681). Mahwah, NJ: Lawrence Erlbaum.
Olweus, D. (2001). Olweus' core program against bullying and antisocial behavior: A teacher handbook. Bergen, Norway: Author.
Ortiz, M. A. C., & Gandara, V. D. B. (2006). Studies on the relation between temperament, aggression, and anger, in children. *Aggressive Behavior, 32*, 207–215.
Panskepp, J. (1986). The neurochemistry of behavior. *Annual Review of Psychology, 37*, 77–107.

Panskepp, J. (1993). Neurochemical control of moods and emotions: Amino acids to neuropeptides. In M. Lewis & J. M. Haviland (Eds.), *Handbook of emotions* (pp. 87–107). New York: Guilford Press.

Panksepp, J. (1998). *Affective neuroscience: The foundations of human and animal emotions*. New York: Oxford University Press.

Paterson, G., & Sanson, A. (1999). The association of behavioral adjustment to temperament, parenting and family characteristics among 5-year-old children. *Social Development, 8*, 293–309.

Pellegrini, A. D., & Bartini, M. (2000). A longitudinal study of bullying, victimization, and peer affiliation during the transition from primary school to middle school. *American Educational Research Journal, 37*(3), 699–725.

Pellegrini, A. D., Bartini, M., & Brooks, F. (1999). School bullies, victims, and aggressive victims: Factors relating to group affiliation and victimization in early adolescence. *Journal of Educational Psychology, 91*, 216–224.

Pepler, D., Jiang, D., Craig, W., & Connolly, J. (2008). Developing trajectories of bullying and associated factors. *Child Development, 79*, 325–338.

Posner, M. I., & Rothbart, M. K. (2007). Research on attention networks as a model for the integration psychological science. *Annual Review of Psychology, 58*, 1–23.

Posner, M. I., Rothbart, M. K., Sheese, B. E., & Tang, Y. (2007). The anterior cingulate gyrus and the mechanism of self-regulation. *Cognitive, Affective, and Behavioral Neuroscience, 7*(4), 391–395.

Poulin, F., & Boivin, M. (2000). Reactive and proactive aggression: Evidence of a two-factor model. *Psychological Assessment, 12* (2), 115–122.

Pulkkinen, L. (1996). Proactive and reactive aggression in early adolescence as precursors to anti- and prosocial behavior in young adults. *Aggressive Behavior, 22*, 241–257.

Putnam, S. P., Ellis, L. K., & Rothbart, M. K. (2002). The structure of temperament from infancy through adolescence. In A. Eliasz & A. Angleitner (Eds.), *Advances in research on temperament* (pp. 165–182). Lengerich, Germany: Pabst Science.

Raine, A., Reynolds, C., Venables, P. H., Medrick, S. A., & Farrington, D. P. (1998). Fearlessness, stimulation-seeking, and large body size at age 3 years as early predispositions to childhood aggression at age 11 years. *Archives of General Psychiatry, 55*, 745–751.

Raine, A., Dodge, K., Loeber, R., Gatzke-Kopp, L., Lynam, D., Reynolds, C., et al. (2006). The reactive-proactive aggression questionnaire: Differential correlates of reactive and proactive aggression in adolescent boys. *Aggressive Behavior, 32*, 159–171.

Rigby, K. (2001). Health consequences of bullying and its prevention in schools. In J. Juvonen & S. Graham (Eds.), *Peer harassment in school: The plight of the vulnerable and victimized* (pp. 310–331). New York: Guilford.

Rothbart, M. K., Ahadi, S. A., & Evans, D. E. (2000). Temperament and personality: Origins and outcomes. *Journal of Personality and Social Psychology, 78*, 122–135.

Rothbart, M. K., & Bates, J. E. (2006). Temperament. In N. Eisenberg (Ed.), *Handbook of child psychology: Vol. 3. Social, emotional, and personality development.* (6th ed., pp. 99–166). New York: Wiley.

Rothbart, M. K., & Posner, M. I. (2006). Temperament, attention, and developmental psychopathology. In D. Cicchetti & D. J. Cohen (Eds.), *Developmental psychopathology: Vol 2. Developmental neuroscience* (2nd ed., pp. 465–501). Hoboken, NJ: Wiley.

Rubin, K. H., Burgess, K. B., Dwyer, K. M., & Hastings, P. D. (2003). Predicting preschoolers' externalizing behaviors from toddler temperament, conflict, and maternal negativity. *Developmental Psychology, 39*, 164–176.

Rubin, K. H., Hastings, P., Chen, X., Stewart, S., & McNichol, K. (1998). Intrapersonal and maternal correlates of aggression, conflict, and externalizing problems in toddlers. *Child Development, 69*, 1614–1629.

Rutter, M. (1997). Nature-nurture integration: The example of antisocial behavior. *American Psychologist, 52*, 390–398.

Salmivalli, C., Kaukiainen, A., Voeten, M., & Sinisammal, M. (2004).Targeting the group as a whole: The Finnish anti-bullying intervention. In P. K. Smith, D. Pepler, & K. Rigby (Eds.), *Bullying in schools: How successful can interventions be?* (pp. 251–273). Cambridge, UK: Cambridge University Press.

Salmivalli, C., & Nieminen, E. (2002). Proactive and reactive aggression in bullies, victims, and bully-victims. *Aggressive Behavior, 28*, 30–44.

Schmidt, L. A., Fox, N. A., Rubin, K. H., Hu, S., & Hamer, D. H. (2002). Molecular genetics of shyness and aggression in preschoolers. *Personality and Individual Differences, 33*, 227–238.

Schwartz, D., Proctor, L. J., & Chien, D. H. (2001). The aggressive victim of bullying: Emotional and behavioral dysregulation as a pathway to victimization by peers. In J. Juvonen & S. Graham (Eds.), *Peer harassment in school: The plight of the vulnerable and victimized* (pp. 147–174). New York: Guilford.

Shields, A., & Cicchetti, D. (1998). Reactive aggression among maltreated children: The contributions of attention and emotion dysregulation. *Journal of Clinical Child Psychology, 27*, 381–395.

Smillie, L. D. (2008). What is reinforcement sensitivity? Neuroscience paradigms for approach-avoidance process theories of personality. *European Journal of Personality, 22*, 359–384.

Smith, J. D., Stewart, R., & Cousins, B. (2004). Anti-bullying interventions: A survey of Ontario schools. *Canadian Association of Principals Journal, 12*(1), 9–11.

Smith, P. K., Pepler, D., & Rigby K. (Eds.). (2004). *Bullying in schools: How successful can interventions be?* Cambridge, MA: Cambridge University Press.

Unnever, J. D. (2005). Bullies, aggressive victims, and victims: Are they distinct groups? *Aggressive Behavior, 31*, 153–171.

van Aken, C., Junger, M., Verhoeven, M., van Aken, M. A. G., & Dekovic, M. (2007). The interactive effects of temperament and maternal parenting on toddlers′ externalizing behaviours. *Infant and Child Development, 16*, 553–572.

Vitaro, F., Barker, E. D., Boivin, M., Brendgen, M., & Tremblay, R. E. (2006). Do early difficult temperament and harsh parenting differentially predict reactive and proactive aggression? *Journal of Abnormal Child Psychology, 34*, 685–695.

Vitaro, F., Brendgen, M., & Tremblay, R. E. (2002). Reactively and proactively aggressive children: Antecedent and subsequent characteristics. *Journal of Child Psychology and Psychiatry, 43*, 495–506.

Watson, M. W., Fischer, K. W., Andreas, J. B., & Smith, K. W. (2004). Pathways to aggression in children and adolescents. *Harvard Educational Review, 74*, 404–430.

Zhou, Q., Eisenberg, N., Wang, Y., & Reiser, M. (2004). Chinese children's effortful control and dispositional anger/frustration: Relations to *parenting* styles and children's social functioning. *Developmental Psychology, 40*, 352–366.

The Intentional Personal Development of Mind and Brain Through Education

Michel Ferrari and Ljiljana Vuletic

Our particular focus in this chapter is on the intentional development of oneself as a person, and how this relates to both brain and education. In this we aim to promote a person-centered developmental science such as Bronfenbrenner and Morris (2006), Magnusson and Stattin (2006) and Rathunde and Csikszentmihalyi (2006) have recently called for, one that has long-standing roots in psychology (Rogers, 1961). Developing individual persons are often trichotomized into the following: (1) a biological body (including especially its *brain*) and its physical environment; (2) a biological body and an experiencing self (conscious and unconscious *mind*); and (3) an experiencing self and other selves (sociocultural or symbolic environment) that has its own institutions and practices (including *educational* institutions and practices). These divisions are conceptually rich, but we argue they are best understood in a way that is emergent and relational. In other words, because persons are at once biological, social, and cultural actors, considering the development of "personal selves" allows us to span this Cartesian divide between mind, body, self and environment, inherited from the 19th century, that still haunts developmental psychology. Furthermore, it allows us to address an issue often sidelined: how people make deliberate efforts to develop themselves in ways that are personally meaningful to them (see also Blasi, 2004 and Foucault, 1994, 2004).

The developmental relations between mind, brain, and education are a particularly fruitful framework for understanding personal development; however, this ambitious task is fraught with problems. Let's lay out the problems before us:

1. What it means to be and become a person and how this relates to notions of self-identity.
2. The place of autonomy and intentionality in personal development.
3. Relation of mind, brain, and education to intentional personal development.

M. Ferrari (✉)
Department of Human Development and Applied Psychology, Ontario Institute for Studies in Education, University of Toronto, Toronto, ON, Canada
e-mail: mferrari@oise.utoronto.ca

M. Ferrari, L. Vuletic (eds.), *The Developmental Relations among Mind, Brain and Education*, DOI 10.1007/978-90-481-3666-7_13, © Springer Science+Business Media B.V. 2010

One might despair of making any headway with such a list, and this chapter just sketches out a few suggestions of promising directions that integrate the work of Francesco Varela, Antonio Damasio, Paul Ricoeur, and Jochen Brandtstädter.

Being and Becoming a Person

Before we begin, it is important to consider what we mean by a person and how this relates to the notion of self. These concepts have a rich and linked history in philosophy, linguistics, and the law, as one can see by consulting the Oxford English Dictionary entry for person. Among the principal meanings of concern to us in this context are the following:

1. In *grammar*, person is a category used to classify pronouns, possessive determiners, and verb forms: More specifically, person is used to denote whether one indicates the speaker (first person), the addressee (second person), or someone or something spoken of (third person). As we will see, this is important to the work of theorists like Rom Harré and Paul Ricoeur, in particular to the relation between the self and the other in personal development.
2. In a general *philosophical* sense, a person is a conscious or rational being; that is, an individual human being, as distinguished from another kind of animal or thing.[1] In this sense, a human person is characterized in part by their neurobiology. More specifically, the term person refers to the self, or individual personality, as distinct from their occupation or created works. In this chapter, self and person will be considered synonyms—although self is perhaps more closely identified with the psychological experience of being an individual actor, while person often refers to the sociocultural aspect of identity.
3. Person also refers to individuals considered with regard to their outward appearance, or to a social or cultural *role or character* assumed in real life or in a literary narrative. Carl Jung (1953) contrasted *persona* (the social masks we don to hide our true self) with anima or *soul* (the authentic desires and possibilities we find socially difficult to express). Erwin Goffman (1959) developed an entire dramaturgical theory of self, in which people compete to assume roles that they believe have the greatest advantage. This notion of character or role relates to the legal sense of the term person, in which a person—whether an individual (i.e., a natural person) or corporate body (artificial person)—is recognized as having certain rights and duties; artificial persons are beyond the scope of our chapter.

---

[1] For Locke (1690/1997), a person "is a thinking intelligent Being, that has reason and reflection, and can consider itself as itself, the same thinking thing in different times and places; which it does only by that consciousness, which is inseparable from thinking, and as it seems to me essential to it." [*Essay* II xxvii 9]

For Mihaly Csikszentmihalyi and Kevin Rathunde (1998), persons are not born but made through their cultural participation. They propose six features of personal development that are particularly important:

1. being healthy and fit of body;
2. sustaining an alert, active, and open mind, and an interest in life;
3. having and sustaining a vocation or other meaningful social roles;
4. sustaining and nurturing relationships with family and friends;
5. involvement in one's community; and
6. gaining wisdom, defined as holistic thinking that discerns the essence of problems; an equanimity that accepts oneself and the world; an ability to act gladly to do one's part for the common good, or as Baltes and colleagues say, an expertise in the "fundamental pragmatics of life" (Ardelt, 2004; Baltes & Smith, 2008; Baltes & Staudinger, 2000).

While these six points are important, we believe this list is incomplete because it fails to include one's efforts to intentionally develop oneself into a particular kind of person, in particular a good person. As Taylor (1989) proposes:

> We are selves only in that certain issues matter for us. What I am as a self, my identity, is essentially defined by the way things have significance for me.[. . .] To ask what a person is, in abstraction from his or her self-interpretations, is to ask a fundamentally misguided question, one to which there couldn't in principle be an answer.[. . .] We are not selves in the way that we are organisms, or we don't have selves in the way that we have hearts and livers. We are living beings with these organs quite independently of our self-understandings or -interpretations, or the meaning things have for us. But we are only selves insofar as we move in a certain space of questions, as we seek and find an orientation to the good. (p. 34)

What is appealing about the concept of person, then, is that it spans biological, experiential, and cultural senses of human self and identity and promises to allow us to bridge very different discourses about these various aspects of human life. This, in turn, will allow a way to overcome a long-standing problem—some have called it a crisis—that dates to the very origins of psychology as a science.

An Enduring Crisis in the Scientific Study of Psychology

When Wundt (1863) founded psychology as a discipline in the late 19th century, he immediately identified a problem for the emerging field—namely, that two quite separate aspects of psychology need to be addressed by this science. On the one hand, psychology is an extension of biology and physiology, and the task of a science of psychology is to explain how the human body can have various psychological functions, such as perception, rationality, consciousness, and other capacities that connect and distinguish us from other living things. On the other hand, psychology must also explain how people come to have a personal identity within the cultural, social, and historical context into which they are born as infants and to which they contribute as adults; this second sort of psychology requires an understanding of cognitive science as it relates to language and education—both informal education, and formal education as mandated within cultural institutions designed to educate children or adults in special skills. Wundt called the first kind of science "physiological psychology" (Wundt, 1911) and the second "cultural psychology" (*Völkerpsychologie*) (Wundt, 1900–1920). He believed that each required its own distinct methods of investigation, but did not build a clear bridge between them. The only proposal he advanced was to consider spoken language as a personal expression of historically developing cultural laws, myths, and customs, but their specific link (e.g., through autobiographical narratives) was never formally studied.

Over the years, others have continued to point to this crisis in the science of psychology (Snow, 1959, 1964; Vygotsky, 1927). Most notably, Vygotsky (1927) considered the split between physiological and cultural psychology to be the defining crisis in psychology. His efforts to resolve this crisis led him to propose that personal development requires mastery of cultural symbol systems (e.g., language) that generate higher mental functions (such as higher memory or higher attention) by building on and transforming our basic biological capacities. For Vygotsky, education in the use of such cultural tools was essential to becoming fully human. Piaget's (1968/1995) sociological writings and those on education (Piaget, 1998) make a very similar point, adding that such social interactions must allow individuals to develop increasingly complex and coherent cognitive structures that make sense of the world.

These points are not merely of historical interest. Neo-Piagetians like Robbie Case and Kurt Fischer (whose work in many ways bridges the ideas of Vygotsky and Piaget) have refined earlier insights noting that Central Conceptual Structures (Case, 1992, 1998) or Skills (Fischer & Bidell, 2006) emerge out of personal efforts to master knowledge domains developed within a particular subculture, with more or less support from significant social others. But neo-Piagetian theories do not build a bridge from neuroscience all the way to the humanities as Wundt and Vygotsky had hoped, and in considering developmental relations between brain, mind, and education today, we find that the crisis in psychology still endures—as seen in the debate between Jean-Pierre Changeux and Paul Ricoeur (1998/2000) that could as easily be held today. As Ricoeur points out in this debate, the difficult task is to create a "third discourse," in which biological, phenomenological, and cultural aspects of human experience are integrated (and not merely correlated). Ricoeur doubted such a discourse was even possible, but we believe that the most promising example of a third discourse is the enactive approach championed by Maturana and Varela and their colleagues.

Experienced Bodies and Their Physical and Symbolic Environment

The enactive approach is a contemporary effort to bridge this divide between biology and culture in a way that also integrates the phenomenology of personal experience, as well articulated in the work of Maturana and Varela (1980, 1992; Varela,

1987, 1992/1999) and Thompson (2007; see also Varela, Thompson & Rosch, 1991). The enactive approach acknowledges Piagetian genetic epistemology as a direct predecessor (Varela et al., 1991, Chapter 1), and so it is easy to imagine it would have been of interest to Robbie Case, who was master at synthesizing various competing approaches to developmental psychology (see Case, 1998, for example).

According to the enactive approach, autonomy is integral to life from its earliest and most basic forms. In their remarkable book, *The Tree of Knowledge,* Maturana and Varela (1992) illustrate the importance of considering the relation between brain and mind—and more generally between biology and knowing—as a circle rather than as a line (an approach also adopted by Piaget). In this way, Maturana and Varela propose to resolve the crisis in psychology that dates back to Wundt's original division of psychology into physiological psychology and *Völkerpsychologie*. (How the circle between the individual knower and his symbolic environment involves education is shown later in this chapter.)

The idea that there is a circle between biology and knowing is motivated by certain experiences that are clearly explained by our biological history. For example, Maturana and Varela (1992) begin their book by allowing the reader to personally experience colored shadows and how our visual blind spot is filled in, such that we have no perception of it without special effort such as they propose. The point of staging these first-person conscious experiences is to show unequivocally that our experience is bound to our biological structure, such that "we live our field of vision [and] our chromatic space" (p. 23). This leads to the further point that we cannot separate the history of our biological and social actions from how the world appears to us (a point also made by Lewin (1939)). Facts are not independently "out there" in the world and then represented internally "in our brain," rather they are meanings that emerge from our human interaction with the world that has both an evolutionary and a personal history. They make the strong claim that "every act of knowing brings forth a world" (p. 26) summed up by the following aphorisms: (1) "All doing is knowing, and all knowing is doing" (p. 26) and (2) "Everything said is said by someone" (p. 26).

The *validity* of this is shown by considering the very origins of life on earth, as it emerged from the world before life existed. Most particularly, we recognize living things by a particular kind of organization they exhibit. Maturana and Varela (1992) propose that what characterizes living things is that they are literally "self-producing," or as they put it, "the organization that defines them [is] an autopoietic organization" (p. 43), something that is true of all living things from single-celled organisms to multicellular organisms like human beings. The defining feature of an autopoietic organization is that the system is involved in "a network of dynamic transformations that produces its own components and that is essential for a boundary [itself] essential for the operation of the network of transformations that produce it as a[n autonomous] unity" (p. 46). In this sense, organisms specify their own laws proper to their functioning (and in so doing call forth an environment).[2]

---

[2]Thus, to speak of individual, we need to identify both (1) what remains invariant in their organization and (2) what structural changes they undergo, to sustain that organization. In the most basic

For Maturana and Varela, the history of life on earth is the history of autopoietic forms that have descended throughout their histories with modification that allowed structural change without loss of unity, but also provided new possibilities of coupling with their environment—a structural drift that resembles natural selection, but is better thought of as co-creation of self and environment. Individuals are distinct from their environment, but the very distinction defines both the organism and its environment.

What this framework highlights is that, for all biological systems with an autonomous identity, interactions with the environment are perceived as perturbations for which the system must compensate by changing its structure to preserve its identity (if severe enough, perturbations can destroy it). The entire developmental history of the organism is the history of these environmental couplings—not merely its own, but those of its historical lineage. Each such history is unique and not predetermined; rather it is the active expression of individual behavior that acts to preserve and enhance its own identity. For Varela (1987), the history of these environmental couplings is an internal project that the system manifests in light of environmental perturbations it encounters—perturbations it also provokes. In this light, it is important to distinguish between determinism and predictability. Living beings always function in their structural present because of their structural coupling, itself a result of their biological and individual history; in the present moment they have a range of options allowed by this history. Thus, representation is the wrong metaphorical model; rather it is better to think of skilled behavior. The nervous system expands the range of interactions of an organism by coupling its sensory and motor surfaces through a network of neurons—most particularly, in humans, the brain.[3] "The nervous system, therefore, by its very architecture does not violate but enriches the operational closure that defines the autonomous nature of the living being" (p. 166). By its very plasticity, the nervous system (through its sensory and motor organs) participates in the structural drift of the organism in ways that help conserve its structure. An organism's range of possible behaviors is determined by its structure, both innate and as acquired through learning, at the most fundamental level.

---

sense, living things are characterized by their organization, not their specific structure. According to Varela (1987), the minimal organization required to create and sustain life is already seen in the way cells produce themselves through a network of processes that loop back on themselves, producing the very components that generate a distinct separate unit from the environmental background. A living system must thus have two properties that act together: (1) a network of processes that create and destroy its components, which in turn continually regenerate that network, (2) and a structural barrier consisting of elements created by the network that make possible the network's own operation. In other words, to maintain their autonomy from the environment, individuals actively strive to create and recreate themselves. Thus, for Varela, the mechanism that characterizes living individuals (from the simplest cell to animals, including human beings) is a particular organization by which they produce themselves, for which Maturana and Varela coined the Greek term, *autopoiesis*.

[3] In human beings, 100 billion interneurons connect 1 million motor neurons (connected to a few thousand muscles) to 10 million sensory cells; some respond to stimulation within the system and others to stimulation outside of it (Maturana & Varela, 1987/1992, p. 159).

Social phenomena arise spontaneously in what Maturana and Varela (1992) call "third order couplings" that create social systems.[4] In this view, communication most fundamentally allows coordinated behavior that is mutually triggered in members of any such social system—whether insect or human—such that it acts like a new unity.[5]

Human linguistic activity in particular is central to the operation of the human social system. Language appears when operations appear in the linguistic domain that result in the coordination of actions that pertain to the linguistic domain itself; thus, as languages arise, so do objects that reflect "linguistic distinctions of linguistic distinctions" (Maturana and Varela, 1992, p. 210).[6]

In this sense, language is reflexive, allowing the emergence of new phenomena such as psychological reflection and consciousness. In other words, language enables those who speak it to describe themselves and their circumstances through "linguistic distinction of linguistic distinctions" (Maturana & Varela, 1992). According to Maturana and Varela, with the emergence of linguistic distinctions there also arises ability to distinguish oneself and others linguistically as languaging entities by virtue of participating in the linguistic domain. Furthermore, recurrent individual interactions that linguistically personalize other individuals (e.g., by identifying them by name), may allow the emergence of the notion of self—a point further articulated by Paul Ricoeur (1992). All of this suggests to Maturana and Varela (1992), that

> It is in language that the self, the I, arises as the social singularity defined by the operational intersection in the human body of the recursive linguistic distinction in which it is distinguished. This tells us that in the network of linguistic interactions in which we move, *we maintain an ongoing descriptive recursion which we call the "I". It enables us to conserve our linguistic operational coherence and our adaptation in the domain of language* (p. 231; italics in the original)

Thus, the conscious mind and the self are better thought of as belonging to a realm of social coupling than as residing within an individual brain: "it is by languaging that the act of knowing [...] brings forth a world [...] because we are constituted in language in a continuous becoming that we bring forth with others" (Maturana and Varela, 1992, pp. 234–235); for Maturana and Varela social coupling

---

[4]No mention is made of coupling with artifacts and tools, but we believe that Maturana and Varela might agree with Latour (1999) in proposing that these artifacts themselves become actors (albeit, not conscious actors) in these systems.

[5]Components of higher-order unities can themselves have various degrees of autonomy. Thus, the individual cells of organisms, once fully developed, have only a limited degree of autonomy, whereas the human beings considered as components of society have much greater degree of autonomy (they have more degrees of interdependent existence outside their roles in particular social systems).

[6]While linguistic behavior is acquired ontogenetically through dynamic interaction within a linguistic community, Maturana and Varela call this cultural behavior when it remains stable across generations. Specific linguistic domains arise as a cultural drift within linguistic communities, without pre-established design (e.g., German *Tafel* —> French *Table*—>English *Table* [pronounced with harder "a"]).

supports (even compels) an ethics of mutual love and charity, in the hope of creating a world that we all can share and enjoy together, rather than fight over whose ideology or worldview is true.

Thus, in the more complex case of human experience, our environment involves both physical and personal and autopoiesis. Personal autopoiesis involves determining how best to live a good life, in which one can flourish both biologically and personally as a member of one's cultural community (Brandtstädter, 2006). Indeed, as the original Greek term implied, personal autopoiesis involves intentionally crafting oneself to meet challenges and opportunities that arise in our life as part of a historical community. But this capacity to intentionally develop ourselves is itself a developmental accomplishment.

The Biological Bases of Self and Personal Identity

The ideas of Maturana and Varela (1992, see also Thompson, 2007) are supported, but also challenged, through the work of Damasio (1999), who proposes three layers to the self, as understood in contemporary neuroscience: the proto-self, core self, and autobiographical self. According to Damasio, these three levels support an ever more articulate experience of personal consciousness.

The *proto-self* is a "preconscious biological precedent" (Damasio, 1999, p. 153) to the sense of self that consists of "a coherent collection of neural patterns which map, moment by moment, the state of the physical structure of the organism in its many directions" (p. 154). A number of brain structures are required to implement the proto-self including the several brain-stem nuclei, the hypothalamus, the insular cortex, the cortices known as S2, and the medial parietal cortices. According to Damasio, the proto-self supports the emergence of the core self and core consciousness.

The *core self* is generated for any object that incites core consciousness, and is considered "an imaged, nonverbal account of how the organism's own state is affected by the organism's processing of an object, and when this process enhances the image of the causative object, thus placing it saliently in a spatial and temporal context" (Damasio, 1999, p. 169). The core self generates a transient experience of knowing that is the object of experience and requires the presence of the proto-self. The neuro-anatomical structures that support core consciousness and core self include those that support the proto-self mentioned earlier, as well as the cingulate cortices, the thalamus, and the superior colliculi. Core consciousness and core self, in turn, allow for the emergence of extended consciousness and an autobiographical self (Damasio, 1999). The core self is an agent and object of linguistic designators such as "I," identified by Maturana and Varela (1992) as essential to a sense of self, but it cannot sustain a personal narrative of events extended in time. The proto and core self together seem to capture what Ricoeur (1987) calls "Mimeses_1"—or the implicit organization of events that might be rendered as a narrative about a particular person, but has not yet been articulated as such.

The *autobiographical self* (or we would say personal identity) is based on "the permanent but dispositional records of core self-experiences" (Damasio, 1999, p. 175). The sustained display of autobiographical self requires the presence of a core self and core consciousness and is the key to the experience of extended consciousness (i.e., a sense of self that is connected to the lived past and anticipated future). Extended consciousness is generated by accumulating autobiographical memories and occurs when working memory simultaneously holds in mind the object known and the objects constituting the autobiographical self for that time. The neuro-anatomical structures that support autobiographical self and extended consciousness include the early sensory cortices (also referred to as the limbic cortices), subcortical nuclei, and higher-order cortices. Ultimately, extended consciousness allows for distinctive human mental abilities (e.g., the ability to value self and life) and supports human conscience (Damasio, 1999). The autobiographical self, to the extent that it is articulated as a self-concept or a personal narrative, captures what Ricoeur (1988) calls Mimesis_2—the actual historical or fictional personal narratives that organize events into life stories.[7]

What Damasio's (1999) work shows is that the self needs to be considered in a more complex way than Maturana and Varela had imagined; we need to consider not only the biological and autobiographical self, but also a core self that precedes our ability to describe ourselves linguistically. However, as Robbie Case's work and others have shown, the ability to sustain an autobiographical self, and associated personal narratives, is itself a developmental accomplishment.

Development of the Autobiographical Self

The work of Damasio (1999) and that of Maturana and Varela (1992) both suggest that an autobiographical self should itself emerge through ontogenetic development, specifically, as brain systems that support more complex sociocultural interactions become available. This is in fact the position of neo-Piagetians like Case and Fischer: Case (1991) explored the possibility that Self is a Central Conceptual Structure essential to social life, one that develops in complexity as persons themselves develop. Work by Fischer has also fruitfully explored this idea (see Fischer & Bidell, 2006).

Along these lines, Habermas and Bluck (2000) consider the autobiographical self an increasingly coherent integration of (1) neo-Piagetian structures allowing

---

[7] For Ricoeur, Mimesis_1 refers to the prenarrative structure of experience; Mimesis_2 refers to the self-structuring of stories on the basis of narrative codes internal to discourse; Mimesis_3 refers to the encounter between the world of the text and the world of the reader or listener (Abel & Porée, 2007). Ricoeur (1987) proposes that Mimesis_3, in which historical or literary narratives themselves shape the kinds of narratives articulated in Mimesis_2 or embodied in Mimesis_1. Mimesis_3 is important in providing educational models for intentional personal development, as will be discussed later in the chapter.

increasing cognitive competence and (2) of sociohistorical norms expressed or institutionalized in different historical times and cultures.[8] They propose four kinds of coherence by which to judge life narratives, suggesting that "*Temporal* coherence and the *cultural* concept of biography are used to form a basic, skeletal life narrative consisting of an ordered sequence of culturally defined, major life events. *Causal* and *thematic* coherence express the unique interpretative stance of the individual." (Habermas & Bluck, 2000, p. 750, italics added). Only life narratives that are causally and thematically coherent will be recognized as good life narratives; nevertheless, temporal ordering—which can be linear, circular, or involve multiple timelines, depending on the cultural expectations governing such stories—provides a fundamental coherence in life narratives and appears early in childhood (Brockmeier, 2000; Lalonde & Chandler, 2004; Habermas & Bluck, 2000).

Studies of children's earliest autobiographical memories in natural contexts show that the earliest verbal remembering starts around 16 to 20 months and extends to distal events around 30 months when a familiar adult helps the child to remember (Fivush, Gray, & Fromhoff, 1987). (At this age, the degree of children's elaboration is predicted by adult scaffolding.) Katherine Nelson (1988, 1993) found that generalized scripts describing normative action sequences (i.e., specifying actors, locations, and objects) evolve between ages 2 and 3; these become structurally more complex and hierarchical (e.g., with nested and subordinate actions) by age 4–5.

Young children can order some events in time: For example, 3-year-olds can embed events into daily and weekly routines (Nelson, 1988) and by early school age children have a linear transitive sense of time (McCormack & Hoerl, 1999; Piaget, 1946); however, studies suggest that the ability to order remote events into a series develops later (Habermas & Bluck, 2000; also see Friedman, 1986, 1992, 1993).

According to McKeough and Griffiths (Chapter "Adolescent Narrative Thought: Developmental and Neurological Evidence in Support of a Central Social Structure"), the ability to temporally sequence distant experiences (what Ricoeur (1988) calls "emplotment" essential to all forms of mimesis) begins to develop around age 6: The ability to tell stories with subplots seems to emerge around age 8, but Habermas and Bluck (2000) claim that a cultural concept of biography only emerges around age 10. Other researchers have arrived at slightly different ages for these abilities. For example, some claim that about age 4 or 5, children begin to tell stories in terms of initiating problems and their resolution, reaching almost adult levels of performance around age 9–11, but all agree that these narratives are not integrated into an account of their life as a whole (Applebee, 1978; Botvin & Sutton-Smith, 1977; Case & McKeough, 1990; Habermas & Bluck, 2000; Chapter "Adolescent Narrative Thought: Developmental and Neurological Evidence in Support of a Central Social Structure").

---

[8] Daston and Galison (2007) provide an interesting account of scientific selves as being transformed across centuries, especially under the influence of the philosophical writings of Locke and Kant.

Habermas and Bluck (2000) detail many studies that suggest that the emergence of an integrated personal identity (whether a self-concept or a personal narrative able to integrate diverse episodes in ways that generate causal coherence) does not occur before early adolescence, when children become able to integrate characters' actions and their mental states into a single story: By age 12, early adolescents begin to interpret the intentions of characters in terms of lasting mental states and character traits that transcend the particular situation recounted (Chapter "Adolescent Narrative Thought: Developmental and Neurological Evidence in Support of a Central Social Structure"). Only in mid- to late adolescence does evidence support the emergence of biographical conceptions of a self capable of change through life experiences. Likewise, the ability to thematically interpret complex texts and an awareness of the need to interpret past personal events in light of the present develop simultaneously (as predicted by Ricoeur, 1992); this occurs in mid- to late adolescence—an ability that may continue to develop into adulthood.

For example, in a study comparing 12-, 15-, and 18-year-olds, Habermas and Paha (1999; cited in Habermas and Bluck, 2000) note that it is more difficult to establish global thematic coherence across stories in an individual's life than it is to find local coherence within a story. Supporting this intuitive claim, they found that efforts to explain action according to general personality and developmental status were present only in 15- and 18-year-olds, while explanations of personal discontinuity as due to particular biographical experiences were found only among 18-year-olds. Likewise, McKeough and Griffiths (Chapter "Adolescent Narrative Thought: Developmental and Neurological Evidence in Support of a Central Social Structure") found that by age 18, adolescent narratives can contain a coherent and coordinated dialectic tension between a character's internal and external struggles. These findings concord well with findings by Harter (1999) that late adolescence is associated with a more integrated self-conception used to explain a variety of events and actions more coherently. As McKeough's work shows (see Chapter "Adolescent Narrative Thought: Developmental and Neurological Evidence in Support of a Central Social Structure"), these changes in narrative capability are well explained by Robbie Case's (1985, 1992) theory of cognitive and self-development. Marini and Case (1994) conducted a study in which they gave five tasks of increasing difficulty to adolescents between the ages of 11 and 19. Participants read vignettes containing several situations and then inferred the protagonist's traits and predicted their behavior in a new situation. Most 13-year-olds gleaned one personal trait from a vignette when predicting the protagonist's behavior in the new situation. Most 16-year-olds gleaned two possibly contradictory traits and used them both to predict new behavior. Most 19-year-olds considered mood as a situational modifier.

Causal coherence does more than link life episodes; it also explains how one's values or personality change over time. Thematic coherence requires establishing thematic identity among disparate life events; sometimes this is implicit to the stories told, but sometimes links are made explicit by narrators who describe abiding metaphors of their life experience, or describe evaluative trajectories often associated with declared turning points in people's lives (Bruner, 1990, 2001, 2002). Organizing life narratives is not merely a matter of cognitive skill in coordinating information about one's life. Understanding of a normatively typical life varies according to culture, and within cultural groups, according to class and gender, and awareness of these norms can provide an "advance organizer" of personal autobiography (Botvin & Sutton-Smith, 1977; Peterson & McCabe, 1983, 1994; Schutze, 1984).

Development of Self-Concept

Selman (1980), Damon and Hart (1988), and McKeough and Griffiths have all documented the development of self-concept. Habermas and Bluck (2000) characterized the development of children's conceptions of self- and other as falling into the following five levels[9]:

- *Level 0*: preschool children describe themselves and other people in terms of their physical appearance, and make general evaluations about them such as being "good" or "nice."
- *Level 1*: young schoolchildren describe self and other people in terms of simple feelings and preferences, or in terms of specific abilities, like "She's good at swimming."
- *Level 2*: older schoolchildren compare their own skills to a reference group, describing their personality as unrelated but fairly stable habits and attitudes that explain a variety of actions and feelings.
- *Level 3*: early to mid-adolescents develop psychological concepts of personality able to integrate and coordinate a wide range of emotions, motivations, and action in relationships. Thus, the notion of a consistent personality or self emerges that makes sense of a disparate set of characteristics in light of underlying personality traits—sometimes over-generalized into thinking of others stereotypically as a "jock" or some other summative label.
- *Level 4*: mid- to late adolescents develop self-concepts that begin to acknowledge potential conflict between aspects of one's personality and realize that some aspects may not be fully articulated or even accessible to personal awareness; evaluations of people are sometimes made in light of particular belief systems, including religious or philosophical systems.

Once one reaches level 4, one is capable of engaging in intentional efforts to craft one's life to conform to particular ideals, or to make plans that allow one to tell certain kinds of stories characteristic of adult conceptions of self (Brandtstädter, 2006; Ferrari & Mahalingam, 1998). The importance of intentionally crafting life stories

---

[9]See Fischer and Bidell (2006; Chapter "Interviewing: An Insider's Insight into Learning") and McKeough and Griffiths (Chapter "Adolescent Narrative Thought: Developmental and Neurological Evidence in Support of a Central Social Structure") for a more complex developmental sequence.

relates to what we deeply care about in our lives—how we make sense of our lives and shape them so that we can talk about ourselves or live as a certain sort of person (Blasi, 1983, 2004; Frankfurt, 1988, 2004; Taylor, 1977, 1989)—a long-standing concern that can be traced to autopoietic practices of the Ancient Greeks (Foucault, 1978, 1994, 2004). It is in this sense that we can understand well-documented abilities for life plans, life guides, and life review (Staudinger, 2005; Staudinger, Dörner, & Mickler, 2005) in light of possible and feared selves (Markus & Nurius, 1986; Oyserman, Bybee, Terry & Hart-Johnson, 2004; Oyserman, Bybee, & Terry, 2006).

As Brandtstädter (2006) notes in writings about intentional self-development, adults intentionally plan and manage their self-concept throughout life—and particularly in old age, as physical resources begin to fail. To do so requires constantly balancing between assimilative and accommodative modes of self-development. Assimilative processes are involved in preventative or corrective action (problem solving), compensating actions (especially for highly valued aspects of one's personal narrative) and self-verification (when one selects social contexts and information to validate personally meaningful self-conceptions). When the "production possibility frontier" diminishes, people eventually accommodate (that is, change their story), through devaluing, re-interpreting, or redeploying their attention:

> The distinction between assimilation and accommodation processes ...may recall traditional distinctions between active and passive concepts of happiness; philosophical notions of wisdom have emphasized the importance of finding the right balance between these stances. ...Intentional self-development across the life span is based on this interplay between engagement and disengagement; between tenacious goal pursuit and flexible goal adjustment (Brandtstädter, 2006, p. 555)

Thus, empirical evidence suggests that our sense of self gains in complexity from childhood to adolescence, and that full-fledged autobiographical reasoning that relates life events into a globally coherent "autobiographical self," such as Damasio describes, does not appear before adolescence. However, it is important to remember that our sense of self is a product of our cultural participation, not an inherent essence (Varela et al., 1991). Indeed, Michael Chandler and his associates (1987) note that any conception of self must also be able to deal with change in the self and self-understanding over time. Indeed, one is always poised between personal sameness and personal change—a tension Ricoeur (1992) has captured wonderfully in his discussion of "oneself as another."

Oneself as Another

Ricoeur (1987, 1992) sets out to explain how self as both what is identical and what is constantly changing over time develops out of our linguistic resources. Ricoeur makes the important point that neuroscience is concerned with the questions of "*how* mind relates to brain," or "*what* part of the brain relates to what function of the mind," but the narrative is essentially concerned with the question "*who?*"

(who speaks? who acts? who narrates? who is responsible?). Ricoeur explores two contrasting notions of self and personal identity:

a. Self-identity as an identical core that remains unchanged, or whose elements can be substituted one for the other (from the Latin *idem*, which means "same"); psychological studies of self-concept also often emphasize sameness.
b. Self-identity of the same object that has undergone a series of transformations (from the Latin *ipse*); thus an oak tree is the same (the Latin *ipse*) as the acorn from which it developed.

These two senses of self-identity are not opposed, but rather are dialectically engaged with each other in any discussion of self or personal identity. While Ricoeur (1987, 1992) agrees with Varela and colleagues (1992) and Dennett (1991) that there are no core or essential elements of self that remain identical over the lifespan, he echoes Maturana and Varela (1992) in defending an "ipsitive" sense of identity, constructed and maintained through our use of language to express and talk about our individuality. Ricoeur presents his views in three steps (individualization, identification, and imputation) that he claims allow us to go systematically from the *idem* to the *ipse* notions of personal identity by means of two transitions (pragmatics and narrativity).

The *first step* concerns the epistemological problem of how an individual is *individuated* as distinct within a species by an identifying phrase (e.g., the discoverer of neurons), a proper name (e.g., Broca), or an indicator (e.g., "he," "you," "I," "then," "there"). The *pragmatics* of language takes up the same problem, but in such a way that speaking distinguishes the individual human being who is speaking from people in general; any statement one makes implies the phrase "I say [that statement]." In this initial step, we are concerned with the issue of determining of whom one speaks in designating a person, or who speaks when addressing someone else (all such speech acts are subsets of a broader consideration of identifying actors through their actions).

Ricoeur constructs his theory around language use and builds a strong separation between the discourses associated with language and those of biology and the natural sciences. However, when considered in light of Maturana and Varela's (1992) point about the emergence of personal experience out of our primate heritage, our ability to communicate through language seems a clear case of a natural drift of primate communication, as Maturana and Varela would say, which explains the relation between Ricoeur's (1988) spoken narrative and Mimesis$_1$—something that Tomasello, Gust, and Frost (1989) have shown distinguishes even very young children from chimpanzees and other primates of comparable linguistic ability using sign systems.[10]

[10]The question of whether chimpanzees and other primates actually possess language is much debated and beyond this chapter. For how language emerged from gesture, see Donald (1991, 2001).

The *second step* (*identification*) involves separating the "I" from "I say": In this way, someone is self-identified by saying "I," which generates a second transition to *narrative identity*: Narratives operate to configure the pragmatic engagement of someone in space and time. For Ricoeur, narrative identity is not distinct from experience and need not be accompanied by an explicit narrated story about an "I." Rather, the history of a life is the identity of a character with that life. What matters is that life events are (or could be) emploted into a narrative, an idea taken up by many psychologists (Gergen, 1991; McAdams, 1990, 1993; McLean, 2005. Variations between sameness and self are attested to by imaginative narrative variations; narrative seeks out and engenders such variations, and fiction is a vast laboratory for thought experiments—or as Oatley (1999) says, "simulations"— designed to test them and determine their merits. Narratives of personal identity thus oscillate between two extremes: At one extreme are characters who have a set role in a plot (the wise man, or villain); at the other are characters portrayed through their stream of consciousness, in which plot is put at the service of character. In limit cases, such as Musil's (1953) *The man without qualities*, we seem to have reached the point in which there is no longer a character. But even here, Ricoeur (1987) reminds us, we can always ask "Who is without qualities?" And that "who" remains a character within the narrative.[11]

On this view, narratives are essentially a mimesis of action and life, not of persons. Here Ricoeur (1992) joins Fischer and Bidell (2006) in claiming that the development of a sense of self depends on skilled practices that are developed, coordinated, and subordinated within the context of constitutive rules established by others within a culture. Thus, we need to consider how specific practices (skills)—and the self-regulation needed to employ those skills—are related to general life projects (involving e.g., family, profession, community, and political action). Ricoeur (1992) proposes that skills and projects are coordinated through life plans. Charles Taylor (1989), echoes this important connection between narrative, personal meaning making, and human agency. Our sense of our lives as expressed in a narrative, or a life story, is bound up with our notion of what it means to be a person. For Taylor (1985), as for Ricoeur, "a person is a being with a certain moral status, or a bearer of rights"—a moral status that depends on one's having certain capabilities:

> A person is a being who has a sense of self, has a notion of the future and the past, can hold values, make choices; in short, can adopt life plans. [. . .] A person must be a being with his own point of view on things. The life plan, the choices, the sense of self must be attributable to him as in some sense their point of origin. A person is a being who can be addressed, who can reply. (p. 97)

---

[11] So Dennett (1991) is right to claim that self is a "center of narrative gravity," but he is wrong to believe this makes self a fiction. For Ricoeur, it means that even the literary thought experiments of the most avant-garde novels, like Robert Musil's *The man without qualities* concern characters: literary characters are fictions, but lived characters are a dialectic construction of fictional and historical possibilities. As Fingarette (1963) said, we become historians of our own lives, even if we cannot step outside of a narrative, broadly understood.

Indeed, evidence shows that *future orientation*, in the form of life plans (Lachman & Burack, 1993), ideal selves (Higgins, 1987, 1991), and possible selves (King & Raspin, 2004; Markus & Nurius, 1986; Oyserman, Bybee, Terry, & Hart-Johnson, 2004; King & Raspin, 2004) are crucial to understanding personal narrative and personal development. One of the most significant achievements of adolescence is the acquisition of formal operations, which allow going beyond the world of concrete experience and mentally travel through the world of ideas and ideals—the world of possibilities and necessities (Case, 1998, Fischer & Bidell, 2006; Chapter "Mental Attention, Multiplicative Structures, and the Causal Problems of Cognitive Development"). This achievement, together with a general increase in working memory capacity allows new kinds of self-examination more specifically, it allows the simultaneous consideration of remembered past, known current events (actual self), and imagined future events (possible and ideal selves), and their integration into a coherent view of oneself as one would want to be (Allport, 1937; Damon & Hart, 1988; Higgins, 1987; Inhelder & Piaget, 1958; McLean, 2005; Sullivan, 1953; Thorne, McLean, & Lawrence, 2004).

Ricoeur's *third step* (*imputation*) in the development of a personal identity is ethical and moral: promises, for example, by committing someone to acting toward another in the future make individuals "self-constant." Self-constancy means that one can be counted on and is accountable for one's actions, that one is responsible. This sets up a fruitful dialectic between constancy and change. One can ask oneself, "Who am I, so inconstant, who nevertheless remains someone you can still count on?" Here we see that possession of unchanging experiences is not essential to self, for Ricoeur, but rather the ethical primacy of the other by which the self makes itself available to others (and so making us co-authors, not authors or the stories of our lives). The ethical and moral determinants of action become important (i.e., what is considered good and obligatory, respectively): Here the dialectic of self and other is developed further and the autonomy of the self is shown to be tightly bound to solicitude for one's friends and neighbors. Ricoeur ultimately proposes another transition, *cosmopolitical*—in which one acknowledges that obligations are always set within a sociohistorical framework that implies some idea of justice; we must keep our promises not only to one another, but to sustain a society in which promises matter and we do our fair share for ourselves and for others. Thus, justice becomes central both for individuals to whom one is personally committed, as well as to others in one's society and culture (justice as a personal obligation, and justice as fair institutions and laws).

Self-Fashioning and Intentional Personal Development

Promises are made not only to others, but also to ourselves. These promises are integral to our assessment of our lives, and to our efforts to intentionally author, fashion, or develop ourselves (Baxter Magolda, Creamer, & Meszaros, 2010; Blasi, 2004; Stanovich, 2004). This ability to intentionally develop ourselves into persons able to live a good life has long been a hallmark of wisdom (Foucault, 2004; Plotzek, Winneskes, Kraus, & Surmann, 2002; Ricoeur, 1992).

What Is Intentional Personal Development?

Intentional personal development highlights the openness and plasticity of human development. The importance of self-development is a very old idea.[12] In discussions of the Renaissance, intentional self-development has been called "self-fashioning" and includes both instrumental and aesthetic considerations (Greenblatt, 1980). Contemporary philosophers refer to processes of self-development as "taking ourselves seriously" (Frankfurt, 1971, 1988, 2004), "care for the self" (Foucault, 1978, 2004), or "self-improvement" in which one "work[s] on oneself with the regard to the possibilities of [...] becoming something different from what we have been made" (Hacking, 1986, p. 233). This notion continues to find voice in contemporary psychology in recent discussions of intentional self-development (Brandtstädter, 2006) and of student "self-authorship" (Baxter Magolda et al., 2010; King et al., 2009).

For Frankfurt (1988, 2004), "caring for oneself" and "taking oneself seriously" highlight the importance of adopting a caring relationship and require taking a stand on one's life and oneself as a person that necessarily *incorporates values* and is closely tied to one's understanding of meaning of one's life. Not only of what is possible, but what one desires to be, which necessarily includes one's understanding of what constitutes a good life (King & Napa, 1998; Plotzek, Winneskes, Kraus, & Surmann, 2002; Seligman & Csikszentmihalyi, 2000; Taylor, 1989; Varela, 1992/1999). Deep insight into what it means for oneself to live a good life has been called personal wisdom—wisdom not in the form of general understanding or advice about human life, but wisdom about one's own life and how to live it well, which studies show is harder to come by (Staudinger et al. 2005).

Intentional personal development and associated concepts (e.g., free will, agency, and self-actualization), remain a central notion of existential philosophy (e.g., Sartre, 1956) and psychology (e.g., Maslow, 1943, 1954, 1962; Rogers, 1961). Goldstein's (1939/1995) and Maslow's concept of *self-actualization* (1954, 1962) helps articulate the aim of intentional personal development as personal flourishing. Following a very long philosophical tradition, these and other authors argue that all beings, including human beings, have a natural tendency to actualize their potential. However, potential includes not only existing biological capacities but also possibilities that are dynamically shaped by choices people make and the education they receive (Egan, 1997). That is, people not only have personal narratives, but they

[12] The importance of self-development can be traced at least as far back as Pliny and if we consider mere self-improvement, certainly to Seneca and the Socratics and before them to the Pythagoreans—who may have drawn on insights of the Wisdom Schools that spanned the Ancient Middle East, including the Ancient Egyptians (Kugel, 2007).

have second-order evaluations and desires about how to advance or change those stories that are the source of their willed desires to fashion their lives to the extent they can, in conjunction with others with to whose lives they are linked (Blasi, 2004; Frankfurt, 1988; Taylor, 1989).

Following Erikson (1959), Case (1998) and others, we believe that cognitive achievements of adolescence, together with accompanying physical social changes, play an important role in how adolescents understand their lives, as they review their past and plan for the future (Elder, 1999; Hitlin, Brown, & Elder, 2007). As they enter adulthood, adolescents become increasingly able to orchestrate and structure their values and ideals about what a person and what a good life should be. They also engage in new kinds of self-evaluation that lead them to positioning themselves in the world around them (Harré & Moghaddam, 2003; Harré et al., 2009). They, also begin to consider the meaning and purpose of their lives (Damon, Menon, & Bronk, 2003; McAdams, 1990, 1993) and to orient toward the future with an "'I do care' attitude" (Allport, 1937, p. 223). All these changes lead to the formulation of "self-guides" (Higgins, 1991) and life plans that guide efforts at intentional personal development. Likewise, Sternberg and Spear-Swerling's (1998) concept of *personal navigation* connect self-understanding and self-efficacy as "the means by which self-awareness is translated into a plan of action for one's life" (p. 222).

Similarly, "life programs" incorporate future goals for oneself and provide motivation for self-regulation (Steinberg et al., 2006) and self-change (Higgins, 1991; Inhelder & Piaget, 1958). Naturally, self-guides are not produced in a social vacuum. Mentors and models of a particular kind of self-practice—including, e.g., meditative self-practices and other ways of forging a certain kind of self that include schooling—are all critical to the choices people make and to their efforts to develop both general and personal wisdom. All this contributes ability to intentionally develop themselves. Recognizing that to people's merely having a plan and direction is not enough in face of unforeseen obstacles, Ryan and Deci (2000) propose that a desire for *self-determination* is another critical aspect of intentional personal development.

Changes in capacity that occur in adolescence create both opportunities and challenges for a developing individual and can lead to significant alterations of developmental trajectories (Cicchetti & Toth, 1996; Compas, Hinden, & Gerhardt, 1995; Rutter & Rutter, 1993; Steinberg et al., 2006)—for better or for worse. Thus, although adolescence is usually conceptualized as a time of increased vulnerability to the emergence of psychopathology or the worsening thereof (Cicchetti & Rogosch, 2002; Steinberg et al., 2006), it is also recognized as a time of increased opportunity for overcoming, lessening, or controlling an already existing psychopathology (e.g., stuttering; Finn, 2004). Research shows that whether children with an existing psychopathology will get better in adolescence depends on both external and internal resources: For example, the availability and quality of the social support network (Thompson, Flood, & Goodvin, 2006) and the meaning they assign to their experience and their reaction to it (Nolen-Hoeksema, 1991; Rutter, Kim-Cohen, & Maughan, 2006, respectively).

Thus, intentional personal development should be studied by assessing people's self-insight in ways that are both retrospective—life review—and prospective—life planning. Such studies might use methods that resemble those of cultural anthropology. In other words, that study people as they live their lives, and explore how they plan and cope with the events that occur: sometimes tragic events, naturally accompanied by grief, that nevertheless allow an opportunity for personal growth and insight into the deepest values of life. And this is where we believe current models of identity development (e.g., Case, 1996) need some adjustments to allow for a person's own role in developing their identity.

*Intentional Personal Development and Education (***Autopoiesis** *Through Emulation and* **Bildung***)*

As mentioned earlier, our assessment of what it means to develop into a good person necessarily expresses ideals of human development that integrate both biology and culture across the lifespan. One key form of cultural participation is formal education, not only for children and adolescents, but also for adults who continue to educate and develop themselves in pursuit of a better life, a sense of education that is closer to the German notion of *Bildung*[13] than to rote learning.

For Egan (1997), public schools have three competing agendas: Job preparation, teaching truths about the world (e.g., scientific and historical truths), and promoting personal flourishing. Public schools are well equipped students to prepare for jobs, for example by teaching particular skills, such as reading, math, or computer programming. Schools also devote a lot of effort to teaching scientific truths that are not readily apparent—for example, low to overcome deep misconceptions that even advanced students fall into when studying advanced physics or Darwin's theory of evolution by natural selection has been the focus of a huge effort in cognitive science and education. What about personal flourishing?

Certainly there are specialized schools, often religious schools with entire programs for improving one's sense of well-being. These schools can be said to focus on different aspects identified by Damasio as components of the self. Various forms of Yoga, for example, aim to train the body and through it a sense of well-being that encompasses the entire person. Mindfulness meditation, and other spiritual exercises (what is sometimes called "contemplative science") are gaining advocates for their incorporation within the public school system (Rosch, 2008;

[13]The noun "*Bildung*" has several meanings, which is why the term is often left untranslated. Ranner (2008) sums up the range of meanings nicely, stating "Bildung... can be translated into English as 'education'; it equally can be taken to mean 'formation,' 'growth,' 'shaping,' 'cultivation,' 'civilization,' or 'refinement.' *Bildung* is not limited by specific goal-orientation, nor is it passive. *Bildung* is ongoing, unlimited in scope and most importantly, encompasses the whole person. No one leads you anywhere. Material is made available, but it is up to the student to put it to use. *Bildung* is the education you give yourself" (see also Boes, 2006, 2009).

Siegel, 2007; Wallace, 2007; Wallace & Shapiro, 2006), promoting curricula that encourage students to focus on the experience of the present moment, or allow them to heighten the attention and clarity of their experience, or develop greater compassion.

We also find efforts to promote intentional personal development as part of the standard Liberal Arts Curriculum. King and her colleagues (2009) describe efforts to document the development of self-authorship among college students, and provide recommendations for curriculum design to help promote its development. Building on the work of Kegan (1982) they propose four broad themes of developing self-authorship that are manifested differently by students who define themselves by external criteria (e.g., ethnic or religious traditions), internally (e.g., by personal ideals and choices), or a mixture of the two: (1) increasing awareness, understanding, and openness to diversity; (2) exploring and establishing the basis for their beliefs, choices, and actions; (3) developing a sense of personal identity that guides their choices; and (4) increasing awareness of their responsibility for their own learning. They propose that educational strategies be tailored to students' particular style of meaning making (i.e., external, internal, or mixed): In standard classrooms, this implies educators should use a variety of approaches since their classrooms will have students with a range of different meaning-making orientations. Generally, they suggest that educators provide students with the chance to experience and reflect on the diversity and complexity of the world and invite them to make sense of that complexity. Educators should also find ways to help students to make the best sense of different perspectives, in light of their own background and upbringing, and to apply this deeper appreciation of diversity into the choices they make in their own lives. These calls for colleges to provide "developmentally effective experiences" are very much a plea for education as *Bildung*.

The aims toward which one should aspire through intentional personal development, or self-authorship, are often expressed through models to be emulated. This is certainly the approach of character education programs that claim to teach for wisdom, such as *Project Wisdom* and *Wise Skills*. A more fully articulated program was developed by Renaissance humanists: Humanist education in the Renaissance was devoted to learning skills, but also to the emulation of models from antiquity, for example Ovid. But Quintilian (95/2009) had warned long ago that models should not be followed slavishly, but adapted to the rhetorical needs of particular times and circumstances. A recent paper by Dixon (2009) suggests that the point of Shakespeare's *Titus Andronicus* was to show what happens when people draw immoral lessons from historical examples that are meant as cautionary tales. Of course, flourishing also depends on different ideals of a good life, and these can be intimately tied to one's temperament and to other aspects of one's neurobiology (Rothbart, & Bates, 2006; Siegel, 2007).

Unfortunately, most public education, at least in North America, does not concern itself with intentional personal development (*bildung*), something increasingly important given the disproportionate overabundance of negative role models presented through various media.

Alternative Pathways of Intentional Personal Development

All of these points suggest that we need a wide-ranging approach to consider the developmental relations between mind, brain, and education. In particular, any consideration of their developmental relations is most likely to be successful when engaged at the level of persons' own efforts at self-fashioning and intentional development, as opposed to the subpersonal level characteristic of classical cognitive science.

What about atypical development? Here we agree with Fischer and Bidell (2006) that one must be alert to potential alternative pathways to learning and to personal well-being. Consider the case of Asperger syndrome, which characterizes individuals with relatively high intellectual functioning who are nevertheless placed on the autism spectrum due to deficits in social sensitivity. We suggest that such individuals represent an alternative (non-normative) pathway with a unique path to personal flourishing, in school and out. Presumably, individuals diagnosed with Asperger syndrome, even if less social than the average person, will need to develop an expertise in the fundamental pragmatics of *their own* lives characteristic of personal wisdom (Ardelt, 2003; Staudinger et al, 2005), if they are to navigate all of the obstacles they encounter to living a good life on their own terms. And they will need to develop themselves in ways that promote their own personal flourishing.

In fact, several studies/clinical reports indicate that intentional personal development might be a crucial factor in social adjustment of individuals with conduct, autistic, and other disorders. For example, Rogers, Kell, and McNeil (1948) found that the most important predictor of adjustment of adolescents with conduct disorders was self-insight, that included self-understanding, self-acceptance, and taking responsibility for oneself (a notion very similar to intentional personal development). Similarly, based on his follow-up study of the first group of children ever diagnosed as autistic, Leo Kanner (1971) concluded that self-awareness and acting on, it could crucially contribute to good life outcomes of autistic individuals. More recently, Hauser, Allen, and Golden (2006) confirmed the importance of these factors in their study of resilience of adolescents with troubled early lives who, against all odds, became well adjusted (according to their own and others' criteria). More specifically, they showed how self-reflection and agency (along with relatedness) appear to be crucial for overcoming adversity and for positive growth. Our own in-depth case studies (Vuletic, Ferrari, & Mihail, 2005; Vuletic, 2010) have also shown the importance of intentional personal development to quality of life in adolescents and adults with Asperger syndrome.

It seems plausible that an important aspect of education for individuals with Asperger syndrome will include efforts to emulate others with Asperger syndrome who have been successful in crafting a good life—as expressed in their autobiographies (e.g., Temple Grandin [Grandin, 1995; Grandin & Scariano, 1986], Liane Holliday Willey, 1999, Stephen Shore, 2001, John Elder Robison, 2008, Daniel Tammet, 2006, and Donna Williams, 1992, 1994, 1996, 2004). Such emulation would allow them to intentionally develop themselves in the way that knowledge of their cognitive and genetic differences from typical individuals will not.

Self and Will as Illusions?

Intentional personal development is sometimes documented at the biological level in terms of the neuroplasticity of the brain, (Doidge, 2007)—but it is equally well documented at the personal level. It claims that, at least as there the limits of our human potential, our flourishing or suffering, our *bildung*, depends on our own efforts as much as it depends on our environment or our genes (King et al., 2009; Stanovich, 2004). This is a very old idea, best expressed by Pico della Mirandola (1486/1956), who famously wrote in his *Oratio*:

> [God] made man a creature of indeterminate and indifferent nature, and, placing him in the middle of the world, said to him 'Adam, we give you no fixed place to live, no form that is peculiar to you, nor any function that is yours alone. According to your desires and judgment, you will have and possess whatever place to live, whatever form, and whatever functions you yourself choose. All other things have a limited and fixed nature prescribed and bounded by our laws. You, with no limit or no bound, may choose for yourself the limits and bounds of your nature. We have placed you at the world's center so that you may survey everything else in the world. We have made you neither of heavenly nor of earthly stuff, neither mortal nor immortal, so that with free choice and dignity, you may fashion yourself into whatever form you choose. To you is granted the power of degrading yourself into the lower forms of life, the beasts, and to you is granted the power, contained in your intellect and judgment, to be reborn into the higher forms, the divine.' / Imagine! The great generosity of God! The happiness of man! To man it is allowed to be whatever he chooses to be! As soon as an animal is born, it brings out of its mother's womb all that it will ever possess. Spiritual beings from the beginning become what they are to be for all eternity. Man, when he entered life, the Father gave the seeds of every kind and every way of life possible. Whatever seeds each man sows and cultivates will grow and bear him their proper fruit.

Despite the power of this imagery, some contemporary philosophers claim that the idea of a single or enduring self and the notion of free will are illusions. These ideas, they say, are holdovers from a Judeo-Christian understanding of the soul—well expressed by Pico—that modern science has shown to be false. The notion that will is an illusion begets support from empirical reviews purporting to show that there is no one area of the brain devoted to the self, or to capacities that we associate with the ability to have and recognize an enduring sense of self (Gillihan & Farah, 2005). Dan Wegner (2002, 2005) and others have made several studies purporting to show that our sense of free will is an illusion; that our choices are actually influenced by many subpersonal factors of which we are not aware; and that our declarations of having decided to act in a particular way are pure confabulations.[14] However, it is somewhat ironic to consider that these studies are deliberately designed to show that will is an illusion and depend on the willful action of a confederate who steers the subject wrong in order to induce an "illusion of will."

---

[14]Such a way of construing human life flies in the face of how most of us want to narrate our lives (Berlin, 1969). As Angell (1911) said long ago, psychologists can march under any banner, but should not expect most people to always follow them.

Certainly, we are not even always the best judge of our own physical boundaries; in cases of asomatognosia (associated with damage to the right parietal lobe), people feel that parts of their body are not their own, or that they have an ability to move and choose not to when they are clearly unable to do so (Benson, 2003; Feinberg, 2001). Likewise, damage to the corpus callosum, medial frontal cortex, or some other more posterior parts of the brain (Scepkowski & Cronin-Golomb, 2003) leads people not to feel their movements as their own (the alien hand syndrome). Both of these phenomena show dramatically that even our core sense of our immediate selves depends on the proper functioning of our brain.

Likewise, Luria (1972) famously documented the case of brain damage that led a Russian soldier Zazetsky to be unable to emplot the fragments of his life into a coherent narrative, and more recent studies show that the ability to recall and organize our first-person experiences is severely affected by the brain deteriorization associated with Alzheimer's disease or severe traumatic brain injury (Piolino et al., 2003; Piolino, Desgranges, Manning, North, Jokic, Eustache, 2007).

These and other findings lead philosophers like Dennett (1991, 2003) to conclude that self is nothing more than the center of narrative gravity, with no more reality than the earth's physical center of gravity. Even Varela et al. (1991) and Ricoeur (1992) agree that ultimately self-narratives are personal creations that are, in a Buddhist sense, "empty of inherent being"—there is no permanent self-substance and our sense of ourselves can be mistaken, or naïve.

We certainly acknowledge the truth of these claims, as far as they go, as does Brandtstädter (2007): There is no denying that there are many subpersonal influences on our actions. But one of the best defenses of the notion of free will was given by William James, inspired by Renouvier, who wrote in his April 30, 1870, diary entry that his "first act of free will shall be to believe in free will"—precisely because it has such pragmatic importance for our lives; indeed, this affirmation helped lift James out of a personal depression (Richardson, 2007).

This is precisely what we understand Ricoeur to propose when he claims that the reality of identity is not in a constant core of experience—the idea of which is certainly an illusion—but in our imputation of personal responsibility to ourselves and to others. In this way, we construct a personal identity that persists despite lower-level influences that might have derailed it. For example, promises are kept, job obligations are fulfilled, and many other things happen that show people to be dependable and to fulfill important aspects of their social identity.[15] Our identity is intimately bound up with our perceived ability to choose among possible courses of action and the resulting possible selves that we will create by our actions.

Not only promises to others, but promises to ourselves to develop ourselves in particular ways these second-order desires are precisely what guide us and make us

---

[15]Piaget (1962) proposed that will emerges as our values become structured and more important values override the immediate appeal of less important interests—removing the puzzle of James's "fiat" of will. Nicholas of Cusa proposed that the human power of conjecture is at the heart of our ability to fashion ourselves; and knowing or conjecturing this power about ourselves is to live with a philosophy of hope and possibility (see Hopkins, 2002).

alert to subtle influences that weaken or derail our efforts to intentionally develop and fashion ourselves in ways that we value. In other words, our personal identity is not given as our biological or spiritual birthright; it must rather be constructed and co-constructed through our actions as members of a linguistic community of individuals for whom selves matter. But this selfhood is also an expression of basic biological realities, too, in which our continued survival as autonomous beings depends on creating the conditions of our own flourishing and of caring for ourselves in the most basic senses of the term. For this reason, we believe it is better to consider the self a personal creation—more akin to a work of art than to an illusion. As such, it is self-authored (or co-authored) and self-fashioned for the parts we wish to play (and play well). It is in this lived narrative that we fully engage life and avoid a nihilism, sometimes just below the surface of much subpersonal cognitive science (Ricoeur, 1992; Varela et al., 1991).

Thus, the reality of self is not attested to by some inner certainty of our existence that seems to characterize Damasio's core self, for example. Rather, we propose that the kind of certainty to which the hermeneutic approach to personal identity advocated by Maturana and Varela, and Ricoeur, can aspire is one of "attestation"—a conjunction of analysis and reflection. For Ricoeur (1992), attestation requires less than the Cartesian exaltation of the ego but more than its Nietzschean annihilation. Attestation is fundamentally opposed to the notion of science as ultimate and self-founding knowledge—whether subjective or objective—and in this sense it joins the Buddhist notion of self as "empty" of inherent being. Attestation is belief—not a doxic "I believe—that ..." but, rather, the credence of "I believe—in ..." (Ricoeur, 1992) that echoes James' (1897) "will to believe." Attestation links to testimony about which there is no absolute certainty, because the questions "who speaks?" "who acts?" and "who is responsible?" can be answered in many different ways. But the best answer to false testimony is not to declare that all testimony is an illusion; rather, it is to seek better testimony (Ricoeur, 1992). Thus, an essential aspect of credence in self-testimony is trust and, ultimately, it is this trust that allows us all to believe that we are real, that our lives matter, and that we can intentionally make life better for ourselves and our community.

References

Abel, O., & Porée, J. (2007). *Le vocabulaire de Paul Ricoeur*. Paris: Ellipses

Allport, G. W. (1937). *Personality: A psychological interpretation*. New York: Henry Holt.

Angell, J. R. (1911). Philosophical and psychological usages of the terms mind, consciousness, and soul. *Psychological Bulletin, 8*(2), 46–47.

Applebee, A. N. (1978). *The child's concept of story.* Chicago: University of Chicago Press.

Ardelt, M. (2003). Empirical assessment of a three-dimensional wisdom scale. *Research on Aging, 25*(3), 275–324.

Ardelt, M. (2004). Wisdom as expert knowledge system: A critical review of a contemporary operationalization of an ancient concept. *Human Development, 47*(5), 257–285.

Baltes, P. B., & Smith, J. (2008). The fascination of wisdom: Its nature, ontogeny, and function. *Perspectives on Psychological Science, 3*(1), 56–64.

Baltes, P. B., & Staudinger, U. M. (2000). Wisdom: A metaheuristic (pragmatic) to orchestrate mind and virtue toward excellence. *American Psychologist, 55*(1), 122–136.

Baxter Magolda, M. B., Creamer, E. G., & Meszaros, P. S. (Eds.). (2010). *Development and assessment of self-authorship: Exploring the concept across cultures*. Sterling, VA: Stylus.

Benson, C. (2003). The unthinkable boundaries of self: The role of negative emotional boundaries in the formation, maintenance and transformation of identities. In R. Harré & F. M. Moghaddam (Eds.), *The self and others: Positioning individuals and groups in personal, political, and cultural contexts* (pp. 61–84). Westport, CN: Praeger.

Berlin, I. (1969). *Four essays on liberty*. London: Oxford University Press.

Blasi, A. (1983). Moral cognition and moral action: A theoretical perspective. *Developmental Review, 3*(2), 178–210.

Blasi, A. (2004). Neither personality nor cognition: An alternative approach to the nature of the self. In C. Lightfoot, C. Lalonde, & M. Chandler (Eds.), *Changing conceptions of psychological life* (pp. 3–25). Mahwah, NJ: Erlbaum.

Boes, T. (2006). Modernist studies and the Bildungsroman: A historical survey of critical trends. *Literature Compass, 3*(2), 230–233.

Boes, T. (2009). Teaching & learning guide for: Modernist studies and the Bildungsroman: A historical survey of critical trends. *Literature Compass, 6*(1), 249–252.

Botvin, G. J., & Sutton-Smith, B. (1977). The development of structural complexity in children's fantasy narratives. *Developmental Psychology, 13*(4), 377–388.

Brandtstädter, J. (2006). Action perspectives on human development. In W. Damon & R. M. Lerner (Series Eds.) & R. M. Lerner (Vol. Ed.), *Handbook of child psychology: Vol. 1. Theoretical models of human development* (6th ed., pp. 516–568). New York: Wiley.

Brandtstädter, J. (2007). Causality, intentionality, and the causation of intentions: The problematic boundary. In M. Ash & T. Sturm (Eds.), *Psychology's territories: Historical and contemporary perspectives from different disciplines* (pp. 51–66). Mahwah, NJ: Erlbaum.

Brockmeier, J. (2000). Autobiographical time. *Narrative Inquiry, 10*(1), 51–73.

Bronfenbrenner, U., & Morris, P. (2006). The ecology of developmental processes. In W. Damon & R. M. Lerner (Series Eds.) & R. M. Lerner (Vol. Ed.), *Handbook of child psychology: Vol. 1. Theoretical models of human development* (6th ed., pp. 793–828). New York: Wiley.

Bruner, J. (1990). *Acts of meaning*. Cambridge, MA: Harvard University Press.

Bruner, J. (2001). Self-making and world-making. In J. Brockmeier & D. Carbaugh (Eds.), *Narrative and identity: Studies in autobiography, self, and culture* (pp. 25–37). Amsterdam: John Benjamins.

Bruner, J. (2002). *Making stories: Law, literature, life*. New York: Farrar, Strauss and Giroux.

Case, R. (1985). *Intellectual development: Birth to adulthood*. New York: Academic Press.

Case, R. (1991). Stages in the development of the young child's first sense of self. *Developmental Review, 11*(3), 210–230.

Case, R. (1992). *The mind's staircase: Exploring the conceptual underpinnings of children's thought and knowledge*. Hillsdale, NJ: Erlbaum.

Case, R. (1996). *Stages in the formation of an adult social identity*. Unpublished manuscript, Toronto: University of Toronto.

Case, R. (1998). The development of conceptual structures. In W. Damon (Series Ed.) & D. Kuhn & R. S. Siegler (Vol. Eds.), *Handbook of child psychology: Vol. 2. Cognition, perception, and language* (5th ed., pp. 745–800). New York: Wiley.

Case, R., & McKeough, A. (1990). Schooling and the development of central conceptual knowledge structures: An example from the domain of children's narrative. *International Journal of Education, 13*(8), 835–855.

Chandler, M. J., Boyes, M., Ball, L., & Hala, S. (1987). The conservation of selfhood: A developmental analysis of children's changing conceptions of self-continuity. In T. Honess & K. Yardley (Eds.), *Self and identity: Perspectives across the life-span* (pp. 108–119). London: Routledge.

Changeux, J. P., & Ricoeur, P. (2000). *What makes us think?* Princeton, NJ: Princeton University Press.

Cicchetti, D., & Rogosch, F. A. (2002). A developmental psychopathology perspective on adolescence. *Journal of Consulting and Clinical Psychology, 70*(1), 6–20.

Cicchetti, D., & Toth, S. L. (Eds.). (1996). *Adolescence: Opportunities and challenges*. Rochester, NY: University of Rochester Press.
Compas, B. E., Hinden, B. R., & Gerhardt, C. A. (1995). Adolescent development: Pathways and processes of risk and resilience. *Annual Review of Psychology, 46*, 265–293.
Concise Oxford English Dictionary (11th, rev. ed.). (2008). Oxford: Oxford University Press.
Csikszentmihalyi, M., & Rathunde, K. (1998). The development of the person: An experiential perspective on the ontogenesis of psychological complexity. In W. Damon (Series Ed.) & R. M. Lerner (Vol. Ed.), *Handbook of child psychology: Vol. 1. Theoretical models of human development* (5th ed., pp. 635–684). New York: Wiley.
Damasio, A. (1999). *The feeling of what happens: Body and emotion in the making of consciousness*. Orlando, FL: Harcourt.
Damon, W., & Hart, D. (1988). *Self-understanding in childhood and adolescence*. New York: Cambridge University Press.
Damon, W., Menon, J., & Bronk, K. C. (2003). The development of purpose during adolescence. *Applied Developmental Science, 7*(3), 119–128.
Dennett, D. C. (1991). *Consciousness explained*. Boston: Little, Brown.
Dennett, D. C. (2003). *Freedom evolves*. New York: Viking.
Dixon, V. G. (2009). "A pattern, precedent, and lively warrant": Emulation, rhetoric, and cruel propriety. *Titus Andronicus. Renaissance Quarterly, 62*, 376–409.
Doidge, N. (2007). *The brain that changes itself: Stories of personal triumph from the frontiers of brain science*. New York: Viking.
Donald, M. (1991). *Origins of the modern mind: Three stages in the evolution of culture and cognition*. Cambridge, MA: Harvard University Press.
Donald, M. (2001). *A mind so rare: The evolution of human consciousness*. New York: Norton.
Egan, K. (1997). *The educated mind: How cognitive tools shape our understanding*. Chicago: University of Chicago Press.
Elder, G. H., Jr. (1999). *Children of the great depression: Social change in life experience*. Boulder, CO: Westview Press. (Originally published 1974).
Erikson, E. (1959). Identity and the life cycle: Selected papers. *Psychological Issues, 1*, 1–171.
Feinberg, T. (2001). *Altered egos: How the brain creates the self*. Oxford: Oxford University Press.
Ferrari, M., & Mahalingam, R. (1998). Personal cognitive development and its implications for teaching and learning. *Educational Psychologist, 33*(1), 35–44.
Fingarette, H. (1963). *The self in transformation: Psychoanalysis, philosophy, and the life of the spirit*. New York: Basic Books.
Finn, P. (2004). Self-change from stuttering during adolescence and adulthood. In A. K. Bothe (Ed.), *Evidence-based treatment of stuttering: Empirical bases and clinical applications* (pp. 117–136). Mahwah, NJ: Erlbaum.
Fischer, K. W., & Bidell, T. R. (2006). Dynamic development of action, thought, and emotion. In W. Damon & R. M. Lerner (Series Eds.) & R. M. Lerner (Vol. Ed.), *Handbook of child psychology: Vol. 1. Theoretical models of human development* (6th ed., pp. 313–399). New York: Wiley.
Fivush, R., Gray, J. T., & Fromhoff, F. A. (1987). Two-year-olds talk about the past. *Cognitive Development, 2*(4), 393–409.
Foucault, M. (1978). *The care of the self*. New York: Vintage.
Foucault, M. (1994). L'éthique du souci de soi comme pratique de la liberté. In D. Defert, F. Ewald, & J. Lagrange (Eds.), *Dits et écrits IV* (pp. 708–729). Paris: Gallimard. (Original interview given in 1984).
Foucault, M. (2004). *The hermeneutics of the subject: Lectures at the Collège de France, 1981–1982*. (A. I. Davidson, English Series Ed.; G. Burchell, Trans.). New York: Macmillan.
Frankfurt, H. G. (1971). Freedom of the will and the concept of person. *Journal of Philosophy, 68*(1), 5–20.
Frankfurt, H. G. (1988). *The importance of what we care about: Philosophical essays*. Cambridge: Cambridge University Press.

Frankfurt, H. G. (2004). Taking ourselves seriously. In G. B. Peterson (Ed.), *Tanner lectures on human values* (pp. 169–185). Salt Lake City, UT: University of Utah.
Friedman, W. J. (1986). The development of children's knowledge of temporal structure. *Child Development, 57*(6), 1386–1400.
Friedman, W. J. (1992). Children's time memory: The development of a differentiated past. *Cognitive Development, 7*(2), 171–187.
Friedman, W. J. (1993). Memory for the time of past events. *Psychological Bulletin, 113*(1), 44–66.
Gergen, K. J. (1991). *The saturated self: Dilemmas of identity in contemporary life*. New York: Basic Books.
Gillihan, S., & Farah, M. J. (2005). Is self-related processing special? A critical review. *Psychological Bulletin, 131*(1), 76–97.
Goffman, E. (1959). *The presentation of self in everyday life*. Garden City, NY: Doubleday.
Goldstein, K. (1995). *The organism: A holistic approach to biology derived from pathological data in man*. New York: Zone Books. (Original work published 1939)
Grandin, T. (1995). *Thinking in pictures: And other reports from my life with autism*. New York: Doubleday.
Grandin, T., & Scariano, M. M. (1986). *Emergence: Labeled autistic*. New York: Warner Books.
Greenblatt, S. (1980). *Renaissance self-fashioning: From More to Shakespeare*. Chicago: University of Chicago Press.
Habermas, T., & Bluck, S. (2000). Getting a life: The emergence of the life story in adolescence. *Psychological Bulletin, 126*(5), 748–769.
Habermas, T., & Paha, C. (1999). *The development of the ability to create causally coherent life stories in adolescence*. Paper presented at the 3rd Biannual Meeting for the Society for Applied Research in Memory and Cognition, Boulder, CO.
Hacking, I. (1986). Self-improvement. In D. Hoy (Ed.), *Foucault: A critical reader* (pp. 235–240). Oxford, UK: Basil Blackwell.
Harré, R., & Moghaddam, F. M. (2003). *The self and others: Positioning individuals and groups in personal, political, and cultural contexts*. Westport, CN: Praeger.
Harré, R., Moghaddam, F. M., Cairnie, T. P., Rothbart, D., & Sabat, S. R. (2009). Recent advances in Positioning theory. *Theory and Psychology, 19*(1), 5–31.
Harter, S. (1999). *The construction of the self: A developmental perspective*. New York: Guilford Press.
Hauser, S. T., Allen, J. P., & Golden, E. (2006). *Out of the woods: Tales of resilient teens*. Cambridge, MA: Harvard University Press.
Higgins, E. T. (1987). Self-discrepancy: A theory relating self and affect. *Psychological Review, 94*(3), 319–340.
Higgins, E. T. (1991). Development of self-regulatory and self-evaluative processes: Costs, benefits, and tradeoffs. In M. R. Gunnar & L. A. Sroufe (Eds.), *Self processes and development. The Minnesota symposia on child psychology* (Vol. 23, pp. 125–165). Hillsdale, NJ: Erlbaum.
Hitlin, S., Brown, J. S., & Elder, G. H., Jr. (2007). Measuring Latinos: Racial vs. ethnic classification and self-understandings. *Social Forces, 86*(2), 587–611.
Holliday Willey, L. (1999). *Pretending to be normal: Living with Asperger's syndrome*. London: Jessica Kingsley.
Hopkins, J. (tr.), 2001, *Complete Philosophical and Theological Treatises of Nicholas of Cusa*, Minneapolis: Banning.
Inhelder, B., & Piaget, J. (1958). *The growth of logical thinking from childhood to adolescence: An essay on the construction of formal operational structures* (A. Parsons & S. Milgram, Trans.). New York: Basic Books.
James, W. (1897). *The will to believe and others essays in popular philosophy.* New York: Holt.
Jung, C. G. (1953). *The collected works* (Bollingen Series XX, Vol. 1–20, R. C. F. Hull, Trans.). Princeton: Princeton University Press.
Kanner, L. (1971). Follow-up study of eleven autistic children originally reported in 1943. *Journal of Autism and Childhood Schizophrenia, 1*(2), 119–145.

King, P. M., Baxter Magolda, M. B., Barber, J. P., Kendall Brown, M., & Lindsay, N. K. (2009). Developmentally effective experiences for promoting self-authorship. *Mind, Brain, and Education, 3*(1), 108–118.
King, L. A., & Napa, C. K. (1998). What makes a life good? *Journal of Personality and Social Psychology, 75*(1), 156–165.
King, L. A., & Raspin, C. (2004). Lost and found possible selves, subjective well-being, and ego development in divorced women. *Journal of Personality, 72*(3), 603–632.
Kugel, J. (2007). *How to read the Bible: A guide to Scripture, then and now*. New York: Free Press.
Lachman, M. E., & Burack, O. R. (1993). Planning and control processes across the life span: An overview. *International Journal of Behavioral Development, 16*(2), 131–142.
Lalonde, C., & Chandler, M. (2004). Culture, selves, and time: Theories of personal persistence in native and non-native youth. In C. Lightfoot, C. Lalonde, & M. Chandler (Eds.). *Changing conceptions of psychological life* (pp. 207–229). Mahwah, NJ: Erlbaum.
Latour, B. (1999). *Pandora's hope: Essays on the reality of science studies*. Cambridge, MA: Harvard University Press.
Lewin, K. (1939). Field theory and experiment in social psychology: Concepts and methods. *American Journal of Sociology, 44*(6), 868–896.
Locke, J. (1997). *An essay concerning human understanding* (6th, rev. ed.). London: Penguin Books. (Original work published 1690)
Luria, A. R. (1972). *The man with a shattered world*. New York: Basic Books.
Magnusson, D., & Stattin, H. (2006). The person in context: A holistic-interactionistic approach. In W. Damon & R. M. Lerner (Series Eds.) & R. M. Lerner (Vol. Ed.), *Handbook of child psychology: Vol. 1. Theoretical models of human development* (6th ed., pp. 400–464). New York: Wiley.
Marini, Z., & Case, R. (1994). The development of abstract reasoning about the physical and social world. *Child Development, 65*(1), 147–159.
Markus, H., & Nurius, P. (1986). Possible selves. *American Psychologist, 41*(9), 954–969.
Maslow, A. H. (1943). A theory of human motivation. *Psychological Review, 50*(4), 370–396.
Maslow, A. H. (1954). *Motivation and personality*. New York: Harper.
Maslow, A. H. (1962). *Toward a psychology of being*. Princeton, NJ: Van Nostrand.
Maturana, H. R., & Varela, F. J. (1980). *Autopoiesis and cognition: The realization of the living*. New York: Springer.
Maturana, H. R., & Varela, F. J. (1992). *The tree of knowledge: The biological roots of human understanding* (R. Paolucci, Trans.). Boston: Shambhala. (Original work published 1987)
McAdams, D. P. (1990). Unity and purpose in human lives: The emergence of identity as a life story. In A. I. Rabin, R. A. Zucker, R. A. Emmons, & S. Frank (Eds.), *Studying persons and lives* (pp. 148–200). New York: Springer.
McAdams, D. P. (1993). *The stories we live by: Personal myths and the making of the self*. New York: The Guilford Press.
McCormack, T., & Hoerl, C. (1999). Memory and temporal perspective: The role of temporal frameworks in memory development. *Developmental Review, 19*(1), 154–182.
McLean, K. C. (2005). Late adolescent identity development: Narrative meaning making and memory telling. *Developmental Psychology, 41*(4), 683–691.
Musil, R. (1953). *The man without qualities*. London: Minerva.
Nelson, K. (1988). The ontogeny of memory for real events. In U. Neisser & E. Winograd (Eds.), *Remembering reconsidered: Ecological and traditional approaches to the study of memory* (pp. 244–276). New York: Cambridge University Press.
Nelson, K. (1993). The psychological and social origins of autobiographical memory. *Psychological Science, 4*(1), 7–14.
Nolen-Hoeksema, S. (1991). Responses to depression and their effects on the duration of depressive episodes. *Journal of Abnormal Psychology, 100*(4), 569–582.
Oatley, K. (1999). Why fiction may be twice as true as fact: Fiction as cognitive and emotional simulation. *Review of General Psychology, 3*(2), 101–117.

Oyserman, D., Bybee, D., & Terry, K. (2006). Possible selves and academic outcomes: How and when possible selves impel action. *Journal of Personality and Social Psychology, 91*(1), 188–204.

Oyserman, D., Bybee, D., Terry, K., & Hart-Johnson, T. (2004). Possible selves as roadmaps. *Journal of Research in Personality, 38*(2), 130–149.

Peterson, C., & McCabe, A. (1983). *Developmental psycholinguistics: Three ways of looking at a child's narrative.* New York: Plenum.

Peterson, C., & McCabe, A. (1994). A social interactionist account of developing decontextualized narrative skill. *Developmental Psychology, 30*(6), 937–948.

Piaget, J. (1946). *The child's conception of time.* London: Routledge.

Piaget, J. (1995). *Sociological studies* (L. Smith, Ed.). London: Routledge. (Original work published 1928–1977)

Piaget J. (1998). *De la Pédagogie* [On pedagogy]. Paris: Odile Jacob. (Original work published 1930–1970)

Pico della Mirandola, G. (1956). *Oration on the dignity of man* (A. R. Caponigri, Trans.). Chicago: H. Regnery. (Original work published 1486)

Piolino, P., Desgranges, B., Belliard, S., Matuszewski, V., Lalevée, C., De la Sayette, V. et al. (2003). Autobiographical memory and autonoetic consciousness: Triple dissociation in neurodegenerative diseases. *Brain, 126*(10), 2203–19.

Piolino, P., Desgranges, B., Manning, L., North, P., Jokic, C., & Eustache, F. (2007). Autobiographical memory, the sense of recollection and executive functions after severe traumatic brain injury. *Cortex, 43*(2), 176–95.

Plotzek, J. M., Winneskes, K., Kraus, S., & Surmann, U. (Eds.). (2002). *Ars vivendi ars moriendi: Die Kunst zu leben; die Kunst zu sterben.* Munchen: Hirmer-Verlag.

Quintilian, M. F. (2001). *The orator's education* (D. A. Russell, Trans.). Cambridge: Harvard University Press. (Original work written ca. 95 AD).

Ranner, L. (2008). *'Bildung' a new meaning of education.* Retrieved June 4, 2009, from http://www.loyolamaroon.com/2.8031/bildung-a-new-meaning-of-education-1.1125137.

Rathunde, K., & Csikszentmihalyi, M. (2006). The developing person: An experiential perspective. In W. Damon & R. M. Lerner (Series Eds.) & R. M. Lerner (Vol. Ed.), *Handbook of child psychology: Vol. 1: Theoretical models of human development* (6th ed., pp. 465–515). New York: Wiley.

Richardson, R. D. (2006). William James: In the maelstrom of American modernism. New York; NY: Houghton Mifflin.

Ricoeur, P. (1987). Individu et identité personnelle. In P. Veyne, J.-P. Vernant, L. Dumont, P. Ricoeur, F. Dolto, F. Varela, & G. Percheron (Eds.), *Sur l'individu, Contributions au colloque de Royaumont* (pp. 55–72). Paris: Seuil.

Ricoeur, P. (1988). *Time and narrative* (Vol. 3). Chicago, IL: University of Chicago Press.

Ricoeur, P. (1992). *Oneself as another*. Chicago, IL: University of Chicago Press.

Robison, J. E. (2008). *Look me in the eye: My life with Asperger's.* New York: Crown.

Rogers, C. R. (1961). *On becoming a person: A therapist's view of psychotherapy.* Boston, MA: Houghton Mifflin.

Rogers, C. R., Kell, B. L., & McNeil, H. (1948). The role of self-understanding in the prediction of behavior. *Journal of Consulting Psychology, 12*(3), 174–186.

Rosch, E. (2008). Beginner's mind: Paths to the wisdom that is not learned. In M. Ferrari & G. Potworowski (Eds.), *Teaching for wisdom* (pp. 135–162). Amsterdam: Springer.

Rothbart, M. K., & Bates, J. E. (2006). Temperament. In N. Eisenberg (Ed.), *Handbook of child psychology: Vol. 3. Social, emotional, and personality development* (6th ed., pp. 99–166). New York: Wiley.

Rutter, M., Kim-Cohen, J., & Maughan, B. (2006). Continuities and discontinuities in psychopathology between childhood and adult life. *Journal of Child Psychology and Psychiatry, 47*(3–4), 276–295.

Rutter, M., & Rutter, M. (1993). *Developing minds: Challenge and continuity across the lifespan.* New York: Basic Books.

Ryan, R. M., & Deci, E. L. (2000). Self-determination theory and the facilitation of intrinsic motivation, social development, and well-being. *American Psychologist, 55*(1), 68–78.
Sartre, J. P. (1956). *Being and nothingness: An essay on phenomenological ontology* (H. E. Barnes, Trans.). New York: Washington Square Press.
Schütze, F. (1984). Kognitive Figuren des autobiographischen Stegreiferzahlens [Cognitive structures of improvised personal narratives]. In M. Kohli & G, Robert (Eds.), *Biographie und soziale Wirklichkeit* (pp. 78–118). Stuttgart, Germany: Metzler.
Scepkowski, L. A., & Cronin-Golomb, A. (2003). The alien hand: Cases, categorizations, and anatomical correlates. *Behavioral and Cognitive Neuroscience Reviews, 2*(4), 261–277.
Seligman, M. E. P., & Csikszentmihalyi, M. (2000). Positive psychology: An introduction. *American Psychologist, 55*(1), 5–14.
Selman, R. (1980). *The development of social understanding*. New York: Academic Press.
Shore, S. M. (2001). *Beyond the wall: Personal experiences with Autism and Asperger syndrome*. London: Jessica Kingsley.
Siegel, D. J. (2007). *The mindful brain: Reflection and attunement in the cultivation of well-being*. New York: Norton.
Snow, C. P. (1959). *The two cultures and the scientific revolution*. Cambridge, UK: Cambridge University Press.
Snow, C. P. (1964). *The two cultures: A second look*. Cambridge: Cambridge University Press.
Stanovich, K. E. (2004). *The robot's rebellion: Finding meaning in the age of Darwin*. Chicago, IL: University of Chicago Press.
Staudinger, U. (2005). Weisheit, Lebens- und Selbsteinsicht [Wisdom, life insight and self insight]. In H. Weber & T. Rammseyer (Eds.), *Handbuch der Psychologie*. Göttingen: Hogrefe.
Staudinger, U. M., Dörner, J., & Mickler, C. (2005). Wisdom and personality. In R. J. Sternberg & J. Jordan (Eds.), *A handbook of wisdom: Psychological perspectives* (pp. 191–219). New York: Cambridge University Press.
Steinberg, L., Dahl, R., Keating, D., Kupfer, D., Masten, A., & Pine, D. (2006). The study of developmental psychopathology in adolescence: Integrating affective neuroscience with the study of context. In D. Cicchetti, & D. Cohen (Eds.), *Developmental psychopathology* (2nd ed., Vol. 2, pp. 710–741). New York: Wiley.
Sternberg, R. J., & Spear-Swerling, L. (1998). Personal navigation. In M. D. Ferrari & R. J. Sternberg (Eds.), *Self-awareness: Its nature and development* (pp. 219–245). New York: Guilford Press.
Sullivan, H. S. (1953). *The interpersonal theory of psychiatry*. New York: Norton.
Tammet, D. (2006). *Born on a blue day*. London: Hodder & Stoughton.
Taylor, C. (1977). What is human agency? In T. Mischel (Ed.), *The self: Psychological and philosophical issues* (pp. 103–135). Oxford: Blackwell.
Taylor, C. (1985). Human agency and language. *Philosophical papers* (Vol. 1). Cambridge, MA: Cambridge University Press.
Taylor, C. (1989). *Sources of the self: The making of the modern identity*. Cambridge, MA: Harvard University Press.
Thompson, E. (2007). *Mind in life: Biology, phenomenology, and the sciences of mind*. Cambridge, MA: Harvard University Press.
Thompson, R. A., Flood, M. F., & Goodvin, R. (2006). Social support and developmental psychopathology. In D. Cicchetti & D. J. Cohen (Eds.), *Developmental psychopathology: Vol. 3. Risk, disorder, and adaptation* (2nd ed., pp. 1–37). Hoboken, NJ: Wiley.
Thorne, A., McLean, K. C., & Lawrence, A. M. (2004). When remembering is not enough: Reflecting on self-defining memories in late adolescence. *Journal of Personality, 72*(3), 513–541.
Tomasello, M., Gust, D., & Frost, G. (1989). A longitudinal investigation of gestural communication in young chimpanzees. *Primates, 30*(1), 35–50.
Varela, F. (1987). Les racines biologiques de la individualité. In P. Veyne, J.-P. Vernant, L. Dumont, P. Ricoeur, F. Dolto, F. Varela, & G. Percheron (Eds.), *Sur L'Individu, Contributions au* colloque *de Royaumont* (pp. 88–95). Paris: Seuil.

Varela, F. J. (1999). *Ethical know-how: Action, wisdom, and cognition*. Stanford, CA: Stanford University Press. (Original work published 1992)
Varela, F. J., Thompson, E., & Rosch, E. (1991). *The embodied mind: Cognitive science and human experience*. Cambridge, MA: MIT Press.
Vygotsky, L. S. (1997). The historical meaning of the crisis in psychology: A methodological investigation. In R. W. Rieber & J. Wollock (Eds.), *The collected works of L. S. Vygotsky* (Vol. 3. Problems of the theory and history of psychology, pp. 233–344). New York: Plenum Press. (Original work published 1927)
Vuletic, L. (2010). *Living in two worlds: Intentional personal development of autistic individuals*. Doctoral dissertation. University of Toronto.
Vuletic, L., Ferrari, M., & Mihail, T. (2005). *Transfer boy: Perspectives on Asperger syndrome*. London: Jessica Kingsley.
Wallace, B. A. (2007). *Contemplative science*. Chicago: University of Chicago Press.
Wallace, B. A., & Shapiro, S. L. (2006). Mental balance and well-being: Building bridges between Buddhism and Western psychology. *American Psychologist, 61*(7), 690–701.
Wegner, D. M. (2002). *The illusion of conscious will*. Cambridge, MA: MIT Press.
Wegner, D. M. (2005). Who is the controller of controlled processes? In R. Hassin, J. S. Uleman, & J. A. Bargh (Eds.), *The new unconscious* (pp. 19–36). New York: Oxford University Press.
Williams, D. (1992). *Nobody nowhere: The extraordinary autobiography of an autistic*. New York: Times Books.
Williams, D. (1994). *Somebody somewhere: Breaking free from the world of autism*. New York: Times Book.
Williams, D. (1996). *Like color to the blind*. New York: Times Books.
Williams, D. (2004). *Everyday heaven: Journeys beyond the stereotypes of autism*. London: Jessica Kingsley.
Wundt, W. (1900–1920). *Völkerpsychologie: Eine Untersuchung der Entwicklungsgesetze von Sprache, Mythus und Sitte*. Leipzig: Engelmann.
Wundt, W. (1911). *Grundzüge der physiologischen psychologie* (6th ed., Vol. 3). Leipzig: Engelmann.
Wundt, W. (1990). *Vorlesungen über Menschen- und Thierseele*. G. Eckardt, E. Scheerer, & L. Sprung (Eds.). Berlin: Springer. (Original work published 1863)

Part III
Conclusion

Development and Its Relation to Mind, Brain, and Education: Continuing the Work of Robbie Case

Michel Ferrari and Ljiljana Vuletic

Introduction

This volume, in honor of Robbie Case, fulfills a dual purpose: On the one hand it is a well-deserved tribute to Robbie Case and the ground-breaking work he did in explaining the dynamic relations between mind, brain, and education throughout development; on the other hand, it shows the achievements and promise of recent efforts to integrate cognitive neuroscience into education, and the challenge of doing so in ways that are sensitive to issues of development. This concluding chapter discusses selective themes presented in the volume by considering some commonalities and differences among the ideas of different contributors. We first provide an overview of Robbie's work, and then consider answers to three questions: How does mind develop? How does neuroscience add to cognitive and behavioral models of development? What are the implications of cognitive neuroscience for education?

Robbie Case's Inspiring Work on the Development: Implications for Integrating Mind, Brain, and Education

Okamoto's chapter highlights two central questions of concern to Robbie Case:

(1) How does knowledge develop in children?
(2) How can this inform educational programs for all children, including those who are disadvantaged?

M. Ferrari (✉)
Department of Human Development and Applied Psychology, Ontario Institute for Studies in Education, University of Toronto, Toronto, ON, Canada
e-mail: mferrari@oise.utoronto.ca

M. Ferrari, L. Vuletic (eds.), *The Developmental Relations among Mind, Brain and Education*, DOI 10.1007/978-90-481-3666-7_14, © Springer Science+Business Media B.V. 2010

Knowledge Development

Robbie developed his answer to the first question across several major publications. In the first, *Intellectual Development: Birth to Adulthood* (Case, 1985), he proposed four stages of cognitive development, roughly corresponding to Piaget's stages, but understood from an information-processing perspective:

- the *sensorimotor* stage (birth to 1½ years),
- the *relational* stage (1½–5 years),
- the *dimensional* stage (5–11 years),
- the *vectorial* stage (11–19 years).

Case hypothesized executive control structures as special sorts of mental units for habitual ways of representing and dealing with problems through four stages of integration. Development within each stage depended upon the growth of working memory that itself depended on increasing operational efficiency (i.e., speed of information processing), which, in turn, depended on maturational factors (e.g., neuronal myelination, practice). Robbie proposed that new, more complex structures emerge at each stage of development and that development between stages resulted from integration of two qualitatively different structures (see Chapters "Children's Developing Understanding of Number: Mind, Brain, and Culture"; "Mental Attention, Multiplicative Structures, and the Causal Problems of Cognitive Development").

In his second book, *The Mind's Staircase: Exploring the Conceptual Underpinnings of Children's Thought and Knowledge* (Case, 1992a), the general structure of his stage model was retained, but Robbie introduced the notion of central conceptual structures (CCS) within broadly defined knowledge domains (e.g., numerical, spatial, social). Still broadly Piagetian (the same four stages and three substages re-occur, as do executive control structures), central conceptual structures were now considered to involve children's central processing—system-wide principles and constraints that change predictably with age. These structures were defined within a knowledge domain as a "network of semantic nodes and relations" (Case, 1992a) and considered central to successful performance within that domain (Chapter "Children's Developing Understanding of Number: Mind, Brain, and Culture"). As such, central conceptual structures differ significantly from Piaget's syntactic structures, even though both Piaget's structures and Robbie's central conceptual structures are symbolic and are a product of cultural learning.

Robbie continued to develop these ideas in *The Role of Central Conceptual Structures in the Development of Children's Thought* (Case & Okamoto, 1996). He now incorporated innate structures operating to set up domains in the first months of life. Robbie was always sensitive to cultural influences and conceptual structures became a "focal hub" for children's understanding of a broad set of culturally defined activities (Chapter "Children's Developing Understanding of Number: Mind, Brain, and Culture").

Lewis and Granic's chapter highlights Robbie's interest in the development of the "whole child," not just cognitive development. In his effort to understand human development, Robbie was particularly interested in the relation between cognitive and emotional development and always emphasized the importance of understanding that cognition does not develop in isolation from emotions or other mental processes (Case, 1985; 1988; Case, Hayward, Lewis, & Hurst, 1988). Robbie maintained that emotions are "intimately related in the development of the child" (Case, 1985, p. 423) and that cognitive and emotional processes have a reciprocal relationship. With regard to emotional development, he developed a specific theoretical proposal, namely, that cognitive development underlies emotional development by influencing the kinds of emotions children are more likely to experience, and suggested ways in which emotional development can influence cognitive processes by influencing their efficiency (Case et al., 1988).

In their chapters, Demetriou and his colleagues (Chapter "A Three-Level Model of the Developing Mind: Functional and Neuronal Substantiation and Educational Implications") and Chapter ("Higher-Order Network Reworking—New Findings") also remind us that Robbie always recognized the importance of understanding brain workings as integral to a complete account of the development of the mind. In 1985 (Case, 1985), when it was uncommon to find references to brain in psychological literature, Robbie postulated that increased mental efficiency depended on neuronal myelinization. As more evidence from neuroscience became available, Robbie incorporated it in his theorizing: In 1992, drawing on Thatcher's (1992) work on age-related increases in EEG coherence in the frontal and posterior cortex, he proposed the neuronal basis of stages of cognitive development (Case, 1992b). Finally, in the late 1990s, in one of his unfinished projects, he started to explore changes in the brain activity as children acquire basic mathematical skills (Case & Mueller, 2001; Mueller, Case, & Pang, 2002).

Educational Programs

More than just a theorist and researcher of child development, Robbie and his students and colleagues worked to implement his ideas in programs designed to enhance academic learning. Based on his theory, several developmentally based instruction programs were designed and empirically tested, most notably in the domains of narrative (Case & McKeough, 1990; Jarvey, McKeough, & Pyryt, 2008; McKeough, Davis, Forgeron, Marini, & Fung, 2005) and early mathematics learning (Griffin & Case, 1996, 1997; Griffin, Case, & Siegler, 1994).

In mathematics learning, Case proposed that basic numerical CCS depended on integrating two essential schemas: *counting* and *global quantity*. In the 1990s, Griffin and Case developed the "Number Worlds" (formerly "Rightstart")—a program specifically designed to teach number sense and build the CCSs foundational to later success in school mathematics through games and activities. For example, one of the games involves cards numbered from 1 to 9 and requires children to figure out how many more cards they need to reach 10. The program succeeded in helping children not only develop an age-appropriate central numerical structure, but also significantly improve their performance on tasks in other domains on which they received no training (e.g., balance scale and money knowledge)—both immediately and 1 year later (Griffin & Case, 1997; Chapter "Children's Developing Understanding of Number: Mind, Brain, and Culture"). Similarly, hypothesizing that understanding of rational numbers develops from essential schemas for halving and doubling and global proportionality (Moss & Case, 1999), Moss and her colleagues successfully implemented an intervention program designed to help students in grades 7 and 8 to understand rational numbers (Moss, London-McNabb, & Vuletic, 2004). Griffin (2009) continues this work, showing the power of learning sequences in the acquisition of mathematical CCS in children from pre-kindergarten to grade 6.

All of this work informs and advances key questions of concern to Robbie and all those continuing to do research in this area, as we show in the following sections.

How Does Knowledge Develop in the Mind?

Agreeing with Robbie, authors in the volume seem unanimous that knowledge develops through active efforts to construct it by engaging the world, although they differ in how exactly they believe this might occur.

For Pascual-Leone and colleagues knowledge develops through a "dialectical relation of complementarity" between maturation and learning (this idea is consistent with Robbie's thinking, who had been a student of Pascual-Leone). They posit two types of constructs to explain development: non-informational and general-purpose, functional "hardware" resources of the brain (content-free *hidden or silent operators*) and information-bearing, context- and experience-dependent knowledge structures (*schemes of different complexity levels*). Maturation is responsible for the growth of hidden operators—including mental attentional capacity—needed to learn increasingly complex subjects. Growth of hidden operators prompts development of knowledge structures, which develop locally with experience in particular contexts (unlike hidden operators that are context-free and work across knowledge domains). Thus, qualitative stages of cognitive development are themselves situated and not general.

Demetriou and his colleagues (Demetriou, Efklides, & Platsidou, 1993; Chapter "A Three-Level Model of the Developing Mind: Functional and Neuronal Substantiation and Educational Implications") propose a functional shift model consistent with both Robbie's and Pascual-Leone's models. Demetriou's model presumes that when the mental units of a given level reach a maximum degree of complexity, the mind tends to integrate them at a higher level of representation to make them more manageable. Having created a new mental unit, the mind prefers to work with this unit (rather than previous units) due to its functional advantages. For example, we find a shift from words to sentences in the verbal domain, and a shift from natural numbers to algebraic representations in the quantitative domain. According to Demetriou's studies, self-awareness and self-evaluation of cognitive processes also develop in three major cycles around the ages 3–7, 8–12, and 13–18. Self-development is also integral to the chapter "The Intentional Personal Development of Mind and Brain Through Education" by Ferrari and Vuletic (this volume).

What Develops?

Knowledge Development

For most of the contributors to this volume, what develops is knowledge, or perhaps knowledge structures. However, there are noticeable differences among the chapter authors in the kind of knowledge structures they consider.

Demetriou and colleagues, Pascual-Leone and colleagues, McKeough and Griffiths, Porath, and Okamoto, consider the development of knowledge structures associated with an increasingly complex understanding of particular task domains. McKeough and Griffiths (Chapter "Adolescent Narrative Thought: Developmental and Neurological Evidence in Support of a Central Social Structure") show how narrative understanding develops alongside social conceptual understanding through central narrative structures that underpin CCS across the social and linguistic domains involved in story composition, story interpretation, moral reasoning, and social decision making. Following Bruner (1986, 1990), McKeough and Griffiths see narrative as one of two main ways that human beings make sense of their experience (the other being paradigmatic thought). While paradigms organize the world into concepts and categories and are particularly well suited to understanding math and science, narrative thought addresses the vicissitudes of human actors and their intentions.

McKeough and Griffiths and Porath propose that children's understanding of social world progresses from simple understanding of actions in early childhood, through understanding of others' intentions in middle childhood, to complex social–psychological interpretations in adolescence (McKeough, 1992; McKeough & Genereux, 2003; Porath, 2003). Porath (as well as Chapter "Phases of Social–Emotional Development from Birth to School Age") also emphasizes that social competences are intrinsically related to emotional competence, and to understanding of others' emotions in particular.

For Lewis and Granic, knowledge necessarily involves both cognition and emotion, with children's cognitive gains underpinning their social–emotional development at every age. Building on Case's ideas about social–emotional development (Case, 1985; Case et al., 1988), Lewis and Granic propose that Case's model of early cognitive development can explain "*why* social–emotional functions appear when they do" by specifying the cognitive tools children have or have not yet developed for interpreting the world that evoke particular emotions (appraisal functions) or ways of coping with those emotions (regulatory functions).

While Pascual-Leone and others postulate two levels of mental organizations, one general and one domain specific, Demetriou and his colleagues—including

Robbie (e.g., Case, Demetriou, Platsidou, & Kazi, 2001)—believe that a third level is needed. Thus, they propose two general-purpose levels and one level of specialized, functionally distinct, systems of thought. Developing an understanding or performing any particular task integrates processes from all three levels. Demetriou and colleagues also propose that the most basic general level of information processing involves three dimensions of processing potential: *speed of processing*, *control of processing*, and *representational capacity*. Processes at this general level constrain the functioning of the systems at the other two levels that support all knowing about the environment or about the self.

More specifically, knowing about the environment involves specialized cognitive capacities for processing different aspects of the physical and the social world. Demetriou's research has found six such domains of thought (i.e., categorical, quantitative, spatial, causal, social, and verbal thought) that emerge as distinct factors in confirmatory factor analysis. Demetriou notes that all of them more or less coincide with Case's (1992a) analysis of central conceptual structures.

Most recently, self-knowing has been proposed as a distinct level of mental organization whose processes support explicit consciousness, intentionality, and self-control. For Demetriou and colleagues, having a *mind* necessarily involves a conscious self-mapping that implies a second-order level of knowing—the *hypercognitive system*—engaged both in the moment (as an awareness needed to pursue goals, self-monitor, and self-evaluate cognitive processes), and in long-term self-representation. Ferrari and Vuletic go further and note that the self-awareness must be extended to include Damasio's core and autobiographical selves, stressing the importance of personal narratives that are both descriptive and prescriptive, and include life plans and life projects that extend self-awareness and self-control beyond mere task monitoring.

Stages of Development

Cognitive development has traditionally been characterized by typical performance patterns at specific periods of children's growth. Neo-Piagetians, led by Pascual-Leone, propose two key assumptions about stages of development:

(1) stages of development are not universal, rather they are developed locally through experience, with the support of biological mechanisms and cultural practice and
(2) the reflective abstraction needed to move to a new stage relies on emerging biologically based capacity for greater mental attention (Chapters "Children's Developing Understanding of Number: Mind, Brain, and Culture," "Mental Attention, Multiplicative Structures, and the Causal Problems of Cognitive Development").

Substages. Pascual-Leone was first to identify substages as the focal point for assessing development, arguing that cognitive development is not caused by qualitative patterns of performance but by quantitative growth of mental attention and other "brain hardware"—an idea later picked up by Robbie Case and other neo-Piagetians.

According to Lewis and Granic, cognition and emotion also maintain a "dialectical relation of complementarity" during development, to borrow a Pascual-Leone phrase, with emotion directing attention in the service of knowledge development, but also responsive to previously developed cognition. In this view, affect is critical to understanding the shift from one substage to the next, especially in terms of gaining deeper understanding how individuals relate to significant others in their social world.

How Is Knowledge Development Supported by Specific Brain Mechanisms?

The relation of mind to brain is much discussed in recent philosophy of mind, with many books coming out each year that aim to explain how cognitive functioning, and by extension cognitive development, is embodied. However, as many contributors point out, we still have no paradigmatic understanding of how environmental factors contribute to neurological developmental trajectories (Chapters "Typical and Atypical Development of Basic Numerical Magnitude Representations: A Review of Behavioral and Neuroimaging Studies"; "A Three-Level Model of the Developing Mind: Functional and Neuronal Substantiation and Educational Implications"; "Children's Developing Understanding of Number: Mind, Brain, and Culture"; "Mental Attention, Multiplicative Structures, and the Causal Problems of Cognitive Development"), nor do we know how developmental trajectories interact with cultural expectations and personal choice across the lifespan (Chapters "The Intentional Personal Development of Mind and Brain Through Education"; "Children's Developing Understanding of Number: Mind, Brain, and Culture"; and "Mental Attention, Multiplicative Structures, and the Causal Problems of Cognitive Development").

Still, Ansari, Price, and Holloway note that neuroimaging methodologies have increasingly been used to understand the temporal and spatial organization of the neural basis of cognitive functions. For example, studies using this methodology unequivocally point to the parietal region of the brain (inferior parietal regions in and around the bilateral intraparietal sulcus [IPS], in particular) as important for representing numerical magnitudes. Although few studies have been specifically developmental, several recent studies found evidence of age-related shifts in neural activity from prefrontal to parietal areas in response to numerical visual stimuli (Ansari & Dhital, 2006; Ansari, Garcia, Lucas, Hamon, & Dhital, 2005). Such characterizations of the functional neuroanatomy underlying the typical developmental trajectory of specific cognitive capacities are important—not only for describing developmental change, but for understanding the nature of dysfunction in atypical populations (Ansari & Karmiloff-Smith, 2002).

Similarly, Porath reviews neural correlates of the "social brain" that include the prefrontal cortex, amygdala, premotor cortex, orbito-frontal cortex, insula, and superior temporal gyrus. She emphasizes the inseparability of social cognition and emotional processes at both the neural level and psychological level, noting that social competences do not just depend on brain structures but on their associated cognitive and emotional processes.

But even if such correlations among mind, brain, and behavior can be documented, how can they be explained? What sort of model is envisioned that would allow mind and behavior to be embodied in this way?

Demetriou and colleagues consider the human mind and brain two sides of the same coin, with the brain providing the underlying biological mechanism that generates the experience of mind at another level of analysis: The brain–mind itself is a product of human evolution. Like Ricoeur (Changeux & Ricoeur, 1998/2000), Demetriou notes that brain functions and psychological experiences exist at different levels of analysis and involve different "research objects." The objects of psychological research include observable responses (e.g., reaction times, problem solving), subjective experiences, and reports about those experiences. The objects of neuroscientific research include biological entities, such as neuronal matter and the responses that correlate with its activity, including blood supply, glucose consumption, electrical and chemical responses. Nevertheless, Demetriou is more optimistic than Ricoeur that brain development can help explain the increasing speed and control observed during psychological development. For example, neuronal pruning should enable faster and more efficient psychological processing; likewise, changes in neural interconnectivity should allow an ever-greater intertwining of neural networks and the ever-greater storage and integration of knowledge, and the greater reasoning capabilities observed during psychological development (Chapter "A Three-Level Model of the Developing Mind: Functional and Neuronal Substantiation and Educational Implications").

Case (1985) suggested that increased myelination of neuronal axons can explain enhanced information-processing efficiency and working memory capacity associated with the transition to higher stages of cognitive development. And indeed, McKeough and Griffiths cite recent neuroimaging studies of the developing brain that provide evidence for non-linear decreases in gray matter and increases in white matter volume (i.e., myelin) with age (Jernigan & Tallal, 1990; Paus et al., 2001; Pfefferbaum et al., 1994; Steen, Ogg, Reddick, Kingsley, 1997), providing support for Robbie's original proposal.

Thatcher (1992, Chapter "Higher-Order Network Reworking—New Findings") shows that increases in neuronal connections *within* brain regions are associated with changes occurring within stages of cognitive development, whereas increases in neuronal connections *between* brain regions are associated with transitions between stages. As Demetriou and colleagues point out, these findings agree with connectionist models of cognitive development, in which acquiring a particular cognitive skill is associated with local changes that strengthen existing connections between units in the model.

Pascual-Leone and colleagues apply Luria's (1973) and Eccles' (1980) models of brain functional organization to explain levels of information processing in different content domains. Following Luria, they suggest that *primary cortical areas* (i.e., areas where sensory and motor information enter and leave the cortex) are where particular modalities of information processing are defined. More specialized *secondary areas* coordinate information within particular content domains (e.g., shape, depth, color, or movement); *tertiary areas* are involved in coordinating information across content domains (e.g., vision, hearing, motor, etc.) as well as in creating new information, action procedures, and accessing information unrelated to immediate experiences. Finally, Pascual-Leone and colleagues propose that the highest integration of information takes place in *quaternary areas*; they consider likely sites for embodying executive processes and complex knowledge (e.g., of cities or technology) to be the prefrontal areas (associated with operative or "motor" functions), the superior temporal sulcus and the occipital-temporal-parietal junction (associated with the figurative or "sensorial" functions).

Pascual-Leone and colleagues suggest that the levels in Case's "spiral staircase" model of cognitive development broadly correspond to these four kinds of brain areas. They also suggest that as children move from one developmental stage to another, their interests and the main focus of their cognitive growth become increasingly abstract, shifting from (1) the immediate present (i.e., sensory perception and motor action) to (2) the inferred present (inferred through analysis, synthesis, and interpretation) to (3) the inferred future to (4) the inferred possible (based not on direct experience but on rational analysis).

In support of this claim, Pascual-Leone and colleagues refer to Thatcher's (1997) data showing a "spiral staircase" of development in the connectivity of brain regions in which the rate of change in EEG coherence roughly corresponds to the rate of *M-capacity* growth.[1] According to Pascual-Leone, *M*-capacity increases at two different "hidden" rates, that of the sensorimotor unit (*e*-scale) and of the mental, symbolic units (*k*-scale). The sensorimotor rate occurs in a phase in which change occurs in frequent and small amounts; the mental or symbolic rate of *M*-growth occurs slowly—every 2 years and in ever-larger amounts up to adolescence. Overall, Pascual-Leone and associates claim that transitions tend to occur every 4 months in the first year, every 8 months in the second year, and every 24 months after the third year. This developmental pattern is consistent with Thatcher's two phases of the development of EEG coherence: The first phase (from about 1.5 to 5 years) characterized by a slow decrease in coherence, has a high coherence point at age 3, and the second phase (from about 6 to 16 years) also characterized by a slow decrease in coherence, has a high coherence point at about age 6 and oscillations about every 2 years.

In their chapter, Demetriou and colleagues show how two major organizational principles of brain organization and functioning, segregation and integration (see Sporns, Chialvo, Kaiser, & Hilgetag, 2004), also describe the organization and functioning of the mind. Hence Pascual-Leone, Demetriou (and perhaps all the volume's authors) might agree with Piaget's (1950) prediction of an eventual coordination and integration of biology and psychology into a new discipline.[2] In fact, contemporary developmental cognitive neuroscience is such an integration and this may be why it has many implications for education and other applied disciplines.

---

[1] EEG coherence is a measure of "shared activity" between spatially separated brain regions (see Chapter "Higher-order network reworking—New findings").

[2] see Ferrari (2009a) for an overview of Piaget's writings on this topic.

Finally, Ferrari and Vuletic (The Intentional Personal Development of Mind and Brain Through Education, this volume) propose an enactive approach in which brain development has co-evolved with the environments to which it is adapted. While this approach does not contradict the position of other authors, we believe it avoids many problems associated with a classical information-processing view of human development and is one that Case would have endorsed as he continued to develop the dynamic systems perspective on cognitive development in his later work (e.g., Case, 1998).

What Are the Implications of Considering the Development of the Embodied Mind for Education?

The relevance of neuroimaging results to educational interventions is clear. Results of such studies can help educators understand brain-based constraints to learning and behavior that help them better understand students and better design curricula (Ansari & Coch, 2006). By providing novel insights about learning beyond those available from developmental and cognitive psychology, neuroscience can influence how teachers think about teaching and learning. As Ansari and colleagues (Chapter "Typical and Atypical Development of Basic Numerical Magnitude Representations: A Review of Behavioral and Neuroimaging Studies") show, understanding the neural basis of atypical developments is particularly important, both in understanding the atypical trajectories needed to develop interventions for students with special needs, and to determine whether networks associated with specific academic difficulties (e.g., in literacy or math) change after remediation. For example, functional neuroimaging has helped evaluate the success of remediation in children with reading difficulties (e.g., Shaywitz et al., 2004; Temple et al., 2003). As already mentioned, this was one of Robbie's unfinished projects: he and his colleagues had just begun to explore the effects of math training on brain activity (Mueller et al., 2002).

But Porath and Ansari urge caution when considering how neuroscience can inform education (see also Ferrari, in press b). Likewise, Ansari and Coch (2006) and Fischer and Daley (2007) suggest that cognitive neuroscience should be responsive to the needs of teachers and policy makers in education: developmental science, neuroscience, and education must reciprocally inform and learn from each other. This is a suggestion that Robbie Case would have applauded, and his own work was refined in light of its real-world usefulness to children in classrooms. However, since we are still at the beginning stages of developmental neuroscience and there is still no consensus on the biological indicators of cognitive development, this important suggestion will probably generate productive debate for some time.

In this way, recent efforts to integrate mind, brain, and education are a natural extension of a long-standing effort to integrate scientific understanding of biology and psychology into educational practice. Educational psychology has been concerned with the relation of mind to education since its early beginnings—dating at least from James' Talks for Teachers in America (1899) and even earlier to the work of Johann Herbart (1816/1891).[3] The relation of mind to brain specifically can be found in the writings of both Piaget and Vygotsky, who proposed theoretical models of an embodied mind and its implications for classroom education. These models integrate mind, brain, and education at a level of theoretical sophistication that still challenge the best contemporary formulations, many of which have been proposed by contributors to this volume.

But the relationship between brain science and education has often been problematic. James' (1899) talks to teachers were about the pragmatics of engaging young minds in school learning. He was skeptical of any direct relevance of psychology to education, telling teachers.

> you make a great, a very great mistake, if you think that psychology, being the science of the mind's laws, is something from which you can deduce definite programmes and schemes and methods of instruction for immediate schoolroom use. Psychology is a science, and teaching is an art; and sciences never generate arts directly out of themselves. An intermediary inventive mind must make the application, by using its originality.

This sentiment echoed even more strongly by Bruer (1997) claims that efforts to link education to neuroscience were "a bridge too far." Among chapter authors, Ansari and colleagues (Chapter "Typical and Atypical Development of Basic Numerical Magnitude Representations: A Review of Behavioral and Neuroimaging Studies") agree that the relevance of neuroscience to education is still unknown—even in the area of numerical cognition, one of the most researched domains to date—precisely because there are few developmental neuroscientific studies. Consequently, neuroscience is still far behind behavioral research in characterizing how children learn about numbers (e.g., how perceived numerosity is mapped onto cultural symbol systems) leading to difficulties in interpreting findings of neuroscientific research about numerical cognition; for example, although we find a developmental shift from frontal to parietal activations during magnitude comparison, the functional implications of this shift are still unknown. Still, James (1899) at least was positive that science could be of real value to teachers, even if they must make intelligent use of scientific results

> if the use of psychological principles thus be negative rather than positive, it does not follow that it may not be great use, all the same. It certainly narrows the path for experiments and trials. We know in advance, if we are psychologists, that certain methods will be wrong, so our psychology saves us from mistakes. It makes us, moreover, more clear as to what we are about. We gain confidence in respect to any method which we are using as soon as we believe that it has theory as well as practice at its back. Most of all, it fructifies our independence, and it reanimates our interest, to see our subject at two different angles,—to get a stereoscopic view, so to speak

[3] Of course, these relations of deep knowledge of human nature and its physical embodiment have been of concern to educators from the beginning of recorded history of philosophy, especially if we count proverbial advice and religious teachings about how to learn from others and from experience associated with the ancient wisdom schools of the ancient Middle East (Kugel, 2007) and ancient Greece (Hadot, 2002).

In just this spirit, Robbie's theory was always closely linked to instruction and several instruction programs developed based on his theory are equally applicable to typical and at-risk students in a particular domain. As McKeough and Griffiths (Chapter "Adolescent Narrative Thought: Developmental and Neurological Evidence in Support of a Central Social Structure"; see also Griffin, 2009) point out, perhaps the success of these programs lies in their sound developmental theoretical foundation supported by neuroscientific research. Furthermore, McKeough and Griffiths suggest, knowing the neuropsychological underpinnings of narrative thought encapsulated in central social structures offers educators the security that teaching will support students' continuing brain development—perhaps an illusory security, as shown by people's greater willingness to support circular logic when couched in neuroscientific terms (Weisberg, Keil, Goodstein, Rawson, Gray, 2008).

How can contemporary cognitive neuroscience add to James' (1899) claims that teachers can benefit from knowing the findings of psychological science? One possibility is that "evolutionary engineering" has shaped the development of both mind and brain over the millennia in ways useful to consider when designing instruction programs, and that the correspondence between brain structures and the psychological structures associated with mental development constrain what can be learned at any particular moment. Demetriou and colleagues show how complex skills based on core processes are difficult to learn and teach, suggesting that teaching in any domain should start from that domain's core elements. Pascual-Leone and colleagues and Schwartz and Fischer reach similar conclusions when discussing studies of how students learn complex math or physics concepts. For example, in their chapter, Pascual-Leone and colleagues show that training is only effective when students have the requisite *M*-capacity (constrained by biological maturation) to simultaneously track and manipulate the elements needed to solve problems at a given level of complexity.

Thatcher (Chapter "Higher-Order Network Reworking—New Findings") believes that evidence about the existence of cyclic reorganization and growth spurts in specific regions of the brain at specific ages have important educational implications. For example, his evidence suggests that the phases of the growth spurts may be associated with "critical periods" in which educational intervention might have the greatest impact. If so, Thatcher suggests, we can use the rising and falling phases of growth spurts as guides for choosing optimal time windows when educational programs will have a maximal impact. For example, educational programs aimed at developing social skills may have greater benefit if implemented at times of right frontal developmental growth spurts because they coincide with the development of social skill and of the awareness of self and others. Similarly, language and reading programs will have a maximal impact if implemented at times of growth spurts in the left temporal lobes (between ages 5 and 7). Thatcher also suggests that measures of EEG coherence and phase in short- and long-distance neural connection systems can be used in evaluating the effectiveness of educational programs.

Neuropsychological models based on evidence from already developed adult brains may not be very useful for understanding typical and atypical development, and developmental trajectories themselves must be investigated (Karmiloff-Smith,

1998), however, Ansari and colleagues point to an area where neuroscientific understanding has already demonstrated its important educational implications—early identification of learning disabilities. They show how improved understanding of the basic features of Developmental Dyscalculia allowed for the development of a screening tool—the "dyscalculia screener" (Butterworth, 2003)—to identify children with problems in basic numerical processing.

Fischer and Bidell (1998, 2006) and Schwartz and Fischer (Chapter "Interviewing: An Insider's Insight into Learning") propose that Fisher's skill theory provides a useful tool for quantifying students' understanding in any knowledge domain. By using skill theory to operationalize students' level of understanding of a particular knowledge domain, teachers can better evaluate both students' initial understanding and the changes in their understanding. Moreover, because which skills students display depends not only on their skill level but also on the context, the interview process itself can provide a special context from which both the student and the teacher can benefit.

Schwartz and Fischer emphasize that the goal of teacher interviews such as they describe in their chapter is twofold: to discover students' current understanding of the subject matter and to help students arrive at a better understanding (that includes motivating the student through the interview itself). The goal for students is to integrate new experiences into their existing understanding so as to acquire a more sophisticated understanding. Schwartz and Fischer argue that without teacher support, new understandings are often short lived, but that with adequate support, students can acquire long-lasting understanding. For this reason, curriculum planning needs to address the ongoing support of student's new understandings.

Also, as Schwartz and Fischer (Chapter "Interviewing: An Insider's Insight into Learning") point out, stages do not merely develop across the lifespan, but also as one gains mastery over particular tasks: the student Eve quickly acquires higher stages of skill as the physics lesson unfolds, but sometimes falls back to a lower level when she encounters difficulty that requires a reorganization of her knowledge. Schwartz and Fischer show that interviewing by teachers sensitive to stages is a good way to assess students' level of sophistication in their understanding of physics. Educators must assess both what children can do on their own, and what they can do with support. In a very real sense, teachers' interview questions are a form of scaffolding that, ideally, lead students to form more coherent explanations that reflect higher stages of understanding. In her studies, Chi has found that students who self-explain problems to themselves achieve the same effects through self-scaffolding as the teacher interviews Schwartz and Fischer describe (see Roy & Chi, 2005 for a review).

As Okamoto reminds us, mature understanding in any knowledge domain involves mastery of culturally shared meaning and practice—so learning symbol systems, even when based on evolved core capacities, fundamentally involves shared intentionality and a sense of self that is socio-historical in its development (Daston & Galison, 2007; Hammack, 2008). Okamoto suggests that recent research into the neural underpinnings of cross-cultural social communication point to a special neuronal network—the mirror neuron system—that is involved in culturally learned motor responses such as those used in social communication (Molnar-Szakacs, Wu, Robles, & Iacoboni, 2007).

Indeed, as Okamoto (Chapter "Children's Developing Understanding of Number: Mind, Brain, and Culture") notes, for all students learning number words and how to map them onto items counted are early cultural activities that young children in industrial nations must master if they are to succeed in school and in society. Mastering these practices requires readjusting how numbers and quantities are mentally represented. At the synaptic and neuronal levels, this requires what Dennett (1991, p. 183) calls "postnatal design-fixing." In other words, it requires that practices valued in a culture are trained repeatedly until corresponding neural connections become stronger. This, in turn, results in the formation of neural networks (or, at the mind level, CCSs) that can respond to cultural expectations. Therefore, the importance of cultural inputs in guiding the development of the brain is especially significant in the first years of life (Nelson, Zeanah, & Fox, 2007; Scherf, Behrmann, Humphreys, & Luna, 2007; Wexler, 2006). Developmental constraints on core capacities help explain why stages limit the ability to work with numbers at roughly the same ages across cultures (Chapter "Children's Developing Understanding of Number: Mind, Brain, and Culture").

This relates to Farah's point (Chapter "Mind, Brain, and Education in Socioeconomic Context") that the impact of SES on brain development (though a variety of factors related to the psychosocial and physical environment) can have a huge impact on academic ability even at the level of basic processing that Demetriou and colleagues show to be critical. Farah argues that good neurocognitive development is necessary for good intellectual and educational attainments which are, in turn, necessary for upward socioeconomic mobility. Ultimately, these concerns about development extend to what Farah calls "cognitive developmental neuro-sociology." In essence, she argues that cognitive neuroscience may offer a new perspective on development by revealing how the experience of growing up in low SES environments limits people's ability to leave such environments. She points to neuroscientific evidence from animal research that suggests that poverty in early life constrains brain development. Two aspects of early life poverty—decreased opportunities for positive stimulating experience and increased negative experiences such as stress—have particularly negative influence on neurocognitive development.

As Farah points out, not much is currently known about the relationship between SES and brain development. Nevertheless, she argues that because cognitive ability is a function of brain development, the correlations between SES and performance on standardized tests (like IQ tests) show that such a relationship exists. Her own research has addressed the specific neurocognitive systems that correlate with SES, as well the impact of neurocognitive disparities on school readiness and school achievement. Her findings show that children from low SES environments perform less well on tests of three neurocognitive systems: language, executive function, and memory (corresponding to the left perisylvian, the medial temporal, and the prefrontal neuronal systems respectively). Farah argues that it is reasonable to assume that these SES disparities have important implications for academic achievement in a variety of ways. For example, she points to research evidence documenting the importance of executive function for school readiness and academic achievement (e.g., Blair & Razza, 2007; Case, 1992b; McClelland et al., 2007; Mischel, Shoda, & Rodriguez, 1989; Posner & Rothbart, 2005).

Importantly, though, Demetriou and colleagues show how effective learning environments can help remediate some of these deficits. As their studies suggest, a refined understanding of development within specific knowledge domains can aid learning, especially for disadvantaged children. In their math training study (Demetriou, Christou, Spanoudis, Pittalis, & Mousoulides, 2007), one group received instructions by specifically trained teachers who used specifically designed developmentally sensitive training material, while a second group studied from standard training material only. Both groups significantly improved their performance at the post-test; however, after the effect of processing speed and working memory were partialed out, only the group that received the developmentally sensitive instruction still showed significant pre- and post-test differences. This study clearly shows that "when the learning environment is well structured and systematic even students with processing deficits can profit because structuring the learning environment compensates for weakness in processing efficiency" (Chapter "A Three-Level Model of the Developing Mind: Functional and Neuronal Substantiation and Educational Implications"). Moreover, Demetriou and colleagues found that the gains in math learning were transferred to general inferential processes. In another study, in which they explored the impact of self-awareness on learning, Demetriou and colleagues also found that more reflective and self-aware students profit more from educational training, as suggested by Chi's work mentioned earlier. These studies show that when properly designed, educational programs for particular knowledge domains can impact general-purpose learning mechanisms, including executive functions. Thus, a well-scaffolded learning environment allows disadvantaged students to learn regardless of deficits associated with a low SES environment that Farah is rightly concerned to document.

Informal Education

These points extend beyond formal education to informal education through parenting or emulation of others. People are not only educated in school, but more generally learn to become well-socialized members of their families and society. Several authors have focused on how informal education interfaces with individual development of both cognition and emotion.

In their chapter, Lewis and Granic identify two alternating periods during stages of emotional development: one characterized by more resilience, stability, and self-reliance, the other by more vulnerability, sensitivity, and dependency. They suggest that knowledge about the characteristics of these periods has important consequences for parenting. Thus, periods of vulnerability correspond to important developmental transitions that transform children's cognitive and emotional worlds, when children are preoccupied with internal reorganizations (i.e., coordinations of new understandings and capacities). Additional challenges during such periods may not only make development more difficult, but may also increase children's negative emotional reactions. Lewis and Granic recommend that, to the extent possible, parents should spare children challenging life events (e.g., the start of daycare, extended parental leaves, and major changes to daily sleeping or feeding routines) during periods of vulnerability and wait until a new period of resilience.

In their efforts to understand bullying in light of the biological basis of emotion regulation and empathy, Marini, Dane and Kennedy (Chapter "Multiple Pathways to Bullying: Tailoring Educational Practices to Variations in Students' Temperament and Brain Function") also stress that parents and teachers need to be sensitive to the temperament of the child and not just to their general stage of development. Their chapter helps us see that cognitive capacities are reciprocally engaged with emotions as they come online, and how development of cognitive structures is important for the moral reasoning needed to deal with problems in social interaction, like bullying, that involve the reciprocal engagement of cognition, emotion, and temperament. More specifically, Marini and colleagues note very different sources for what on the surface appear to be very similar bullying behavior, pointing to the need for different interventions to deal with them. Specifically, they describe two different pathways to bullying that stem from two different types of temperament: callous-unempathic and emotionally dysregulated. Callous-unempathic temperament is characterized by low negative emotionality (e.g., low fear, anxiety, and sadness) and low affiliation, and such children are prone to proactive (i.e., planned or instrumental) aggression, including bullying; emotionally dysregulated temperament is characterized by high negative emotionality (e.g., high fearfulness, anger, frustration, and irritability), high approach, and low deliberate control, and such children are thus more prone to reactive (i.e., emotional, provoked, or defensive) aggression. Marini and colleagues further propose that individual differences in neuronal systems that underlie fear and affiliativeness are key to understanding callous-unempathic temperament (prone to bullying). More specifically, neuronal systems involved with fear—the amygdala in particular—might be underactive in children with a callous-unempathic temperament, resulting in reduced fearfulness and greater insensitivity to negative consequences of their aggressive behavior, making them more likely to use aggression as a tool to accomplish their goals. Likewise, feelings of social connectedness, normally engendered by opiate projections from the amygdala and cingulate cortex to the hypothalamus, are relatively absent in these children. Whereas feelings of friendliness and warmth generally suppress aggressive tendencies, this self-regulatory mechanism is underdeveloped in children with callous-unempathic characteristics.

Children with different temperaments necessarily respond differently to the same behavior management strategies and so Marini's research has important implications for all socialization agents of children, including teachers. Rather than resolving conflicts, parents and teachers can help emotionally dysregulated children by mediating conflict resolution and strengthening self-regulation skills. Given their difficulties controlling emotions, self-regulation skills of emotionally dysregulated students can be improved through directly teaching meditative breathing techniques or emotion regulation techniques (e.g., counting to 10 before acting when angry) as ways to remain calm and to allow more time for reflection. Finally, drawing on research relating parental distress to children's decreasing self-regulation abilities over time (Eisenberg et al., 1999), Marini and colleagues suggest the importance of teachers' modeling appropriate self-control over their own emotions.

Research also shows that temperament can be shaped by parenting and is, therefore, far from being a fixed characteristic amenable to change. Temperament qualities like emotion dysregulation can be either aggravated or diminished by parenting, which, in turn, influences the risk of aggressive behavior (Eisenberg et al., 1999; Finkenauer, Engels, & Baumeister, 2005; Lengua & Kovacs, 2005; Shields & Cicchetti, 1998; Watson, Fischer, Burdzovic Andreas, & Smith, 2004; Zhou, Eisenberg, Wang, & Reiser, 2004). Marini suggests that these studies provide important insights into how parents and teachers can interact with emotionally dysregulated and callous-unempathic children to help them regulate their aggressive tendencies and develop more adaptive functioning.

In her chapter on social giftedness, Porath also recommends educational environments that are rich in opportunities to integrate multiple interpretations of behaviors, characters, and situations. She calls environments that encourage the flexible elaboration of central social structures "smart contexts" and suggests that such contexts are essential to social development. It is important that socially gifted students be provided with learning opportunities to engage in social and emotional reasoning in these kinds of smart contexts. Equally important, Ferrari and Vuletic propose that people can intentionally develop themselves through their own efforts, and that this is especially true when the developmental interplay of mind, brain, and education is considered from a lifespan perspective. They point out that educational contexts can also provide virtual models that point to exemplary aims of personal development that people themselves can seek to emulate.

As all of the work in this volume shows, cognitive neuroscience and education have a lot to offer each other, and a great deal can be learned from considering the developmental relations of mind, brain, and education. Robbie Case was at the cutting edge of efforts to develop this emerging field. We can only regret that he is no longer here to see how far we have progressed, and can only imagine how much more he might have contributed. But the contributors to this volume, many of them friends, students, and close colleagues carry on this important work in ways that would have made him proud.

Acknowledgment Thanks to Juan Pascual-Leone and Martha Farah for comments on an earlier version of this chapter.

References

Ansari, D., & Coch, D. (2006). Bridges over troubled waters: Education and cognitive neuroscience. *Trends in Cognitive Sciences*, *10*, 146–151.

Ansari, D., & Dhital, B. (2006). Age-related changes in the activation of the intraparietal sulcus during nonsymbolic magnitude processing: An event-related functional magnetic resonance imaging study. *Journal of Cognitive Neuroscience*, *18*, 1820–1828.

Ansari, D., Garcia, N., Lucas, E., Hamon, K., & Dhital, B. (2005). Neural correlates of symbolic number processing in children and adults. *Neuroreport, 16*, 1769–1773.

Ansari, D., & Karmiloff-Smith, A. (2002). Atypical trajectories of number development: A neuroconstructivist perspective. *Trends in Cognitive Sciences, 6*, 511–516.

Blair, C., & Razza, R. P. (2007). Relating effortful control, executive function, and false-belief understanding to emerging math and literacy ability in kindergarten. *Child Development, 78*, 647–663.

Bruer, J. (1997). Education and the brain: A bridge too far. *Educational Researcher, 26*, 4–16.

Bruner, J. (1986). *Actual minds, possible worlds*. Cambridge, MA: Harvard University Press.

Bruner, J. (1990). *Acts of meaning*. Cambridge, MA: Harvard University Press.

Butterworth, B. (2003). *Dyscalculia screener*. London, UK: NFER Nelson Publishing.

Case, R. (1985). *Intellectual development: Birth to adulthood*. New York: Academic Press.

Case, R. (1988). The whole child: Toward an integrated view of young children's cognitive, social, and emotional development. In A. D. Pellegrini (Ed.), *The psychological bases for early education* (pp. 155–184). Chichester, UK: John Wiley.

Case, R. (1992a). *The mind's staircase: Exploring the conceptual underpinnings of children's thought and knowledge*. Hillsdale, NJ: Erlbaum.

Case, R. (1992b). The role of the frontal lobes in the regulation of cognitive development. *Brain and Cognition, 20*, 51–73.

Case, R. (1998). The development of conceptual structures. In W. Damon (Series Ed.) & D. Kuhn & R. S. Siegler (Vol. Eds.). *Handbook of child psychology: Vol. 2. Cognition, perception and language* (5th ed., pp. 745–800). New York: Wiley.

Case, R., Demetriou, A., Platsidou, M., & Kazi, S. (2001). Integrating concepts and tests of intelligence from the differential and developmental traditions. *Intelligence, 29*, 307–336.

Case, R., Hayward, S., Lewis, M., & Hurst, P. (1988). Toward a neo-Piagetian theory of cognitive and emotional development. *Developmental Review, 8*, 1–51.

Case, R., & McKeough, A. (1990). Schooling and the development of central conceptual knowledge structures: An example from the domain of children's narrative. *International Journal of Education, 13*, 835–855.

Case, R., & Mueller, M. (2001). Differentiation, integration, and covariance mapping as fundamental processes in cognitive and neurological growth. In J. L. McClelland & R. S. Siegler (Eds.), *Mechanisms of cognitive development: Behavioral and neural perspectives* (pp. 185–219). Mahwah, NJ: Lawrence Erlbaum.

Case, R., & Okamoto, Y. (1996). The role of central conceptual structures in the development of children's thought. *Monograph of the Society for Research in Child Development, 61*(Serial No. 246).

Daston, L., & Galison, P. (2007). *Objectivity*. New York: Zone Books.

Demetriou, A., Christou, C., Spanoudis, G., Pittalis, M., & Mousoulides, N. (2007). Processing, working memory, and problem solving requirements for mathematics learning. In preparation.

Demetriou, A., Efklides, A., & Platsidou, M. (1993). The architecture and dynamics of developing mind: Experiential structuralism as a frame for unifying cognitive developmental theories. *Monographs of the Society for Research in Child Development, 58*(Serial No. 234).

Dennett, D. C. (1991). *Consciousness explained*. Boston, MA: Little & Brown.

Eccles, J. C. (1980). *The human psyche*. Berlin, Germany: Springer-Verlag.

Eisenberg, N., Fabes, R. A., Shepard, S. A., Guthrie, I. K., Murphy, B. C., & Reiser, M. (1999). Parental reactions to children's negative emotions: Longitudinal relations to quality of children's social functioning. *Child Development, 70*, 513–534.

Ferrari, M. (2009a). Piaget's science of consciousness. In U. Mueller, J. Carpendale, & L. Smith (Eds.), Cambridge companion to Piaget. pp. New York: Cambridge University Press.

Ferrari, M. (in press b). Future directions of mind, brain, and education research. *Educational Philosophy and Theory*, (Special issue on Educational Neuroscience).

Finkenauer, C., Engels, R., & Baumeister, R. (2005). Parenting behaviour and adolescent behavioural and emotional problems: The role of self-control. *International Journal of Behavioral Development, 29,* 58–69.

Fischer, K. W., & Bidell, T. R. (1998). Dynamic development of psychological structures in action and thought. In W. Damon (Series Ed.) & R. M. Lerner (Vol. Ed.), *Handbook of child psychology: Vol. 1. Theoretical models of human development* (5th ed., pp. 467–561). New York: Wiley.

Fischer, K. W., & Bidell, T. R. (2006). Dynamic development of action, thought, and emotion. In W. Damon (Series Ed.) & R. M. Lerner (Vol. Ed.), *Handbook of child psychology. Vol.1. Theoretical models of human development* (6th ed., pp. 313–399). New York: Wiley.

Fischer, K. W., & Daley, S. G. (2007). Connecting cognitive science and neuroscience to education: Potentials and pitfalls in inferring executive processes. In L. Meltzer (Ed.), *Executive function in education: From theory to practice* (pp. 55–72). New York: Guilford.

Griffin, S. (2009). Learning sequences in the acquisition of mathematical knowledge: Using cognitive developmental theory to inform curriculum design for pre-K-6 mathematics education. *Mind, Brain, and Education, 3*, 96–107.

Griffin, S. A., & Case, R. (1996). Evaluating the breadth and depth of training effects when central conceptual structures are taught. In R. Case & Y. Okamoto (Eds.), The role of conceptual structures in the development of children's thought. *Monographs of the Society for Research in Child Development, 61* (Serial No. 246), 83–102.

Griffin, S., & Case, R. (1997). Rethinking the primary school math curriculum: An approach based on cognitive science. *Issues in Education, 3*, 1–65.

Griffin, S., Case, R., & Siegler, R. (1994). Rightstart: Providing the central conceptual prerequisites for first formal learning of arithmetic to students at risk for failure. In K. McGilly (Ed.), *Classroom lessons: Integrating cognitive theory and classroom practice* (pp. 25–49). Cambridge, MA: MIT Press.

Hadot, P. (2002). *What is ancient philosophy*? (M. Chase Trans.). Cambridge, MA: Belknap Press.

Hammack, P. L. (2008). Narrative and the cultural psychology of identity. *Personality and Social Psychology Review, 12*, 222–247.

Herbart, J. F. (1816/1891). *Sämtliche Werke* (Vol. 4). *Lehrbuch zur Psychologie* [Textbook of Psychology], pp. 295–436.

James, W. (1899). *Talks to teachers on psychology: And to students on some of life's ideals*. New York: Holt.

Jarvey, M., McKeough, A., & Pyryt, M. C. (2008). Teaching trickster tales: A comparison of instructional approaches. *Research in the Teaching of English, 43*, 32.

Jernigan, T. L., & Tallal, P. (1990). Late childhood changes in brain morphology observable with MRI. *Developmental Medicine and Child Neurology, 32*, 379–385.

Karmiloff-Smith, A. (1998). Development itself is the key to understanding developmental disorders. *Trends in Cognitive Sciences, 2*, 389–398.

Kugel, J. (2007). *How to read the bible: A guide to scripture, then and now* (Free Press).

Lengua, L. J., & Kovacs, E. A. (2005). Bidirectional associations between temperament and parenting and the prediction of adjustment problems in middle childhood. *Journal of Applied Developmental Psychology, 26*, 21–38.

Luria, A. R. (1973). *The working brain*. Middlesex, UK: MiPenguin Books.

McClelland, M. M., Cameron, C. E., Connor, C. M., Farris, C. L., Jewkes, A. M., & Morrison, F. J. (2007). Links between behavioral regulation and preschoolers' literacy, vocabulary, and math skills. *Developmental Psychology, 43*, 947–59.

McKeough, A. (1992). The structural foundations of children's narrative and its development. In R. Case (Ed.), *The mind's staircase: Stages in the development of human intelligence* (pp. 171–188). Hillsdale, NJ: Erlbaum.

McKeough, A., Davis, L., Forgeron, N., Marini, A., & Fung, T. (2005). Improving story complexity and cohesion: A developmental approach to teaching story composition. *Narrative Inquiry, 15*, 96–125.

McKeough, A., & Genereux, R. (2003). Transformation in narrative thought during adolescence: The structure and content of story compositions. *Journal of Educational Psychology, 95*, 537–552.

Mischel, W., Shoda, Y., & Rodriguez, M. L. (1989). Delay of gratification in children. *Science, 244*, 933–938.

Molnar-Szakacs, I., Wu, A. D., Robles, F. J., & Iacoboni, M. (2007). Do you see what I mean? Corticospinal excitability during observation of culture-specific gestures. *PLoS ONE, 2*, e626. doi:10.1371/journal.pone.0000626

Moss, J., & Case, R. (1999). Developing children's understanding of rational numbers: A new model and experimental curriculum. *Journal for Research in Mathematics Education, 30*, 122–147.

Moss, J., London-McNabb, S., & Vuletic, L. (2004, April). *Implementing an experimental rational number curriculum in 7th and 8th grade classrooms in an urban school*. Paper presented at the AERA Annual Meeting in San Diego, California.

Mueller, M. P., Case, R., & Pang, E. W. (2002, August). *Effects of a community-based math intervention program on cognitive and neural development in kindergarten-aged children*. Paper presented at the Poster presented at the Biennial Meeting of The International Society for the Study of Behavioural Development (ISSBD), Ottawa, Ontario, Canada.

Nelson, C. A., Zeanah, C. H., & Fox, N. A. (2007). The effects of early deprivation on brain-behavioral development: The Bucharest early intervention project. In D. Romer & E. F. Walker (Eds.), *Adolescent psychopathology and the developing brain: Integrating brain and prevention science* (pp. 197–215). New York: Oxford University Press.

Paus, T., Collins, D. L., Evans, A. C., Leonard, G., Pike, B., & Zijdenbos, A. (2001). Maturation of white matter in the human brain: A review of magnetic resonance studies. *Brain Research Bulletin, 54*, 255–266.

Piaget, J. (1950). *Introduction à l'Épistémologie Génétique*. Paris: Presses Universitaires de France.

Pfefferbaum, A., Mathalon, D. H., Sullivan, E. V., Rawles, J. M., Zipursky, R. B., & Lim, K. O. (1994). A quantitative magnetic resonance imaging study of changes in brain morphology from infancy to late adulthood. *Archives of Neurology, 51*, 874–887.

Porath, M. (2003). Social understanding in the first years of school. *Early Childhood Research Quarterly, 18*, 468–484.

Posner, M. I., & Rothbart, M. K. (2005). Influencing brain networks: Implications for education. *Trends in Cognitive Sciences, 9*, 99–103.

Roy, M., & Chi, M. T. H. (2005). The self-explanation principle in multimedia learning. In R. E. Mayer (Ed.), *Cambridge handbook of multimedia learning* (pp. 271–286). New York: Cambridge University Press.

Scherf, K. S., Behrmann, M., Humphreys, K., & Luna, B. (2007). Visual category-selectivity for faces, places and objects emerges along different developmental trajectories. *Developmental Science, 10*, F15–F30.

Shaywitz, B. A., Shaywitz, S. E., Blachman, B. A., Pugh, K. R., Fulbright, R. K., Skudlarski, P., et al. (2004). Development of left occipitotemporal systems for skilled reading in children after a phonologically-based intervention. *Biological Psychiatry, 55*, 926–933.

Shields, A., & Cicchetti, D. (1998). Reactive aggression among maltreated children: The contributions of attention and emotion dysregulation. *Journal of Clinical Child Psychology, 27*, 381–395.

Sporns, O., Chialvo, D. R., Kaiser, M., & Hilgetag, C. C. (2004). Organization, development and function of complex brain networks. *Trends in Cognitive Sciences, 8*, 418–425.

Steen, R. G., Ogg, R. J., Reddick, W. B., & Kingsley, P. B. (1997). Age related changes in the pediatric brain: Quantitative MR evidence of maturational changes during adolescence. *American Journal of Neuroradiology, 18*, 819–828.

Temple, E., Deutsch, G. K., Poldrack, R. A., Miller, S. L., Tallal, P., Merzenich, M. M.et al. (2003). Neural deficits in children with dyslexia ameliorated by behavioral remediation: Evidence from

functional MRI. *Proceedings of the National Academy of Sciences of the United States of America, 100*, 2860–2865.
Thatcher, R. W. (1992). Cyclic cortical reorganization during early childhood. *Brain and Cognition, 20*, 24–50.
Thatcher, R. W. (1997). Human frontal lobe development: A theory of cyclical cortical reorganization. In N. A. Krasnegor, G. R. Lyon, & P. S. Goldman-Rakic (Eds.), *Development of prefrontal cortex* (pp. 85–113). Baltimore, MD: Paul H. Brooks.
Watson, M. W., Fischer, K. W., Burdzovic Andreas, J., & Smith, K. W. (2004). Pathways to aggression in children and adolescents. *Harvard Educational Review, 74*, 404–430.
Weisberg, D. S., Keil, F. C., Goodstein, J., Rawson, R., & Gray, J. R. (2008). The seductive allure of neuroscience explanations. *Journal of Cognitive Neuroscience, 20*, 470–477
Wexler, B. E. (2006). *Brain and culture: Neurobiology, ideology, and social change*. Cambridge, MA: MIT Press.
Zhou, Q., Eisenberg, N., Wang, Y., & Reiser, M. (2004). Chinese children's effortful control and dispositional anger/frustration: Relations to *parenting* styles and children's social functioning. *Developmental Psychology, 40*, 352–366.

Author Index

M. Ferrari, L. Vuletic (eds.), *The Developmental Relations among Mind, Brain and Education*, DOI 10.1007/978-90-481-3666-7,

Subject Index

The letters 'f' and 't' following the locators refer to figures and tables respectively.

The manufacturer's authorised representative in the EU is Springer Nature Customer Service Centre GmbH, Europaplatz 3, 69115 Heidelberg, Germany. If you have any concerns regarding our products, please contact ProductSafety@springernature.com

Printed and bound by CPI Group (UK) Ltd, Croydon, CR0 4YY
22/09/2026
02220985-0005